Contents

Preface

This book arose from two social science modules that I co-coordinated with my colleague and friend Christine Grabowska. They concerned the social context in which women give birth. Many students found them inspiring and fundamental to any study of midwifery, but others were more concerned with the biosciences, finding them more relevant to their needs. To them, social sciences were 'woolly' subjects and had little to do with childbirth. It is easy to understand this viewpoint. With the medicalisation of birth, the biosciences have assumed a greater importance. 'A' must equal 'B', and linear thinking abounds – every woman needs a vaginal examination every 4 hours, every woman needs to have syntocinon if she goes right of 'the line', and so on. This is 'authoritative knowledge', the knowledge that reigns supreme and is consciously and often unconsciously accepted, and although we try to think of midwifery care as woman-centred and holistic, in reality it is impossible to practise this way in a scientific environment where thinking is in absolutes and care is usually fragmented.

To me and like-minded midwives, childbirth is much more than a biological event or a set of case-notes with a number. Giving birth to a child *always* occurs within a social context, and this is what this book is all about. Furthermore, the intention is to make the content accessible to everyone. The academic disciplines of anthropology, psychology and sociology have produced copious contributions about women and birth, but are often written in academic language which denies access to students and healthcare workers who do not have a background in the subject. On the other hand, the text needed to be written to some type of framework, and this proved to be a real challenge which I hope we have overcome. The approach of the book is therefore sociocultural, and clinical practice has been left to other publications. All of the areas considered can be applied to the care and support of women when they give birth because they are about women's lives – they are not abstract 'woolly' subjects. They have direct relevance both to childbirth and also to the lives of ourselves as midwives (who are almost always women). The book does not aim to discuss every aspect of women's lives – that would be impossible – but I hope that many key areas have been addressed.

The relationship between midwives and obstetricians has always been problematic, and will doubtless be so for many years to come. Most midwives are women, and for me personally the most difficult chapter by far was that concerning 'Women and Society', which suggests that the development of feminism has mirrored the development of midwifery in this country. For me, how midwives view themselves affects women and their births, and we need to ask ourselves whether we are 'with woman' or 'with institution/obstetrician', or with both? Indeed, can we be with both? Of course, where women (and midwives as women) are in society now is a vexed question, and there is no one answer, just a multiplicity of truths (as postmodernists would tell us). Is it still a man's world? Is being a mother valued? Are we supported as mothers in our society? Are midwives considered to be the helpers of obstetricians?

The concept of 'woman-centredness' or being 'with woman' is bandied around in publication after publication. And so it should be − it is extremely important that childbearing women are *listened to* and *understood* − but the concept is often used with little thought about the complexity of what it really means. It is so difficult in an institutionalised and scientific institution which deals with thousands of women in an objective manner even to approach being 'woman-centred'. It seems to me that being a midwife *and* a woman is challenging to say the least, and it behoves us to have knowledge and understanding of different women leading different lives to our own. Only then can we begin to feel that we are trying to be 'with woman'.

Sandy Nelson considers the fundamental issue of sex in her chapter on 'Women and Sex'. It seems to me that many of us are very ignorant about sex and the sexual lives of other women, yet it is a 'predisposing factor' (as it were) to childbirth! I think it is closely related to breastfeeding, which is discussed in Cathryn Britton's chapter. Having been a midwife since 1981, it has been one of the most frustrating aspects of my career that, despite so much work, so few women breastfeed in the UK. However, if one considers the social context in which women breastfeed one can understand why this is so, and it seems to me that no midwife will be effective in this area who does not have a real understanding of sex, sexuality and how different women lead their lives.

Some of the chapters will test our attitudes to different women. In particular, Dave Sookhoo's consideration of 'Race and Ethnicity', Jo James' account of 'Refugee Women', Comfort Momoh's chapter on 'Female Genital Mutilation' and Kate Beverley's deliberation on 'Women and Poverty' require us to look at our own stereotyping of these women and ourselves. Nicola Winson, in her chapter on 'Transition to Motherhood' and Christine Grabowska, in her chapter on 'Unhappiness after Childbirth', ask us to consider whether we as a society really value mothers and the raising of families. This is related to Val Dunn-Toroosian's account of the family, in which she shows that the family as an institution is often not a safe and loving environment for the mother. Sally Price's chapter on 'Domestic Violence' sadly reiterates and clarifies this. My own chapter considers birth following sexual abuse in childhood, and illustrates that unhappily the same is true for many children as well.

Fortunately, most women love their children, but some have difficulty with this. Cathy Rowan considers 'Maternal Infant Attachment' and, importantly, describes how the scientific technologies have affected this attachment for better or worse. The technologies, of course, are said to be favoured by men ('toys for the boys'). Tim Blackshaw discusses this and other issues in his chapter on 'Fathers and Childbirth', an important area which has seen major changes since the time when I qualified as a midwife. The concept of social support is a fundamental one. I have read on numerous occasions in essays that 'the mother was well supported because her own mother was staying with her'. In contrast, I have visited women at home postnatally, asked them what I can do for them, and some have said to me 'get rid of my mother'. The concept is a difficult one, and every midwife needs to get to grips with it to enable insightful practice.

The key issues concerning medicalisation and the rise of a scientific culture are considered by Alyson Henley-Einion in her chapter on 'The Medicalisation of Childbirth', Marilyn Crawshaw in 'The New Reproductive Technologies' and Christine Grabowska in her chapter on 'Fetal Surveillance'. Clearly there have been many benefits for childbearing women and babies, but there are drawbacks as well.

Many women have felt that they were objectified in hospital births and lost much of their control over themselves and their ability to give birth. Does the fetus have 'rights'? And if so, how do these relate to the way in which we view disabled people in our society? These are key questions which will vex us now and in the years to come.

As I mentioned earlier, this book does not approach all of the key issues relating to women, women as midwives, and childbirth. Hopefully, however, it may help the reader to understand the similarities and differences between women, so that the concept of being 'with woman' becomes a little clearer.

Caroline Squire
January 2003

List of contributors

Kate H Beverley MSc, MA, Cert Ed, RN, RM, RCNT
Senior Lecturer, Faculty of Health and Human Sciences,
Thames Valley University

Tim Blackshaw BSc (Hons), RCNT, RN
Senior Lecturer, Faculty of Health and Human Sciences,
Thames Valley University

Cathryn Britton RN, RM, ADM, PGCEA, MSc, PhD
Lecturer, Department of Health Sciences,
University of York

Marilyn Crawshaw MA, CQSW
Teaching and Research Fellow, Department of Social Policy and Social Work,
University of York, and
Inspector for the Human Fertilisation and Embryology Authority

Val Dunn-Toroosian RN, RNT, BA, MSc
Senior Lecturer, Faculty of Health and Human Sciences,
Thames Valley University

Christine Grabowska MSc, BSc (Hons), RN, RM, ADM, PGCEA, LicAc, LicOHM, DIPCST
Senior Lecturer in Midwifery, Faculty of Health and Human Sciences,
Thames Valley University

Alyson Henley-Einion DipHE (Nursing), BSc(Hons), FAETC
Doctoral student, School of Care Sciences,
University of Glamorgan

Jo James MSc, RGN
Clinical Redesigner, BECaD Project,
Central Middlesex Hospital

Christine McCourt BA, PhD
Reader, Faculty of Health and Human Sciences,
Thames Valley University

Comfort Momoh RN, RM, FPN, BSc
Female Genital Mutilation Specialist Midwife,
Guy's and St Thomas' Hospital Trust

Sandy Nelson BEd, MA
Senior Lecturer, Faculty of Health and Human Sciences,
Thames Valley University

Sally Price BSc, RM, MCGI, NNEB
Consultant Midwife, North Bristol NHS Trust and the University of the West of England, and Member of the South Gloucestershire Domestic Violence Forum, the National Domestic Violence Research Forum and the Women's Aid Federation

Cathy Rowan RM, RN, ADM, PGCEA, MA
Senior Lecturer, Faculty of Health and Human Sciences,
Thames Valley University

Dave Sookhoo MEd, BA, RN, RMN, DipN
Principal Lecturer (Research), Faculty of Health and Human Sciences,
Thames Valley University

Caroline Squire MSc, RM, RN, ADM, PGCEA, LicAc, LicOHM
Senior Lecturer, Faculty of Health and Human Sciences,
Thames Valley University

Nicola Winson MA, SRN, SCM ADM, PGCEA
Senior Lecturer, Faculty of Health and Human Sciences,
Thames Valley University

This book is dedicated to Nick, my sister Mary, Sarah and Vicky

CHAPTER 1

Women and society

Caroline Squire

Pregnancy and childbirth are unique events in the lives of women. Midwives and health professionals need to have knowledge and understanding of the social and cultural context which influences women and their lives, and in which they give birth. Women's subjective and collective experiences of life will depend upon such factors as age, ethnicity, social and economic background and the way in which these factors interrelate, contradict and intersect with each other. The study of women's lives is complex but necessary for midwives and health professionals if they are to be able to practise in a so-called 'woman-centred' manner. This chapter discusses the key feminist theories that have contributed to explanations of the experiences of being a woman, as well as considering the sex/gender debate. The concept of 'woman-centred practice' is also addressed with particular reference to postmodernist feminist theory.

Introduction

'She is defined and differentiated with reference to Man and not he with reference to her; she is the incidental, the inessential as opposed to the essential. . . . He is the Subject, he is the Absolute — she is the Other' (de Beauvoir, 1953: xiv). This extract is taken from the translation of de Beauvoir's ground-breaking text, which was originally published in 1949. There is a popular view that times have changed for the better, and that women have achieved equality. Is this true or is it an illusion? Certainly in the UK, individual women seem to be freer and more powerful than before. They drive fast cars, appear on television interviewing politicians (as opposed to being 'weather girls'), become Members of Parliament (MPs), down pints of beer in the pub, live alone, pay the bills, marry men but do not promise to obey their husbands, have children or decide not to have children, and so the list continues.

However, a brief look at the major systems and structures which underpin our society reveals a very different story. Religion remains a major influence in every society, whether one attends church or not. There are no female Roman Catholic priests, very few female Anglican priests (*see* Table 1.1), and no Islamic, Hindu or Buddhist female clerics.

MPs rule the country politically. There has been but one female Prime Minister (Margaret Thatcher), one Speaker of the House of Commons (Bettie Boothroyd), only a handful of female Secretaries of State, and no Chancellors of the Exchequer or Home Secretaries. In 1999, only 18.43% of MPs were women (120 out of a

Table 1.1 Clergy, readers, licensed ministers and others permitted to officiate in post on 31 December 1997 and 2000 (Archbishops' Council, 2002)

	Male (1997)	Female (1997)	Total	Female (2000)
Bishops	110	–	110	–
Archdeacons	116	1	117	3
Cathedral clergy	153	11	164	10
Vicars	7045	426	7471	618
Assistant curates	1228	433	1661	445
Chaplains and others	1289	233	1522	247
Non-stipendiaries	1332	598	1930	744
Total	11 273	1702	12 975	2067
Active retired clergy			6000	
Readers	5162	3110	8272	
Church Army evangelists	195	86	281	
Grand total			27 528	

total of 651) (British Council, 1999). This woeful under-representation of women within conventional politics is crucial in thinking about democracy and gender (Phillips, 1994).

The legal system within a society may be said to prevent anarchy, and is thus absolutely fundamental to the social cohesion and functioning of any civilised society. The legal profession may profess that more than half of all newly qualified lawyers are women, but where do they go? In England and Wales in April 2001, there were only 11 female judges in the High Court and above. In April 1998, the proportion of women in the main tiers of the judiciary was 10.3%, and in April 2001 this figure had increased to 13.7% (Lord Chancellor's Department, 2001), a staggeringly slow increase. Might this affect the experiences of women in the courts of this land? For example, could it influence the very low rate of conviction for rape?

A look at the research of the Equal Opportunities Commission (EOC) into gender equality in pay practices reveals another depressing picture. Women working full-time currently earn only 81% of the average hourly earnings of men (the 'gender pay gap') (Equal Opportunities Commission, 2002). National Statistics (2002) published the statistics shown in Table 1.2 concerning women's pay in comparison with that of men.

In October 1999, the EOC launched 'Valuing Women', a major three-year campaign for equal pay. Ahead of the campaign launch, the EOC commissioned three studies to assess current attitudes towards and awareness of equal pay. Some of the overall key findings were as follows.

- There is a low level of awareness of the gender pay gap.
- Half of all women and men think that the gender pay gap is unfair.
- Most people do not know what their colleagues earn, and only a minority have ever asked them.

Table 1.2   Average gross weekly earnings (£ per week) (National Statistics, 2002)

| | | Adults whose pay was not affected by absence | | | |
		Full-time	Part-time	All	All employees
Aprill 2001					
	Men	490.5	141.4	462.3	445.5
	Women	366.8	135.6	271.7	260.7
	All	444.3	136.6	370.5	355.6
April 2000					
	Men	464.1	137.8	439.1	423.7
	Women	343.7	129.6	255.2	245.5
	All	419.7	131.0	351.0	337.7
Percentage increase					
	Men	5.7	2.6	5.3	5.2
	Women	6.7	4.6	6.5	6.2
	All	5.9	4.3	5.5	5.3

Interestingly, in research involving line managers, both male and female line managers regarded men as the main breadwinners, whose key role is to provide for their families. Male line managers generally regarded women as secondary earners, a view which some (but not all) women shared. Looking at these comments, it is not difficult to see how men may be reluctant to promote women and give them equal pay.

Many women are, of course, perfectly at ease with never having paid employment during their marriage/partnership, or with interrupted careers. This situation is not problematic unless the partnership breaks up and/or divorce occurs, with children often being involved. Then many women may find themselves experiencing poverty. Furthermore, women who never experience paid employment are often in a situation where the household does not rely financially on two wages. Arguably, women in lower socio-economic groups are never able to experience 'career breaks' or not working for financial gain.

At the top end of the labour market, the situation remains iniquitous, with the so-called 'glass ceiling' remaining evident. Almost half of the top 100 companies have no women on the board. Only eight of them employ female executive directors, and the number is falling, not rising (Connon, 2001). However, on the plus side, the first female chairman of a FTSE 100 company commenced that role in January 2002. Whether this will have any effect on the employment of women in higher or lower paid work is in serious doubt, but remains to be seen.

The picture continues to be disastrous in the fields of obstetrics and gynaecology, surely an area where a preponderance of female practitioners might be expected. In the year 2000, there were 1246 consultants, of whom 274 (24%) were women (Royal College of Obstetricians and Gynaecologists, 2001). This figure seems particularly ironic and contradictory in view of the fact that it is a field of medicine which is directly pertinent to women and which can have dramatic effects on the lives of women, for better or worse.

It would be possible to go on giving examples of women's absence from key positions of power and influence within the social system, but does this actually matter? In this chapter it will be argued that this is a real cause for concern and the key feminist theories that have informed women's thinking will be addressed. Radical feminism and postmodernist feminism will be focused on, and comparisons will be made with the history of midwifery and childbirth in the twentieth century. The sex/gender debate will also be discussed, and it will be concluded that women and men are different and that analyses of the similarities and differences *between women* may be fruitful in the future. The chapter ends with a discussion of postmodern feminist theory and how this contributes to the ways in which the differences and similarities in women's experiences of the complexities and contradictions in their lives can be explained.

Feminist theories

There are a number of feminist theoretical approaches to the explanation of gender inequalities. These theories differ markedly from one another, and therefore it is not possible to consider the socialisation of women from a single feminist perspective. The diverse range of theories mirrors the complexity and variation to be found within women's lives both across one society and between different societies.

The word 'feminism' gives rise to many different but profound feelings among women and men alike (Stephens, 1999). Stereotypes of feminists such as 'butch' and 'man-hater' abound. The following description from a health and beauty magazine in the contemporary media provides an illustration of this:

> For too long women have had to choose the hard or soft option – you were either feminist or feminine, careerist or carer, pinstripes or pincurls, hard-nosed or high-heeled. Thankfully, most of us no longer feel the need to take sides. Our mothers might have had to burn their bras to make a point, but now – with due credit to them and the Battle of the Sexes they fought on our behalf – we can wear an Agent Provocateur push-up balconette to work without feeling like an extra in a *Carry On* movie. (Allen, 2001: 37–8)

So feminists are the 'hard option' – careerist, pinstriped and hard-nosed. The use of these words to describe feminists may seem amusing to some, but in truth they are sexist pejorative labels that are intended to discredit and humiliate women who are perceived by some men and women to be a threat to the patriarchal status quo. Incidentally, the infamous photograph taken in the 1970s of women burning their bras was fallacious. Women were seen to be throwing their bras into a waste bin, but the image of the flames was superimposed.

This section of the chapter seeks to relate the development of feminist theories from the modernist period of the 1960s and 1970s to the contemporary postmodern period. These perspectives are themselves manifestations of the struggle to enable women in academia to have their voices articulated within mainstream (malestream) sociological discourse. Sociology as an academic discipline only acknowledged the 'validity' of feminist theory in the 1970s. Such theories offer particular analyses and explanations with regard to how and why women have less power than men and how this imbalance can be challenged and transformed. Knowledge such as this is clearly of fundamental importance to midwives and healthcare professionals who work with women – indeed, the word 'midwife' means 'with woman'. Midwives are encouraged to practise in a 'woman-centred' manner (House of Commons Select Committee, 1992; Department of Health, 1993), and thus an understanding of how other women live their lives is imperative. Furthermore, the vast majority of midwives and nurses are women themselves, and it is important that such practitioners have insight into and self-awareness of the way in which they view themselves as women, in order to be able to assist different women in childbirth in a sensitive, empathetic and woman-centred manner. Feminist perspectives also may enable midwives to understand differently the constraints and limitations that have been and still are imposed on midwifery practice.

Definitions

Feminism has been referred to as a philosophy, a world view, a theory and a method of analysis (McCool and McCool, 1989). There is no single definition because there are multiple perspectives, but it may be useful to consider the following as a possible baseline:

> At the very least a feminist is someone who holds that women suffer discrimination because of their sex, that they have specific needs which remain negated and unsatisfied, and that satisfaction of these needs would require a radical change (some would say a revolution even) in the social, economic and political order.
>
> (Delmar, 1986: 8)

Thus a feminist is someone who recognises that there is discrimination against women, that their specific needs are unsatisfied and that there is a necessity for radical change in order to meet these needs. However, when seeking the reasons for and solutions to these problems, differing views or perspectives are encountered. The main feminist perspectives will now be considered briefly. It can be seen that they are broadly *social constructionist* in that the role of society is fundamental, the exception being radical feminism.

Radical feminism: its contribution to childbirth and patriarchy

Of all the 'feminisms', radical feminism has been the most misunderstood and the most threatening to men (and to many women). The word 'radical' here means 'the root of' and has a direct relationship to radical midwifery (Klima, 2001). In terms of chronology, it can be seen that the development of women's position in society clearly relates to the recent history of midwifery and women's services, as shown in Table 1.3.

Table 1.3   History of women's position in society related to history of midwifery and women's services

Women's movement		History of midwifery and women's services
1897:	The National Union of Women's Suffrage Societies formed (President: Millicent Fawcett)	1902: The Midwives Act
1903:	The Women's Social and Political Union was formed by the Pankhursts	1918: The second Midwives Act
1928:	The Equal Franchise Act gave all women over 21 years the vote	1929: British College of Obstetricians and Gynaecologists was formed
1937:	The Matrimonial Causes Act extended grounds for divorce to cruelty, desertion and insanity	1936: The third Midwives Act
1964:	The Married Women's Property Act enabled a divorced wife to keep half of anything she had saved from any allowance given to her by her husband	1956: Natural Childbirth Association (NCA) was formed in response to the medicalisation of childbirth which developed rapidly during the 1950s and 1960s
1960s–1970s:	The beginnings of 'second-wave' radical feminism	1961: National Childbirth Trust was formed (name changed from NCA)
1970:	The Equal Pay Act	
1975:	The Sex Discrimination Act The Employment Protection Act	
1976:	The Domestic Violence Act	1981: First march by women on an NHS maternity hospital to protest about its over-medicalised policies
		1986: Foundation of the Association of Radical Midwives
1990s:	The development of postmodernist feminist theory	1992: Publication of House of Commons Select Committee, Second Report
		1993: Publication by Department of Health of *Changing Childbirth. Part 1. Report of the Expert Maternity Group*

Radical feminism developed during the 1960s and 1970s as a theory to explain the oppression of women. It coincided with a surge in the use of science and technology in childbirth, which many women were beginning to rebel against due to their experience of loss of control and invisibility (Donnison, 1977; Stanworth, 1994; Tew, 1998). Radical feminist theorists contend that the oppression of women is primarily based on patriarchy (the domination of women by men). The family is seen as a key instrument of the oppression of women through male control of women and children (with marriage, patrilineal heritage and the taking of the man's name regarded as being central to this control). Men, it is argued, systematically dominate women in every sphere of life, and all relationships between men and women are institutionalised relationships of power and therefore an appropriate subject for political analysis. Thus radical feminists are concerned to reveal how male power is exercised and reinforced in all spheres of life. Included in the thrall of patriarchy are personal relationships, childrearing, housework and marriage and the full range of sexual practices, including rape, prostitution, sexual harassment and sexual intercourse.

An analogy has been drawn between the patriarchal nuclear family and the relationships between doctors, nurses and patients by Littlewood (1991). It can be adapted to midwifery as shown in Figure 1.1.

Here obstetrics is seen as a male-gendered profession – scientific, technological, active and patriarchal in its belief system – and there is no room for women's individual emotional needs. The midwife is viewed as analogous to the 'wife' – necessary and useful, but inferior and therefore passive in the hierarchy. She is there to be kind and caring and to support the obstetrician. And what of the woman? She is portrayed as passive and at the bottom of the hierarchy. If she is 'good', she will book early, make use of all the technology that is offered to her, and give birth in the hospital. The analogy here is with the child in the nuclear family.

Male science has been used to legitimise the ideologies that define women as inferior, and that define women's role as domestic labourer (Stanworth, 1994; Abbott and Wallace, 1997; Kent, 2000). In the field of childbirth, the new reproductive technologies are now very fundamental to maternity services and are becoming increasingly widespread. However, Crozier (2001) questions whether technology should be viewed as a purely masculine domain of knowledge which oppresses women, since many women feel the technology to be empowering and

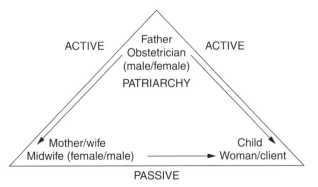

Figure 1.1   Representation of an analogy between the patriarchal nuclear family and relationships between obstetricians, midwives and women.

beneficial in allowing them to make choices. To think otherwise renders women passive and subordinate. Are women, who profess to be in control when they use technology in childbirth, really in control? Or have they been frightened into believing the rhetoric of those whose interests lie in the use of technology, such as obstetricians and pharmaceutical companies? These are vexed questions which will tax midwives and healthcare professionals increasingly in the future.

Patriarchy

To return to the wider field of radical feminism, Mitchell (1974) is a key radical feminist theorist who has made a significant contribution to our understanding of the concept of patriarchy. She views patriarchy as a universal feature of human societies, but argues that its origins are cultural rather than biological, and that it is maintained primarily through ideology. The ideas and beliefs by means of which women make sense of their lived experience are achieved through socialisation and education. Arguably it is men who write the gender socialisation scripts and thus ensure the continual reproduction of dominant masculinity and domi- nated femininity. An example of this would be domestic ideology, which iden- tifies women particularly with the home, and the complementary 'bread-winner' ideology, according to which men are supposed to provide financially for their families (Connell, 1994; Walby, 1994). These ideologies are obviously linked and co-contribute to making sense of the world, usually by supporting the status quo and reinforcing power relationships so that they seem inevitable and 'the way it should be' (Crowley and Himmelweit, 1992). Mitchell (1974) suggests that what is needed is a specific struggle against patriarchy involving a cultural revolution to counter ideological notions of the feminine as being subordinate within society.

However, the concept of patriarchy has not been used within feminist theory in any simple or unified way. Its use ranges from attempts to trace the origins of women's subordination, to the seeking of explanations as to how patriarchy works in terms of the different activities of women and men in society (Stacey, 1993; Connell, 1994).

Delphy (1984) has also made an important contribution to the debate on patriarchy. She considers that there are two modes of production, namely the industrial mode of production, which is the arena of capitalist exploitation, and the family mode of production, in which men exploit women's labour. Men, she says, benefit from women's provision of domestic services and unpaid childrearing within the family, and therefore women's reproductive and productive activities in the household are the main form of women's oppression.

Patriarchy also has an influence over women in that 'motherhood' is set out as the superordinate role for *all* women. The depths of women's identification with this belief are revealed in the agonies which infertility brings. It is threatening the very essence of woman-identity. Furthermore, women who do not 'fit the mould' are disparaged and stigmatised. It may be considered tragic if a woman is unable to bear children, but she is thought to be abnormal if she has chosen not to be a mother.

Walby (1990, 1994) is another feminist writer who has made a major contribution to the debate on patriarchy. She regards patriarchy and capitalism as two distinct systems, so that capitalism may benefit from patriarchy in that female domestic labour is unpaid and sustains male labour (an historical basis). However, she does not view women as victims, and she regards it as mainly due to women's own efforts that, in the UK, they have partially broken out of private patriarchy and achieved a stronger position with regard to paid work.

Walby (1990) has presented six main structures within which patriarchy occurs:

1 paid employment ('glass ceiling', low pay, low status, part-time work)
2 household production (childrearing, housework, production of food)
3 culture (including religion, media and education)
4 sexuality (including definitions of sex as male orientated)
5 male violence (domestic violence – including marital rape, rape, pornography, childhood sexual abuse)
6 the State.

Walby (1990) then suggests that these six main structures of patriarchy are linked to private and public patriarchy. In private patriarchy, male domination occurs directly within the household structure and also by the exclusion of women from public life. In public patriarchy, women play roles within paid employment and in other structures, but their subordination is implemented by segregating them from the main areas of wealth, power and status (e.g. low numbers of female consultant obstetricians, but substantial involvement in clerical work). Importantly, Walby also considers that women have moved from being excluded from the main areas of wealth, power and status to being segregated within these areas. For example, more women work outside the home for money, so they are not excluded from paid work, but they tend to take low-paid, part-time work and may fail to achieve the higher positions.

For midwives and healthcare professionals, patriarchy can be a useful tool for analysis in that it takes the male body as the 'standard, prototype', the female body being seen as 'defective, inferior'. This is particularly relevant to women, reproduction and the negative aspects of the medicalisation of childbirth whereby birth is only viewed as normal in retrospect. Furthermore, it can be argued that much of women's experience of ill health stems from their relationships with men and male-dominated institutions (Doyal, 1995). These experiences of ill health may include the sequelae of domestic violence, stress and poverty, which have profound effects on women and/or fetuses and children (Gary et al., 1998; Lewis, 2001).

Liberal feminism

Historically, liberal feminism has concerned itself with equal opportunities for women and men, and is considered to be reformist in nature. The Equal Pay Act (1970) and the Sex Discrimination Act (1975) could be said to be the results of a widely supported effort to achieve liberal equality between the sexes. Liberal feminists consider a woman's sex to be irrelevant to her rights. They propose that, in western industrial societies, women are discriminated against on the basis of sex in so far as certain restrictions are placed on women as a group without regard to their own individual wishes, interests, abilities and needs (Abbott and Wallace, 1997). Once discrimination is removed, it will be possible for women and men to be treated as individuals, and women will be given the opportunity to show that they are as capable as men in all of the key positions in society that are currently denied them (Crowley and Himmelweit, 1992). This was clearly demonstrated in Britain in the Second World War when women performed men's work (but not political leadership).

Liberal feminism is a useful theoretical approach in that equal opportunities, for example, are important to women. However, it does not address the underlying oppressive ideologies of the status of women in society (Crowley and Himmelweit, 1992). It seeks to reform women's position to that of equality with men without a deconstruction of the pervading masculinist ideologies and their replacement with structures that represent the views and needs of women.

Marxist feminism

In the 1970s, a number of feminist theorists began to draw on the writings of Marx in order to explain the oppression of women. In doing so, they had to extend his theories in order to make women 'visible', because Marxist analysis is *essentialist* in nature in that it assumes a biological basis for gender (power) relationships. Here women's oppression is regarded as being tied to forms of capitalist exploitation of labour, and thus women's paid and unpaid work is analysed in relation to its function within the capitalist economy (Stacey, 1993). Capitalism compounds women's oppression by systematically excluding them from the labour market, thus denying them the opportunity to sell their labour power. Marxist feminists have critiqued the State as not acting in women's interests and as reinforcing relationships of power. They have attempted to analyse the part played by the State in establishing and maintaining women's dependence within the family household and wage labour as interrelated systems (Watson, 1999).

Figure 1.2 sets out the sexual division of labour in diagrammatic form.

Conversations with many women, midwives and healthcare professionals would suggest that such sexual division of labour holds true. Kate Beverley explores this further in Chapter 3 on women and poverty. Letvak (2001) considers that in the UK traditional images of motherhood are enduring, pervasive and incompatible with paid employment. However, in a society with radically reconstructed structures that favour connection and respect between women and men, an alternative model of paid/unpaid work may be represented as shown in Figure 1.3.

Clearly such a model requires a radical ideological change to the structures and systems that make up society. Patriarchy has no place here. The ethos is of mutual respect, sharing and connection. In recent years, some maternity units have become much more flexible with regard to midwives who need career breaks or who wish to work part-time. They have had to be so because of the shortage of midwives rather than because of a radical change in the culture of the workplace.

Black feminism

Black feminists have been critical of the lack of centrality given to issues of ethnic difference, racialisation and racism in feminist theory and research (Abbott and Wallace, 1997). Anthias and Yuval-Davis (1992) go further, stating that black, minority and migrant women have, on the whole, been invisible within the feminist movement in the UK, and they describe the feminist movement as white, middle-class and racist. Although class and gender may be regarded as central to

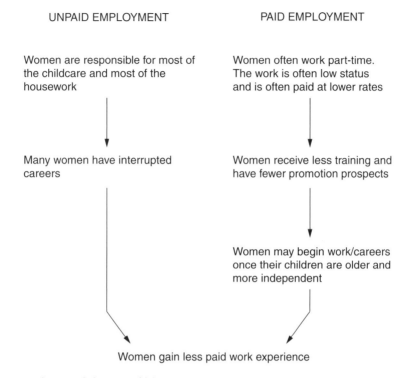

UNPAID EMPLOYMENT   PAID EMPLOYMENT

Women are responsible for most of   Women often work part-time.
the childcare and most of the   The work is often low status
housework   and is often paid at lower rates

Many women have interrupted   Women receive less training and
careers   have fewer promotion prospects

                                           Women may begin work/careers
                                           once their children are older and
                                           more independent

Women gain less paid work experience

Figure 1.2   The sexual division of labour.

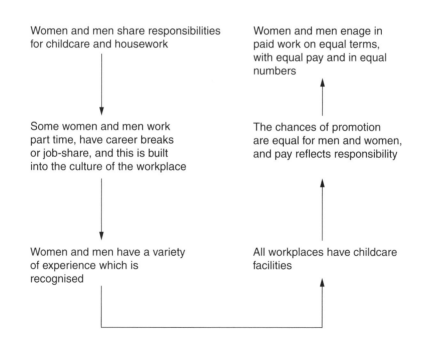

Women and men share responsibilities   Women and men enage in
for childcare and housework   paid work on equal terms,
                                           with equal pay and in equal
                                           numbers

Some women and men work   The chances of promotion
part time, have career breaks   are equal for men and women,
or job-share, and this is built   and pay reflects responsibility
into the culture of the workplace

Women and men have a variety   All workplaces have childcare
of experience which is   facilities
recognised

Figure 1.3   An alternative model of paid/unpaid work for women and men.

women's subordination, race is another form of social exclusion. The ways in which class, race and gender interact with one another may be different for black, minority and migrant women. Women who are oppressed and exploited by racism and/or imperialism have powerful interests in common with their men, and these stand in opposition to those of white men *and* women in western cultures. Therefore the issues here are complex, revealing solidarities, contradictions and struggles with which women globally have to interact in their lives (Aziz, 1992).

In the healthcare literature, stereotypes abound with regard to 'different' women, whether they differ in terms of skin colour, religion, language or between themselves. Asian women are represented as passive and as being controlled within patriarchal family systems. Afro-Caribbean women are viewed as dominating and as running matriarchal family structures. Both stereotypes are devoid of any analysis of class or gender, despite the fact that many black women occupy low-paid, low-status jobs, experience poverty and are particularly vulnerable to oppression (Abbott and Wallace, 1997). Again, despite the fact that there has been development of black and Asian middle-classes, they will nevertheless experience discrimination and prejudice. Bowler (1993), in her study of Asian women who had given birth, found clear evidence of stereotyping and prejudice among the midwives whom she interviewed, including descriptions of lack of maternal instinct, overuse of the service and non-use of contraception. Similarly, Katbamna (2000) found that periods of rest after childbirth can be interpreted as indolence by some midwives. Further examples may be found in Dave Sookhoo's analysis of 'race', ethnicity, culture and childbirth in Chapter 5.

This consideration of black feminism has been brief. However, it is important for midwives and health professionals to develop a real understanding of the complex lives and experiences of black, migrant and minority women to enable them to practise in insightful ways.

Postmodern feminism

Postmodernism constitutes a critique of traditional theorising, and it proposes that there can no longer be a claim that scientific theories actually 'capture' reality. Instead, theories are to be understood as partial representations of or approximations to a reality which is more complex and multifaceted. Central to postmodern theory is the recognition of difference (race, sex and age) and deconstruction (a multiply divided subject in a multiply divided society) (Abbott and Wallace, 1997; Scambler, 1998). Women show similarities and differences to each other, and therefore so do midwives and healthcare professionals. It may be that a postmodern approach is most suitable in terms of contributing to sensitive midwifery practice and trying to understand what it really means to work in partnership *with* women. 'Realities' in childbirth are always too complex for objective understanding, and recognition of this may lead to more sophisticated approaches in an attempt to understand what women want or need. The differing views of women and their relationship with technology and control, as mentioned earlier, are perhaps an example of this.

Postmodern feminists reject biological determinism and the notion of sex differences. Furthermore, they reject the idea of substituting feminist theories for male-stream ones because, they argue, there is no possibility of true knowledge but only a multiplicity of truths. Instead, it is suggested that there is a need to deconstruct truth claims, and to seek knowledge, but to recognise that knowledge is a part of power (Abbott and Wallace, 1997). Flax (1990) has summarised the focus of postmodernism as how to understand and reconstitute the self, gender, knowledge, social relationships and culture without resorting to linear, holistic or binary ways of thinking and being.

However, postmodernism is problematic. It can be argued that difference is a way of not having to think about oppression and subordination, and this makes it possible to ignore the centrality and reality of male power that has been fundamental to other forms of feminism. A politics of difference also aids the rejection of the notion that there is a hierarchy of oppressions, that some such oppressions are more salient than others, or that oppressions are additive. Thus the focus shifts to the ways in which each of these relationships interact, reinforce and contradict each other in specific contexts (McDowell and Pringle, 1992). Patriarchy as 'reality' is denied and oppression is ignored.

Postmodernism is therefore the antithesis of the biomedical system in which midwives work, which encourages binary, linear models of thought. It may be that this form of theorising leads to a more sophisticated understanding of the complexities of different women's lives, and it may be of use to midwives and healthcare professionals in their interactions with different women and their families and with each other. The challenges are enormous. Midwives work in hierarchical institutions which are dominated by men, where both the ethos and the structures are generally highly masculinised (Pringle, 1995), and where binary ways of thinking abound. It would be incredibly difficult to think in terms of a multiplicity of truths in a culture where scientific rigour is supposed to underpin practice. It is not suggested here that patriarchy as a theory should be abandoned, but that postmodernism may contribute to a better understanding of differences. Moreover, it is not suggested that any notion of women having beliefs, values or interests in common should be denied. Indeed, Zadoroznyj (1999), for example, found that social class had a strong effect on the shaping of identity in her study of birthing narratives. Information such as this is useful when one is trying to understand the experiences of different women. In summary, it is a question of balancing the different approaches of patriarchy and postmodernism in the quest for insightful practice.

So far this chapter has focused on the structural issues concerning women and society, and also the contribution of primarily radical and postmodernist feminist theory to midwifery. It will now address the nature–nurture debate and its contribution to the differences between women and men.

Sex and gender

In the study of women and socialisation, the differences between the concepts of 'sex' and 'gender' have been problematic. The term 'sex' relates to nature and biology, and since the 1970s, feminist theory has attempted to explain the differences between being female and being male as being socially constructed. Thus the biologically orientated and determinist theories, which are considered to be patriarchal, have been supplanted by more socio-culturally orientated models (Sebrant, 1998). However, while acknowledging the importance of the concept of social construction in attempting to understand the experiences of being a woman, it would appear reasonable to state that women and men *are* different, but that attention should focus on the unequal power relationships which result from these differences.

Sex

In general, the term 'sex' is used to refer to the chromosomal differences that define male and female bodies. Biologically determinist theories define what women are or can and cannot do because of their sex (Crowley and Himmelweit, 1992). Therefore women have been represented as 'naturally' more caring, nurturing, less aggressive, with smaller brains and ruled by hormones, which is why women tend to look after the home and family while men are more likely to be engaged in activities that require more logical brain activity (Giddens, 2001). Such ideology pervades much of the media in contemporary society, where women are viewed as passive and beautiful and men are regarded as strong, active and muscular. This serves to reinforce the heterosexist notions of femininity and masculinity as a binary divide which in turn supports heterosexual relationships and a patriarchal society (Kent, 2000). It is interesting to note that historically female genitalia were regarded as the same as those of the male, except that they were located inside the body:

> The spermatick vessels (fallopian tubes) in women, called *preparing* because they prepare and convey to the testicles (ovaries) the blood, of which seed is engendered, differ not from those in men, either in number, or use, but only in their insertion and manner of their distribution.
> (Mauriceau, 1697: 22)

Biological determinism can also be applied to men, but it could be argued that the symmetry ends there, because such a theory ultimately valorises existing relationships of power. Male dominance and aggression and female passivity and domesticity are portrayed as biological and therefore as 'natural' and 'normal' (Birke, 1992).

However, some modernist feminist writers do not refute the biological differences, and celebrate the capacity of women's bodies to nurture and reproduce. Assister (1996) argues that there is value in the distinction that is made between gender and sex. With regard to biology and sex, she considers that there is a minimum necessary set of bodily or biological features present in every female (chromosomes, hormones, genitalia and secondary sex characteristics) which forms the 'real essence' of what it is to be a woman and is significant in influencing social and psychological identity. She argues for a universalist basis for feminism, so that a refocusing on nature and the importance of the minimal biological body should provide a basis for a shared identity among women.

However, Annandale and Clark (1996) critique what they call the 'negative consequences' that can arise from feminist thinking which is premised upon a binary division between women and men, male and female, and sex and gender. In their paper on sociology and human reproduction, they propose that these consequences include the following:

- the universalising and valorising of gender differences
- a preoccupation with the abnormalities of women's reproductive health

- a focus on women to the neglect of gender (and men's health) which, it is argued, inhibits the ability truly to understand the experience of being a woman.

Birke (1992) is also uncomfortable about rejecting the biological, but suggests the incorporation of gene theories into postmodernist feminist discourse. She argues that female and male bodies *are* different – and that it is the usage of biological determinism to reinforce inequalities of status and power between women and men that is the problem. She advocates a dynamic interaction between sex and gender as follows:

> What this line of thought emphasises is that what you are now – your biological body, your experiences – is a product of complex transformations between biology and experiences in your past. And those transformations happening now will affect any such transformations in the future. Biology, in this view, does have a role, but it is neither a base to build on, nor determining.
>
> (Birke, 1992: 75)

This theory, which is termed the concept of 'transformative change', would appear to look at women's lives in a more holistic way. It suggests that a woman is affected by the society in which she lives, her particular social and economic background, and by the fact that she carries the XX (female) chromosome. This theory also incorporates the changes that may occur in the future as a result of the complexities of the relationship between social experiences and the experiences of being biologically female. Thus the sense of being female may change through life as a result of the various experiences that may occur. The following list includes examples of such possible experiences:

- poverty or acquiring disposable income
- marriage or deciding not to be married in a relationship
- altered sexual identity
- being homosexual
- the joy or the unhappiness of having children
- making the decision not to have children
- finding that one is unable to have children due to not having a relationship with a man
- finding that one is physically unable to conceive a child
- miscarriage
- termination of pregnancy
- divorce or separation from a partner
- death of a loved adult, stillborn/miscarried baby or child
- a history of sexual abuse as a child and the effects that this has on survivors
- having experienced domestic violence
- relating to and being influenced by the experiences of peers and family.

Many women will experience some of the above, as will midwives and other healthcare professionals.

Gender

In contrast, gender refers to socially constructed notions of femininity and masculinity. Gender theory, especially in the 1970s and 1980s, highlighted the social construction of gender difference and was important for underpinning feminist struggles for equality and liberation. However, social constructions of femininity and the role of women differ according to whether a woman is born in, for example, the UK or Nepal. All countries are stratified, whether by social class, economic class or, for example, the caste system. The way in which women are viewed depends very much on the nature of the system of stratification into which they are born. Furthermore, each individual woman within a given society will experience life in unique ways, making generalisation difficult and invalid. Patterns of behaviour and attitudes can be distinguished, which are normally referred to as 'social norms'. These include norms governing gender identities, and they are transmitted/learned in the course of socialisation. When a midwife assists women who are giving birth to female children, the babies may not look significantly different at birth. However, the midwife will know from her knowledge of social sciences that their lives will vary considerably depending on factors such as social or economic class and attitudes to women held by their parents and the social group with whom they will grow up.

Socially constructed notions of femininity and masculinity in any society are difficult if not impossible to circumvent when bringing up (and therefore socialising) children. They are there in everyday social interactions and in the media, and they begin at birth when considering the differences in the way in which female and male babies are cared for. It may be that male babies are picked up and cuddled less (Nicholson, 1984), and certainly different language is adopted when referring to male or female children, such as 'what a big, strong boy you are', as opposed to 'she's so sweet and pretty'. A recent visit to a department store to look for toys revealed the stereotypes shown in Table 1.4.

Table 1.4 Stereotypes of appropriate toys for boys and girls to play with

Toys for boys	Toys for girls
Military walkie-talkie	Doll like a real baby: • can be fed from her bottle • cries real tears • can have her nappy changed
Battle bashers	Honeymoon nails and rings (age 3+)
Battleline robots	Wedding tiara
Action man	Fashion doll: • goes shopping • goes to the beauty salon
Paratrooper	Nails and jewellery kit
Fireman Sam	
Cowboy	

UK society thus seems to have clearly differentiated views on what are appropriate toys for male and female children to play with (Wajcman, 1994).

The suggestion that gender is more fundamental than other social divisions has been critiqued on the basis of its representation of all women as homogenous (universalist), belonging to the same oppressed group. Doyal (1995) rejects what she calls 'crude universalism'. She points out that women with diverse social contexts and/or lifestyles, such as lesbians, black women, women with disabilities and women from non-industrialised countries, have challenged the white, western, middle-class domination of feminist theory and practice.

Postmodernist feminism has highlighted the limitations of generalisations, emphasising instead the importance of understanding and acknowledging the diversity of the lived experiences of being a woman. A more sophisticated understanding of and emphasis on the relationships between race, class and gender, and a consideration of the differences between women, can be developed from such a perspective. Needless to say, there are problems inherent here. For example, is it appropriate to consider that cultural practices should be respected whatever they are because to do otherwise would denigrate customs and practices that are different from our own? This could lead to a refusal to take action when a female child has been genitally mutilated, out of fear of being considered racist, or a refusal to condemn male violence in cultures where it is widely condoned (Doyal, 1995).

However, Doyal (1995) does not believe that the focus should rest solely on difference. She feels that the possibility of shared beliefs, values or interests should not be denied. For example, many women share the reality of occupying subordinate positions in most social and cultural contexts. There is much commonality in the psychological struggle to make sense of themselves, as women, in the face of strong cultural messages that define women as inferior. For example, women in the UK have the second highest rate in the European Union for participation in employment (Denmark takes the lead), yet 43% are employed on part-time contracts with less pay and fewer employment rights than men (British Council, 1999).

Many women may wish to work part-time, of course, often when they are the prime carers for their children. However, employers and the State do little to facilitate women in these dual roles. A look at some of the letters to the Royal College of Midwives journal, *Midwives*, reveals that some returning midwives are employed at a more junior level than they were when they were employed full-time, surely a state of affairs that is not likely to encourage experienced midwives to return to work after giving birth. Such iniquity is replicated throughout the labour market. The clear message is that these workers are perceived to be of less value than their full-time colleagues. Thus there is a material dimension to women's experiences of subordination, since many women are obliged to deal with the consequences of poverty and economic inequality between the sexes (Doyal, 1995).

Conclusion

This chapter has explored a number of different theories about the socialisation of women which attempt to explain the basis of particular difficulties women face in their lives. Feminist perspectives have been examined in terms of their differing approaches to the explanation of gender inequalities. Radical feminism has been discussed in relation to its influence on evolving approaches to midwifery practice. The various theories offer analyses and explanations with regard to how and why women have less power than men and how this imbalance can be challenged and transformed. Many women are at ease being married, having children and being responsible for childcare, housework and the domestic infrastructure. However, it has been seen that ideologies of women as only being suited to domesticity have been harmful to many women, and their needs should be addressed. The debates concerning sex/gender and nature/nurture are complex and will doubtless continue, but such binary ways of thinking are not sufficiently sophisticated to consider the complexities of interactions and power relationships between men and women.

It is suggested that postmodernism offers a different understanding of women's lives and may be a useful theory for enhancing midwifery practice. Feminism as a 'lay' concept has been much maligned and misunderstood, but can offer relevant insight and understanding to midwives and healthcare professionals who work with women and who profess to be 'woman-centred'. Midwives *as women* have close ties to the patriarchal medical and scientific world. This makes analysis of women's lives all the more pertinent, not just with regard to women who give birth, but also in relation to the lives of midwives and health professionals, most of whom are women themselves. As Elizabeth Davis asks, 'What could be more feminist than the practice of midwifery?' (Davis, 1987: 5).

- Feminist theories enable analysis of women's lives, how and why women have less power than men, and how this situation can be addressed.
- A feminist is not someone who hates men.
- Analysis of the similarities and differences between women would lead to a deeper understanding of what it is to 'be woman'.
- Such analysis is vital for midwives and healthcare professionals, who are mainly women, work with women and sit juxtaposed to a patriarchal medical and scientific community within hierarchical patriarchal institutions.

References

- Abbott P and Wallace C (1997) *An Introduction to Sociology: feminist perspectives.* Routledge, London.
- Allen C (2001) Feel like a woman. *Health and Beauty.* **Winter Issue**: 37–8.
- Annandale E and Clark J (1996) What is gender? Feminist theory and the sociology of human reproduction. *Sociol Health Illness.* **18**: 17–44.
- Anthias F and Yuval-Davis (1992) Contextualizing feminism: gender, ethnic and class divisions. In: L McDowell and R Pringle (eds) *Defining Women: social institutions and gender divisions.* Polity Press, Cambridge in association with the Open University Press, Buckingham.
- Archbishops' Council (2002) *About the Church of England. Key statistics;* www.cofe.anglican.org/about/statistics.html
- Assister A (1996) *Enlightened Women: modern feminism in a postmodern age.* Routledge, London.

- Aziz R (1992) Feminism and the challenge of racism: deviance or difference? In: H Crowley and S Himmelweit (eds) *Knowing Women: feminism and knowledge*. Polity Press, Cambridge in association with the Open University Press, Buckingham.
- Birke L (1992) Transforming biology. In: H Crowley and S Himmelweit (eds) *Knowing Women: feminism and knowledge*. Polity Press, Cambridge in association with the Open University Press, Buckingham.
- Bowler I (1993) 'They're not the same as us': midwives' stereotypes of South Asian descent maternity patients. *Sociol Health Illness*. **15**: 157–78.
- British Council (1999) *Information on Women in the UK: governance*; www.britishcouncil.org/governance/gendev/gadwomuk
- Connell RW (1994) Gender regimes and gender order. In: A Giddens, D Held, D Hillman *et al.* (eds) *The Polity Reader in Gender Studies*. Polity Press, Cambridge.
- Connon H (2001) Old girls' network takes on male bastion. *Observer*. **25 November**: 5.
- Crowley H and Himmelweit S (1992) *Knowing Women: feminism and knowledge*. Polity Press, Cambridge in association with the Open University Press, Buckingham.
- Crozier K (2001) Technology: is it killing the art of midwifery? *RCM Midwives J*. **4**: 410–11.
- Davis E (1987) *Heart and Hands: a midwife's guide to pregnancy and birth* (2e). Celestial Arts, Berkeley, CA.
- de Beauvoir S (1953) *The Second Sex*. David Campbell Publishers Ltd, London.
- Delmar R (1986) What is feminism? In: J Mitchell and A Oakley (eds) *What is Feminism?* Basil Blackwell, Oxford.
- Delphy C (1984) *Close to Home: a materialist analysis of women's oppression*. Hutchinson, London.
- Department of Health (1993) *Changing Childbirth. Part 1. Report of the Expert Maternity Group*. HMSO, London.
- Donnison J (1977) *Midwives and Medical Men: a history of interprofessional rivalries*. Schocken Books, London.
- Doyal L (1995) *What Makes Women Sick. Gender and the political economy of health*. Macmillan, Basingstoke.
- Equal Opportunities Commission (2002) *Research Findings: attitudes to equal pay*; http//www.eoc.org.uk/valuingwomen
- Flax J (1990) *Thinking Fragments: psychoanalysis, feminism and postmodernism in the contemporary west*. University of California Press, Berkeley, CA.
- Gary F, Sigsby LM and Campbell D (1998) Feminism: a perspective for the twenty-first century. *Issues Ment Health Nurs*. **19**: 139–52.
- Giddens A (2001) *Sociology* (4e). Polity Press, Cambridge.
- House of Commons Select Committee (1992) *Maternity Services. Second report*. HMSO, London.
- Katbamna S (2000) *'Race' and Childbirth*. Open University Press, Buckingham.
- Kent J (2000) *Social Perspectives on Pregnancy and Childbirth for Midwives, Nurses and the Caring Professions*. Open University Press, Buckingham.
- Klima CS (2001) Women's health care: a new paradigm for the twenty-first century. *J Midwif Women's Health*. **46**: 285–91.
- Letvak S (2001) Nurses as working women *AORN J*. **73**: 675–82.

- Lewis G (ed.) (2001) *The Confidential Enquiries into Maternal Deaths*. RCOG Press, London.
- Littlewood R (1991) Gender, role and sickness: the ritual psychopathologies of the nurse. In: P Holden and J Littlewood (eds) *Anthropology and Nursing*. Routledge, London.
- Lord Chancellor's Department (2001) *Judicial Appointments in England and Wales: the appointment of lawyers to the professional judiciary. Equality of opportunity and promoting diversity*; http://www.lcd.gov.uk/judicial/judequal.htm
- McCool WF and McCool SJ (1989) Feminism and nurse-midwifery: historical overview and current issues. *J Nurse Midwifery*. **34**: 323–34.
- McDowell L and Pringle R (eds) (1992) *Defining Women: social institutions and gender divisions*. Polity Press, Cambridge in association with the Open University Press, Buckingham.
- Mauriceau F (1697) *The Diseases of Women with Child and in Child-Bed* (trans. H Chamberlen) (3e). Andrew Bell, London.
- Mitchell J (1974) *Psychoanalysis and Feminism*. Penguin, Harmondsworth.
- National Statistics (2002) *New Earnings Survey 2001*. National Statistics, London.
- Nicholson J (1984) *Men and Women: how different are they?* Oxford University Press, Oxford.
- Phillips A (1994) The representation of women. In: A Giddens, D Held, D Hillman *et al.* (eds) *The Polity Reader in Gender Studies*. Polity Press, Cambridge.
- Pringle K (1995) *Men, Masculinities and Social Welfare*. University College London Press, London.
- Scambler A (1998) Gender, health and the feminist debate on postmodernism. In: G Scambler and P Higgs (eds) *Modernity, Medicine and Health. Medical sociology towards 2000*. Routledge, London.
- Sebrant U (1998) Being female in a health care hierarchy. *Scand J Caring Sci.* **13**: 153–8.
- Stacey J (1993) Untangling feminist theory. In: D Richardson and V Robinson (eds) *Introducing Women's Studies*. Macmillan, Basingstoke.
- Stanworth M (1994) Reproductive technologies and the deconstruction of motherhood. In: A Giddens, D Held, D Hillman *et al.* (eds) *The Polity Reader in Gender Studies*. Polity Press, Cambridge.
- Stephens L (1999) Why aren't midwives feminists? *Br J Midwifery*. **7**: 476.
- Tew M (1998) *Safer Childbirth? A critical history of maternity care* (3e). Chapman & Hall, London.
- Wajcman J (1994) Technology as masculine culture. In: A Giddens, D Held, D Hillman *et al.* (eds) *The Polity Reader in Gender Studies*. Polity Press, Cambridge.
- Walby S (1990) *Theorising Patriarchy*. Basil Blackwell, Oxford.
- Walby S (1994) Towards a theory of patriarchy. In: A Giddens, D Held, D Hillman *et al.* (eds) *The Polity Reader in Gender Studies*. Polity Press, Cambridge.
- Watson S (1999) Introduction. In: S Watson and L Doyal (eds) *Engendering Social Policy*. Open University Press, Buckingham.
- Zadoroznyj M (1999) Social class, social selves and social control in childbirth. *Sociol Health Illness*. **21**: 267–89.

Chapter 2

Women and sex

Sandy Nelson

The aim of this chapter is to give the reader a critical understanding of the main theories of female sexuality. The relevance of the concepts of these theories to medicine, midwifery and nursing practice will be explored. The key themes that will be considered include scientific research on sexuality, ideological biases in the research, sexual health, the female body, Freudian theories, current images of female sexuality, heterosexuality and safer sex, pregnancy and sexuality, and cultural differences.

Introduction

Gender and sexuality pervade every aspect of human life, and from childhood onwards we are curious about what it means to be female or male and what attracts us to certain people and not others. A vast amount of money is spent on research that sets out to explore the extent to which sexuality is based on our biological inheritance in the form of hormones, genes or genitals, or whether childhood experience is more important. Other research examines the role of culture. Some studies look at how much influence power, social status and financial independence have on our ability to choose the sexual relationships that we want.

The answers to these questions are not merely academic, but also have important consequences. For example, hormonal explanations of rape and sexual abuse have directly resulted in the use of 'chemical castration' to control sex offenders. Moreover, the law and medicine work hand in hand to judge whether sexual behaviour is natural or unnatural, and consequently whether an individual should be regarded as ill or a criminal, or both. These norms change over time and reflect the cultural values of different periods. For instance, masturbation was believed to be harmful in Victorian England, but today is regarded as a vital part of psychosexual therapy. Women are no longer 'routinely' given hysterectomies, and the National Health Service may provide gender reassignment for transsexuals.

It is ironic, therefore, that a subject of such importance, and one in which medicine plays a central role, is so little dealt with by healthcare workers. Despite the fact that sexuality is regarded as an important aspect of holistic care, sexual issues are rarely addressed with patients. When they are raised, there is a tendency to reduce a person's sexuality to their marital status. This omission is even more astonishing when we consider how ill health can affect feelings of self-esteem and create sexual difficulties in relationships. People with stomas, scars, missing body parts or chronic fatigue may feel anxious about the expression of their sexuality. For many years within midwifery, sexuality was barely mentioned and pregnancy was separated from conception as if all births were virgin births. The sexuality of the elderly was (and often still is) ignored. The specific needs of lesbian and gay patients, and the sexual concerns that people with psychiatric illnesses or learning difficulties may have, seldom appear in either nursing care plans or service provision. Antenatal HIV testing has put sexuality on the agenda for midwives, but whether the test will be discussed within an infection control model or be raised as part of a more open discussion of any sexual concerns remains to be seen.

Perhaps this omission is not so surprising. Many midwives and nurses do not feel confident about their ability to raise the topic of sexuality in discussion, and fear that they may hear disclosures of sexual abuse, sexual assault or homosexuality to which they would not know how to respond. It is difficult to find a language that feels comfortable, and this reflects the conundrum that in the western world there are explicit images of sex everywhere, but little capacity in private to express sexual desires openly, or to communicate and negotiate about sex verbally. Nevertheless, the medical profession is viewed as an appropriate place to turn to for help with sexual difficulties, and people hope that midwives and other healthcare workers will initiate discussions about sex and, by doing so, show them that they have permission to air their concerns. Moreover, sexual health is now regarded as a fundamental component of general health (Baker, 1992), and people believe that they have a right to live sexually fulfilling lives. If people are to be helped to achieve this, and if midwives and other healthcare workers are to feel more comfortable providing information on this subject, an understanding of the complexity of gender and sexuality is needed. Some awareness of the most commonly used theories, as well as a critical appreciation of their limitations, should hopefully provide the basis for this.

Scientific research on sexuality

Since the late nineteenth century, science has been relied upon to describe, define and explain human sexuality. Most research that has been undertaken has adopted the view that sex is a drive or instinct with which every individual is born. The roots of sexuality are thought to reside in biological differences, although there are various theories as to precisely what these differences might be. Researchers tend to divide into two discernible groups, namely those who regard sexuality as a good natural instinct that has been corrupted by society (Kinsey *et al.*, 1953; Masters and Johnson, 1966) and those who view it as a dangerous force that needs to be tamed for the benefit of civilisation (Freud, 1905; Malinowski, 1963). Biological differences and the evolutionary drive to procreate are presented as adequate explanations for all sexual behaviour.

The material body is at the centre of most of the research, the focus being on what can be measured and observed. The type and frequency of sexual activities, the prevalence of male and female homosexuality and the physiological changes that lead to orgasm have all been examined. The search is for facts and objective truth. Sociobiologists have amassed evidence based on animal behaviour to support their theory that women choose their partners on the basis of their superior genes in order to maximise the evolutionary potential of the human race (Dawkins,

1978; Symons, 1979). Homosexual men have been studied to determine whether they have smaller brains, different genes or lower levels of testosterone (Le Vay, 1993; Hamer, 1994). Biological abnormalities in gender characteristics (Money, 1994), the impact of gender reassignment on sexual development (Money, 1975) and the social impact of being raised in a biologically incorrect way (Luria *et al.*, 1987) have all been studied by scientists in an attempt to answer questions about the extent to which human sexuality is dependent on nature and how much it depends on nurture.

Ideological biases in this research

This research is interesting, and much of it may be useful and highlight important aspects of sexuality. However, there is a problem in that it is presented as providing the unquestionable truth about human sexuality. Biological explanations are given the force of moral authority. The assumptions that underpin the research are not regarded as open to question, and although many biologists are less deterministic than was previously the case, the media continue to present reductionist and uncritical 'scientific' versions of sexuality as if they were the absolute truth.

In fact, examination of scientific texts reveals the ideological bias in much of this research. Many of the supposedly neutral scientific descriptions are gender coded in ways that reflect stereotypical definitions of masculinity and femininity. For example, in the 1950s John Money, an influential researcher, described a gene as the 'sex-determining gene' (also known as the 'master-sex-determining gene' (Fausto-Sterling, 1997). In the presence of this gene, the male is formed. The male embryo must *seize* its developmental pathway. The female, on the other hand is formed by the *absence* of the master gene. Recent research has suggested that the ovaries play an active role in conception. This contradicts previous descriptions of conception as a battle involving fighting active sperm gaining access to the passive waiting ovum. Despite this, the 'Body Zone' in the Millennium Dome Exhibition presented conception according to traditional gender stereotypes. Irritating as this may be, of greater concern is the credence given to biologists such as Randy Thornhill, who has written a book arguing that rape is a normal mechanism for spreading genes (Thornhill and Palmer, 2000). His theory is based on his observations of flies (evidence for various theories of human sexuality has been found on the basis of comparisons with monkeys, rats and sparrows, to name but a few, as well as insects!). Thornhill uses the word 'rape' as a scientific term to describe his observations, with no apparent concern that this is a very subjective human term with connotations of consent and conscious choice. This 'scientific' research is thus, in a circular argument, cited as evidence that rape is 'natural' for men. The pernicious effect of this approach can be found in legal arguments, where this and similar theories are used successfully to justify and defend male sexual aggression (Ussher, 1997).

Funded and published research reflects the political and ideological needs of the historical period. Research that highlights the similarities between men and women receives little attention (Unger, 1979, cited by Nicolson and Ussher, 1992), whereas research that demonstrates gender differences receives widespread coverage both in scientific journals and in the popular press. There is a close relationship between current social and political issues and the research that is undertaken and published.

History provides very clear examples of this. For example, in the late eighteenth century a sudden interest developed in the differences between men and women that previously had been regarded as of little importance. This interest was not simply the result of advances in scientific knowledge, but seems to have become important because of the justification that biological explanations could provide for political arguments (Laqueur, 1997). Both feminists and anti-feminists looked to biology to support debates about the role of women in society:

> New claims and counterclaims regarding the public and private roles of women were thus contested through questions about the nature of their bodies as distinguished from those of men.
>
> (Laqueur, 1997: 239)

Moreover, scientific research defines female sexuality in terms of male sexuality. Most of the renowned sex researchers have been male. More than this, men have regarded themselves as the norm for human sexuality, with women being judged in relation to them as lacking, deficient or, at best, the mysterious 'other'. Men are viewed as needing sex, and women are regarded as the passive recipients of that sexual drive. This all-consuming male drive will find expression in 'deviations' or aggressive demands if it is denied legitimate outlets (Jackson, 1987). The penis is regarded as the essential sexual organ. The act of sex itself is defined as penetrative vaginal intercourse (Holland *et al.*, 1998), and anything else is not the real thing, but mere foreplay. The fact that much research indicates that, for many women, orgasm and sexual pleasure in general have less to do with vaginal intercourse and more to do with 'foreplay' is ignored (Segal, 1994). Rarely is sex thought of as being centred around the woman's experience of orgasm.

> The model not only reflects and legitimates the male supremacist myth that the male sexual urge *must* be satisfied; it defines the very nature of 'sex' in male terms. ... Male sexuality has been universalized and now serves as the model of human sexuality.
>
> (Jackson, 1987: 73)

This view has been reinforced by men's political, social and economic power, which has given them a great deal of control over female sexuality. One practical manifestation of this was the practice of stitching women extra tightly after episiotomies in order to increase the male partner's sexual pleasure.

It is not that women have just passively accepted male control of their sexuality. Many of them have actively struggled to define sexuality for themselves, and have found ways to resist and subvert the sexuality that has been imposed on them. Feminists and lesbian and gay writers (Butler, 1990; Rich *et al.*, 1993) have profoundly questioned the prevailing ideas about sexuality and, in recent times, women have claimed their own sexual desires and need for satisfaction. Theories of gender and sexuality have been radically transformed by the critical readings of scientific texts undertaken by contemporary writers (Vance, 1984; Weeks, 1985; Connell and Dowsett, 1992) influenced by feminist and 'gay' perspectives.

Furthermore, scientific research itself provides evidence of the actual complexity of the relationship between gender and sexuality, despite the reductionist versions that have been presented by some scientists and in the popular press. There is no straightforward relationship between biology, gender and sexual orientation. Many people who are born without clearly male or female sexual characteristics grow up with few problems related to their socially (rather than biologically) designated gender. Others, who feel that they have been born in the wrong body and who seek gender reassignment, have no biological abnormalities (Luria *et al.*, 1987). The majority of transvestites have no desire to change from male to female (Blanchard, 1990), and many homosexuals have no problems related to their gender (Luria *et al.*, 1987). Transsexuals and transvestites may or may not remain heterosexual, still choosing partners opposite to their original biological gender, and the majority of us have some degree of bisexuality (Kinsey *et al.*, 1948, 1953). Similarly, interest in sadomasochistic sex, paedophilia, fetishism or any other designated perversions defies biological explanations. The desire to have children can be strong for lesbians and gay men and absent for heterosexuals. In fact, most attempts to categorise and explain human sexuality by reference to biology are undermined by the sheer variety of sexual behaviour.

Sexual health

Medicine is a dominant influence in defining sexuality and judging what is normal and abnormal, healthy and unhealthy, and via midwifery and nursing practice those values are transmitted to individual women. As Frank Mort (cited by Weeks, 2000) convincingly argues, there is a substantial medico-moral tradition linking health and disease to moral and immoral sex. Public hygiene and cleanliness have been closely associated with 'dangerous sexualities'.

> 'Healthy' serves as the modern equivalent to 'normal' in terms of endorsing and recommending sexual scripts for what's done, why it's done, when, where, and with whom it's done. . . . Health is morality nowadays.
> (Tiefer, 1997: 105)

In a recent manifestation of this tradition, hygiene has been replaced by 'concerns about orgasmic efficiency and the management of erotic pleasures' (Hawkes, 1996: 119). Sexual health is now, in practice, regarded as active engagement in a fulfilling sexual relationship, and there are concerns about people who are not interested in sex or who deviate from the norms prescribed by medical experts. Leonore Tiefer, an associate professor in a department of urology and psychiatry, cites an interesting example from a conference on ageing and sexuality. A study had been conducted that involved the measurement of erections during sleep of a group of older male volunteers with no sexual problems. One urologist looking at the results commented as follows: 'So, these men did not have rigid nocturnal erections; they may actually have had disease' (Tiefer, 1997: 108).

The 'epidemic' levels of erectile dysfunction (possibly 50% in men over 40 years of age) and its treatment with Viagra also highlight the medicalisation of sexual desire.

Medical authorities no longer discuss morality, but talk instead of disease (as in the above example) or unhealthy behaviours. However, these descriptions are used in a pejorative way. The prescriptive nature of medical discourse is evident in the way in which being unhealthy can be presented as if it is a personal failing. For example, the sexual activity of young women is no longer presented as morally wrong, but as premature and potentially medically dangerous (Hawkes, 1996), yet the subtext is that it is a problem which ought to be stopped.

In general, midwives and nurses are more tolerant than was previously the case, and they express more awareness of the variety and complexity of sexuality. However, a more thorough examination reveals that sexuality remains bound by ideas of normal, 'good' sexuality positioned above dubious, perverted or socially undesirable sexuality. For example, the contentious and contradictory responses to sex education reveal the actual hierarchical values, as well as the confusion, that underly overt acceptance. Homosexuality should not be 'intentionally promoted' according to Section 28 of the Local Government (Amendment) Act, yet this prohibition should not stop any health education that is necessary to prevent the spread of disease, such as (presumably) safer sex for gay teenagers who are at risk of contracting HIV. Similarly, the difficulties in accessing fertility treatment that are faced by lesbians and HIV-positive women betray the judgements that underpin medical services. Political support for the family reinforces ideas of preferred sexual configurations, and the political will behind attempts to make fathers take financial responsibility for their offspring has restrictive implications for women who choose to be single parents (Weeks, 2000). There was public outrage at the idea that lottery money could be used to support gay and lesbian organisations, prostitutes and drug users, despite the fact that the funds were to be used to work with individuals with HIV and AIDS. Awareness of the power of medical institutions to impose these values on individuals through the sexual healthcare that they offer will hopefully lead to better support for women who are receiving that care, and greater appreciation of the limitations which they may perceive in the care that is offered.

The female body

Women's healthcare needs continue to be assessed on the basis of common-sense assumptions about female bodies and gender differences that are taken from scientific and medical research with little awareness of the values which shape that knowledge and inform apparently objective descriptions of human biology. Far from being described objectively, the female body is presented in medical texts as vulnerable, problematic and generally suspect. 'Raging hormones' take over in premenstrual tension: 'Women are erratic, unreliable and potentially dangerous. Their bodies make them so' (Nicolson and Ussher, 1992: 43).

Menstruation, pregnancy and labour all require the expert attention of the medical profession. Postnatal depression is presented as a definite clinical diagnosis, despite the lack of evidence for a clear biological aetiology. Abortion is justified legally by presenting the woman or her fetus as being vulnerable to medical or mental disorder if the pregnancy continues (Boyle, 1992). In some texts the menopause is described as an oestrogen-deficiency disease (Hunter and O'Dea, 1997). Breast milk has virtually been hijacked by the medical profession, and is increasingly being marketed as a health food or medicine (Auerbach, 1995). Questioning these descriptions because of their negative and derogatory descriptions of women's bodies does not mean that women have no specific concerns related to their experiences of being in female bodies, or that women do not themselves look to medical science to provide relief from debilitating experiences. The material reality of the body is important, but it needs to be understood in relation to the ideological shaping that is provided within purportedly neutral scientific texts, as these descriptions, explanations and theories of the female body profoundly influence women's own understanding of their bodily experiences.

Medical science conceives of the body in mechanistic ways. Consequently, sexual problems are responded to with penile pumps and Viagra. Female sexuality has always posed more problems because it is more difficult to reduce to the specific functioning of one body part. Nevertheless, the quest to measure clitoral swelling, vaginal dryness and orgasmic strength continues. Sex therapists suggest masturbation exercises for women in 'laboratory' conditions to enable them to measure their physical responses to self-stimulation. This ignores the multiple means of achieving sexual satisfaction, and views sexuality in individual rather than social or relational terms. Moreover, people are influenced by the idea that good sex involves penetration and leads to orgasm. It is difficult to define sexual satisfaction for oneself without taking on these stereotyped views about desirable outcomes. Yet there are far more reasons for desiring sex than there are ways of being sexual (Whittier and Simon, 2001), and simply describing sexual behaviour, or counting the number of times that intercourse occurs (Vance, 1991), yields few useful findings about sex.

> Sexology's nomenclature of sexual disorders does not describe what makes women unhappy about sex in the real world, but narrows and limits the vision of sexual problems to failures of genital performance.
> (Tiefer, 1992, cited by Heise, 1995: 110)

Most of us recognise that we have sex for multiple purposes – to try to 'keep' a relationship, to bargain, because it is expected of us, for money, power, self-esteem, protection from violence, social acceptability, intimacy, to conceive, to prove something, as well as for physical pleasure. In these terms, satisfaction, may come in many guises.

Freudian theories

When we consider how broad sexual satisfaction is, the role of the mind and fantasy can be seen to play at least as large a part as biology. The meanings that we give to sexual acts are mediated as much by culture and personal history as by biology. Freud's contribution (Freud, 1905) to our understanding of sexuality was his insight into the role of childhood experience and fantasy in shaping adult sexuality. In his theories, gender identity, heterosexuality and the desire to have children are all achieved through the child's struggle to make sense of his or her sensations, experiences of gender differences and parental sexuality; from this no single developmental path can be guaranteed. The sexual drive dominates the infant's unconscious fantasies, and if 'normal' development is thwarted, alternative outlets will be found. The child's experiences of sucking the breast, the way in which the child is held and touched by both parents, the interactions with the parents during toilet training, and the responses of others to the child's pleasurable genital play all contribute to his or her subsequent sexual preferences. For the child, gender is flexible. It is no more difficult to imagine growing up and turning into the opposite sex than it is to imagine becoming like their mother or father. Primary identification with the mother poses different problems for the boy and girl, but both have to seek ways to separate from her and find their own adult selves. Initially the child is interested in exploring his or her body with anyone and everything, and there is no specific choice of male or female partners. It is only later that desire becomes related to particular genders, age groups or types of sexual activity. Even then it remains fluid for many, and rigid and fixed for some. Finally, there will be fantasies about the capacity to reproduce. There will be fears and anxieties, hopes and dreams about producing babies. For the child these are focused on having babies with their mother or father, and it is only by coming to terms with their exclusion from the parental couple that they become free to go on and find their own partners. All of these aspects live on in adult fantasies, in which humans reveal a capacity to be aroused by a vast range of situations, people, objects and activities.

Freud's theories have been developed (Harding, 2001) and contested by feminist psychoanalysts (Chodorow, 1994; Benjamin, 1998) since he wrote them. However, they continue to be of interest because they offer a means of making sense of the varieties of sexual expression. For example, fetishism, transsexuality, sadomasochism, paedophilia and homosexuality can all be understood using the framework that Freud offered. Nevertheless, they present major problems, particularly for women. Similarly to the theories of the biologists and sexologists, Freud's view of sexuality was phallocentric. Women were viewed as castrated, defective versions of men, consumed with envy for the longed for penis. Various female analysts (Horney, 1932) questioned this and postulated male envy of the female capacity to bear children. Although this provides another useful piece of the whole picture, it focuses attention on women as mothers rather than as sexually desiring beings.

Current images of female sexuality

Female sexuality continues to pose problems for psychoanalysts, biologists and psychosexual therapists, and not least for women themselves. Certainly western women have more choices and freedom sexually than in most periods in history. Yet many women put up with unhappy and frustrating relationships, forego their own sexual satisfaction, gain more pleasure from being an object of desire than from being the author of their own desires, and hope that men will awaken and arouse them in a modern-day version of the old romantic myths.

Language and culture do not present us with images of positive female sexuality. The cultural exaltation of the phallus as the sexual organ par excellence leaves women's sexuality apparently mysterious and lacking to them, despite the distorted reflections that they see everywhere in the ubiquitous images of women's bodies. The language of active desire belongs to the penetrating male: 'our culture presents all agency and power in phallic terms, and there is no equivalent symbol to suggest female desire or potency' (Maguire, 2001: 110).

Women's more diffuse experience of sexual pleasure is lost, absent or misunderstood in cultural representations. Sex scenes in films continue to be genitally driven, and although women initiate sex more readily, they more often remain objects of desire, frequently rewarded by successfully seducing the man who is being pursued, rather than active subjects writing their own sexual scripts. There are now more positive images of women's sexuality available, and a belief that women have as much right to satisfy their sexual needs and desires as men, but this attitude is undermined by more traditional scripts that still have considerable force. The concept of the voracious sexual predator versus the respectable mother, wife and daughter remains alive in our culture, and continues to prescribe female sexuality and rob women of their capacity to define sexual desire for themselves. Despite the rejection of these categories by most women, they continue to be used. For example, courts continue to take into account women's sexual histories when assessing rape charges (Gregory and Lees, 1999), girls judge themselves and their peers on the basis of the number of boys they have 'slept' with, and the term 'slag' is used to control and police teenage female sexuality (Holland *et al.*, 1990). The press presents women with HIV either as innocent victims or as predatory, promiscuous spreaders of the virus.

Although there may be awareness of the unfairness of the double standard, many parents understandably still feel the need to teach young women to protect themselves sexually. Girls are taught that their bodies will turn boys into lustful animals, and that they must be the ones to take responsibility for controlling sexual interactions. Sex is presented as something dangerous to young women, and desire is portrayed as coming from others rather than from within. Women are vulnerable because of the power of the male sexual urge, although if they are very attractive and cunning, they can use their physical attributes to gain sexual power over men. The contradictions within all of these scripts leave girls with a confusing and difficult pathway to a strong sense of their own sexuality.

> Women must, on the one hand, allure, and on the other hand, control and restrain; they must be sensuous, lovable and passionate, but on the other hand, scrupulously chaste.
>
> (Okin, 1980, cited by Seidler, 1987: 89)

The constant threat of sexual violence or social disgrace, and the hierarchies of 'good' and 'bad' sex give women an idea of their sexuality as risky, disturbing and potentially troublesome. It is a very different story from the narratives of pleasure and passion. Moreover, even the more enlightened attitudes that now prevail can turn into injunctions which can be just as oppressive. 'In this brave new age of sex, the greatest sin is sexual boredom' (Hawkes, 1996: 119).

As Hawkes goes on to argue, women's articles leave people with what she calls an 'ignorance anxiety'. She contends that advertisers exploit women's sexual anxieties to sell their products. Their articles claim expertise about sex, and as a result women question their own desires and feel that they ought to be having earth-shattering, adventurous, multi-orgasmic sex regularly. Readers are left insecure and doubting their sexual capacity, as they measure their own experiences against the accounts to which they are exposed.

Heterosexuality and safer sex

In this climate, negotiating safer sex and all kinds of sexual safety and pleasure remains difficult for women. Male-centred definitions of sex continue to dominate, and are actively constructed by women as much as by men. Heterosexuality is rarely questioned or seen as the sexual category and organising principle that it is (Richardson, 2000), yet sexual desire is viewed as distinctly heterosexual. Gay relationships are thought of as 'mimicking' heterosexual ones, and the anus is viewed as taking the place of the vagina in gay male relationships. This can prevent us from identifying the anus as a source of pleasure for all human beings, and it allows us to forget the fact that many heterosexuals also regarded the anus as a site for sex. The 'coital imperative' (Segal, 1994) script is severely limiting. Heterosexual men are still regarded as exempt from the need to change, and suggesting that heterosexual men give up penetrative vaginal sex is unthinkable, whereas gay men are expected to give up penetrative anal sex, as suggested in some safer sex campaigns (Richardson, 2000). The challenge of HIV for hetero-sexual women is to redefine heterosexual sex, expose male control of women's sexuality and produce a female-centred theory of sexuality from which women could insist on pleasurable and safe sex.

Women undermine themselves through ideas about romantic love and trust which supersede any concerns they may have about infections. In relationships, trust is used as a reason why the issue of condom use cannot be raised, either because condoms are regarded as unnecessary or because it is felt that they would jeopardise the relationship by suggesting disease or infidelity (Willig, 1997). In the light of this, it is ironic that 'most women now infected with HIV globally have been infected within a stable, long-term relationship or marriage' (Lewis, 1997: 247).

Women knowingly put themselves at risk because of the idealisation of monogamous, heterosexual relationships – the type of relationship that is thought to bring most status and esteem. The search for intimacy and the sense of being part of a loving relationship overrides sexual health issues (Sobo, 1995). Greater love and intimacy are signified by the lack of a condom, which is why condom use is more likely to be found in casual than long-term relationships (Joffe,1997). I suggest that it is because of an implicit understanding of this that midwives are unwilling to discuss HIV, and in particular to talk about safer sex and condom use during pregnancy.

Pregnancy and sexuality

Pregnancy poses particular challenges in relation to the different constructions of masculinity, femininity and sexuality. At no other time are the differences between men and women so sharply delineated. Envy and resentment of each other's experiences can cause unexpected conflicts between men and women who were previously happy in their relationship. Having a child represents deeply felt hopes, fantasies and fears for those involved. Old anxieties and powerful, primitive emotions are stirred as the expectant parents are reminded of their own early experiences. Long-buried childhood desires and ideas about sexuality and repro-duction rise to the surface in disturbing ways. Childhood experiences of depen-dency and vulnerability, closeness to and separation from their mother are vividly recalled. The way in which their own parents related to their sexual bodies, fertility and the quality of the sexual relationship established by the parents will affect the parents to be. The pregnancy can be viewed as a demonstration of love, as evidence of femininity, potency and virility, as a solution to problems of identity or esteem, or as a route to adult status and social approval. Fertility is an important aspect of sexual identity, and the ability to conceive is highly valued. Consequently, the pregnancy can be seen as a triumphant achievement. Women may feel fascinated and excited, and discontented and exhausted, in confusing combinations. Men may feel envious and excluded, or relieved and guilt-ridden. Such feelings are often only semiconsciously experienced, and can be difficult to talk about, emerging during sex and causing enormous anxiety. Of course, many couples manage these feelings and experience increased tenderness and closeness. Intimacy and sexual passion can be heightened, and women may experience more intense orgasms. However, whether it is enhanced or inhibited, sexuality will be profoundly affected by pregnancy, and in particular by a first pregnancy.

> Pregnancy alters a woman's internal experience of her sexuality, as her spontaneous responses are shaped by unfamiliar bodily sensations and hormonal experiences, as well as by her psychic experience of the pregnancy.
>
> (Raphael-Leff, 1993: 42)

The couple may feel that the baby in the womb represents a third presence in the bed, which must be protected from sex, with the penis viewed as damaging and a potential cause of miscarriage. The baby may be imagined as an audience to the sex, a voyeur or an incestuous partner. Later in the pregnancy the liveliness of the baby may be inhibiting and lead to impotence. The woman may withdraw emotionally from her partner and feel that all of her sexual energy is wrapped up in the baby. She may feel suddenly stripped of her adult independence, or that her swelling body is sexually unattractive. Alternatively, she may feel proud and strong, affirmed in her own identity and confirmed as a sexual woman.

Some women feel invaded, exploited or taken over, and this may culminate in an experience of labour as a kind of rape. The exposure and loss of dignity and control that are experienced when giving birth may leave the woman feeling damaged, helpless and frightened by sex, or the man feeling unable to have sex because of his experience of his partner's labour as damaging and disturbing. Real experiences of rape and sexual abuse may surface and be deeply distressing as the lack of control in labour mirrors the previous violations.

After the birth it may be a long time before the sexual relationship is re-established to the satisfaction of both partners. Psychosexual difficulties can often be traced back to the first pregnancy, and this is thought to be because pregnancy powerfully reactivates unconscious feelings that have been repressed since childhood (Raphael-Leff, 1993).

Cultural ideas about motherhood and social constructions of femininity undoubtedly impact on the woman's experience of herself as a sexual being. The separation of motherhood and madonna images from sexual desire can make it difficult for either or both partners to feel that the 'mother' can still be sexually desiring or desirable. The idealisation and denigration of motherhood exert contradictory pressures on the woman and her concept of herself. Changes in reproductive technology, awareness of the fetus as a separate identity because of scans (Pollack Petchesky, 1997; Piontelli, 2000), the ability of postmenopausal women to have babies, lesbian parents and artificial insemination all radically alter our understanding of parenting, and the relationship between sex and conception seems increasingly tenuous. The lack of a woman-centred perspective on female desire is as evident in discussions of sexuality and pregnancy as it is elsewhere. Books such as *Healthy Pregnancy* by Dr Stoppard (Stoppard, 1998) present sexual activity during pregnancy as being more about heterosexual bonding than about the desire for pleasure.

> Sex becomes another legitimate activity to prime the pregnant body for childbirth, much like aerobics or yoga. Sexual pleasure and activity is legitimate if in the service of hormonal balance, muscular readiness and emotional well-being.
>
> (Huntley, 2000: 357)

As a result of all of these pressures, from social and cultural expectations to primitive anxieties resurfacing from childhood, pregnant women commonly feel a need to talk to someone. They often feel ashamed and disturbed by what they regard as irrational fears, and consequently they feel unable to talk about these matters to friends or partners. Midwives are in an ideal position to listen to these anxieties and provide confidential advice and reassurance.

Cultural differences

This chapter is written from a western perspective. In other cultures, sexuality is conceptualised very differently, and the rules governing sexual interactions are extraordinarily varied, as historians and anthropologists have shown. What is shared across cultures is that 'All societies find it necessary to organize the erotic possibilities of the body – impose who restrictions and why restrictions, provide permissions, prohibitions, limits and possibilities' (Plummer, 1984, cited by Weeks, 2000: 130).

The body is a boundary marker in all cultures, and women's bodies in particular are used to maintain the cultural identity of different groups through rules about marriage, kinship patterns and sexual relationships (Caplan, 1987). There are very diverse ideas about gender roles in different cultures, sexual relationships between men being accepted in some, and the moral judgements that are made about various sexual practices, such as anal sex and masturbation, also differ. The advent of HIV has forced health promotion practitioners to try to find ways of making services, written materials and campaigns more culturally appropriate. Homosexuality, as an identity, is a western category that is rejected in other cultures by men who have sex with men, and consequently materials need to be designed which address sexual practices in culturally sensitive ways. Anthropologists have demonstrated the vast diversity of human sexuality, and as a result have opened our eyes to our own cultural assumptions. However, the other side of this is that our inability to be knowledgeable about what is acceptable and what is taboo in all cultures can seem overwhelming. In fact, all of us accept some aspects of our cultures while resisting and rejecting other aspects, and each of us has a unique relationship with our cultural identities. Furthermore, there are as many differences within cultures as there are between them, and a knowledge of the norms of different groups will not necessarily help us to understand individuals within the group (Pollen, 1993).

Cultural differences are often problematic for us because they make us aware of the values and judgements that we make without conscious thought. One practice that is especially disturbing to the western world is female genital mutilation. Officially it is condemned because of the damage to health, but we know that many women continue to support the practice. In order to work with such women, it may be helpful to be aware of what women relinquish by stopping the practice, as well as what they might gain. A study by Janice Boddy that explored the significance of female genital mutilation for women in Northern Sudan is useful in this respect. She came to understand that the practice was an assertive symbolic act for the women, enhancing their femininity and their social status. In this context, it is easier to relate it to western practices and note similarities in the way 'Feminine selfhood is ... attained at the expense of female well-being' (Boddy, 1997: 322).

Comparisons can be made with cosmetic surgery and the increased number of requests by women for Caesarean births, where the main reason given is the desire to retain an attractive body and maintain self-esteem (Kitzinger, 2000).

Conclusion

This chapter has introduced some of the main theories of sexuality and demonstrated that the assumption that there is a universal natural human sexuality based on gender differences fails to do justice to the complexity of sexual desire. Through greater understanding of the varieties of sexuality, it is hoped that midwives will feel better prepared to initiate discussions about sexuality, or at least will feel interested in learning more about a subject that is of such importance to most of us, and which can contribute so much to our health and happiness.

- In order to deliver appropriate sexual healthcare, it is important to understand theories of sexuality and gender.
- Scientific research has focused on attempts to measure the influences of biology and the environment on human sexuality.
- This research reflects the political and ideological needs of the historical period in which it is undertaken.
- Medicine plays a major role in defining healthy and unhealthy sexuality, and these definitions reflect moral value judgements.
- Freud's theories provide insights into the role of childhood experience and fantasy in sexuality.
- Contemporary images of female sexuality continue to present contradictory scripts. The 'coital imperative' and good/bad girl scripts influence the way in which women feel about their own sexuality.
- Pregnancy has a major impact on sexuality, often stirring up powerful feelings and fantasies.
- Different societies have radically different ways of conceptualising both gender and sex.

References

- Auerbach KG (1995) The medicalization of breastfeeding. *J Hum Lactation.* **11**: 259–60.
- Baker C (1992) Female sexuality. In: P Nicolson and J Ussher (eds) *The Psychology of Women's Health and Health Care.* Macmillan, London.
- Benjamin J (1998) *The Bonds of Love: psychoanalysis, feminism and the problem of domination.* Random House, New York.
- Blanchard R (1990) Gender identity disorders in adult men. In: R Blanchard and BW Steiner (eds) *Clinical Management of Gender Identity Disorders in Children and Adults.* American Psychiatric Press, Washington, DC.
- Boddy J (1997) Womb as oasis. The symbolic context of pharaonic circumcision in rural Northern Sudan. In: RN Lancaster and M di Leonardo (eds) *The Gender/Sexuality Reader.* Routledge, London.
- Boyle M (1992) The abortion debate: an analysis of psychological assumptions underlying legislation and professional decision-making. In: P Nicolson and J Ussher (eds) *The Psychology of Women's Health and Health Care.* Macmillan, London.
- Butler J (1990) *Gender Trouble.* Routledge, London.
- Caplan P (ed.) (1987) *The Cultural Construction of Sexuality.* Routledge, London.
- Chodorow NJ (1994) *Femininities, Masculinities, Sexualities.* Free Association Books, London.
- Connell RW and Dowsett GW (eds) (1992) *Rethinking Sex: social theory and sexuality research.* Melbourne University Press, Melbourne.
- Dawkins R (1978) *The Selfish Gene.* Granada, St Albans.
- Fausto-Sterling A (1997) How to build a man. In: RN Lancaster and M di Leonardo M (eds) *The Gender/Sexuality Reader.* Routledge, London.
- Freud S (1905) Three essays on the theory of sexuality. In: J Strachey (ed.) *The Standard Edition of the Complete Psychological Works of Sigmund Freud. Volume 7.* Hogarth Press and the Institute of Psychoanalysis, London.
- Gregory J and Lees S (1999) *Policing Sexual Assault.* Routledge, London.
- Hamer D (1994) *The Search for the Gay Gene and the Biology of Behaviour.* Simon and Schuster, New York.
- Harding C (ed.) (2001) *Sexuality: psychoanalytic perspectives.* Brunner-Routledge, Hove.
- Hawkes G (1996) *A Sociology of Sex and Sexuality.* Open University Press, Buckingham.
- Heise LL (1995) Violence, sexuality and women's lives. In: RG Parker and JH Gagnon (eds) *Conceiving Sexuality.* Routledge, London.
- Holland J, Ramazanoglu C, Scott S, Sharpe S and Thomson R (1990) *Women, Risk and AIDS Project. Papers 1–8.* Tufnell Press, London.
- Holland J, Ramazanoglu C, Sharpe S and Thomson R (1998) *The Male in the Head.* Tufnell Press, London.
- Horney K (1932) The dread of women. *Feminine Psychology.* Norton, New York.
- Hunter MS and O'Dea I (1997) Menopause bodily changes and multiple meanings. In: JM Ussher (ed.) *Body Talk.* Routledge, London.
- Huntley R (2000) Sexing the belly: an exploration of sex and the pregnant body. In: *Sexualities. Volume 3.* Sage Publications, London.

- Jackson M (1987) 'Facts of life' or the eroticization of women's oppression? Sexology and the social construction of heterosexuality. In: P Caplan (ed.) *The Cultural Construction of Sexuality*. Routledge, London.
- Joffe H (1997) Intimacy and love in late modern conditions. In: JM Ussher (ed.) *Body Talk*. Routledge, London.
- Kinsey AC, Pomeroy WB, Martin CE and Gebhard PH (1948) *Sexual Behaviour in the Human Male*. WB Saunders, Philadelphia, PA.
- Kinsey AC, Pomeroy WB, Martin CE and Gebhard PH (1953) *Sexual Behaviour in the Human Female*. WB Saunders, Philadelphia, PA.
- Kitzinger S (2000) Who would choose to have a Caesarean? *Br J Midwifery*. **9**: 284–5.
- Laqueur T (1997) Orgasm, generation and the politics of reproductive biology. In: RN Lancaster and M di Leonardo (eds) *The Gender/Sexuality Reader*. Routledge, London.
- Le Vay S (1993) *The Sexual Brain*. MIT Press, Cambridge, MA.
- Lewis J (1997) 'So how did your condom use go last night, Daddy?' Sex talk and daily life. In: L Segal (ed.) *New Sexual Agendas*. Macmillan, London.
- Luria Z, Friedman S and Rose MD (1987) *Human Sexuality*. John Wiley and Sons, New York.
- Maguire M (2001) Women's sexuality in the new millennium. In: C Harding (ed.) *Sexuality: psychoanalytic perspectives*. Brunner-Routledge, Hove.
- Malinowski B (1963) *Sex, Culture and Myth*. Rupert Hart-Davis, London.
- Masters WH and Johnson VE (1966) *Human Sexual Response*. Little & Brown, Boston, MA.
- Money J (1975) Ablatio penis: normal male infant sex reassigned as a girl. *Arch Sex Behav*. **4**: 65–72.
- Money J (1994) *Sex Errors of the Body and Related Syndromes: a guide to counseling children, adolescents and their families* (2e). Paul Brookes, Baltimore, MD.
- Mort F (2000) *Dangerous Sexualities* (2e). Routledge and Kegan Paul, London.
- Nicolson P and Ussher J (eds) (1992) *The Psychology of Women's Health and Health Care*. Macmillan, London.
- Piontelli A (2000) 'Is there something wrong?': the impact of technology in pregnancy. In: J Raphael-Luff (ed.) *'Spilt Milk': perinatal loss and breakdown*. Institute of Psychoanalysis, London.
- Pollack Petchesky R (1997) Fetal images. In: RN Lancaster and M di Leonardo (eds) *The Gender/Sexuality Reader*. Routledge, London.
- Pollen R (1993) Cultural perceptions and misconceptions. In: H Montford and R Skrine (eds) *Contraception Care*. Chapman & Hall, London.
- Raphael-Leff J (1993) *Pregnancy. The inside story*. Sheldon Press, London.
- Raphael-Leff J (ed.) (2000) *'Spilt Milk': perinatal loss and breakdown*. Institute of Psychoanalysis, London.
- Rich A, Gelpi BC and Gelpi A (eds) (1993) *Adrienne Rich's Poetry and Prose*. WW Norton, London.
- Richardson D (2000) *Rethinking Sexuality*. Sage Publications, London.
- Segal L (1994) *Straight Sex*. Virago, London.
- Seidler VJ (1987) Reason, desire and male sexuality. In: P Caplan (ed.) *The Cultural Construction of Sexuality*. Routledge, London.
- Sobo EJ (1995) *Choosing Unsafe Sex: AIDS – risk denial among disadvantaged women*. University of Pennsylvania Press, Philadelphia, PA.

- Stoppard M (1998) *Healthy Pregnancy*. Dorling Kindersley, London.
- Symons D (1979) *The Evolution of Human Sexuality*. Oxford University Press, Oxford.
- Thornhill R and Palmer C (2000) *A Natural History of Rape*. MIT Press, Cambridge, MA.
- Tiefer L (1997) Medicine, morality and the public management of sexual matters. In: L Segal (ed.) *New Sexual Agendas*. Macmillan, London
- Unger RK (1979) *Female and Male: psychological perspectives*. Harper and Row, London.
- Ussher JM (1997a) *Fantasies of Femininity*. Penguin, Harmondsworth.
- Vance CS (ed.) (1984) *Pleasure and Danger: exploring female sexuality*. Routledge and Kegan Paul, London.
- Vance CS (1991) Anthropology rediscovers sexuality: a theoretical comment. *Soc Sci Med*. **33**: 875–84.
- Weeks J (1985) *Sexuality and its Discontents: meanings, myths and modern sexualities*. Routledge and Kegan Paul, London.
- Weeks J (2000) *Making Sexual History*. Polity Press, Cambridge.
- Whittier DK and Simon W (2001) The fuzzy matrix of 'my type' in intrapsychic sexual scripting. In: *Sexualities. Volume 4*. Sage Publications, London.
- Willig C (1997) Trust as risky practice. In: L Segal (ed.) *New Sexual Agendas*. Macmillan, London.

CHAPTER 3

Women and poverty

Kate H Beverley

Far from being consigned to history, poverty remains a fact of life for millions of people living in the UK in the twenty-first century. Although the relationship between poverty and poorer health and life expectancy has been known for around 160 years, progress towards its eradication has arguably been faltering and fragmented because of differing political interpretations of the causes of poverty. This chapter focuses on material explanations of poverty, and analyses the issues and limitations inherent in policy approaches, both in the recent past and contemporaneously. The impact of poverty on the health of poor mothers and their babies is explored, together with the challenges presented for midwifery practice. The chapter concludes with a review of some innovative approaches to practice.

Introduction

Around 250 years ago in Britain, poverty was a crime punishable by death in some circumstances. The poor fared little better in the nineteenth and twentieth centuries, as industrialisation and capitalism brought their emphasis on competition and success in an increasingly complex world of work. The expectation was that an individual should 'work to live'. If a person did not work, or their work did not pay enough, they could not expect to have the means to live, or to live well. In a less direct way than was the case during the eighteenth century, poverty was 'punishable' by suffering and even death, as poverty-related diseases and illnesses took their toll. This legacy has persisted into the twenty-first century.

How can differences in life outcomes, such as wealth and health, among people living in a society be understood and explained? Is it a matter of genetics and biology, consistent with Darwin's theory of natural selection, where all species, including humans, evolve and refine themselves through a process which guarantees the survival of the fittest? Do the weak and flawed who cannot 'keep up' simply die off, incrementally creating a gene pool which grows stronger and healthier in the course of successive generations? Such an approach arguably presents a rather gloomy view of human life, suggesting that there is little to be done to improve the life circumstances and health chances of the members of human societies. According to this view, poverty would be regarded as a 'fault' located within the poor person, attributable to some moral or genetic flaw. Either way, the cause of poverty would be seen as resting with the individual.

There are signs that this viewpoint has some influence in our times. During the campaign leading up to the last general election, there was much debate about the extent to which the State should help people who were poor or unemployed, including 'lone mothers'. One of the accusations made by some politicians was that the UK was becoming too much of a 'nanny state'. In other words, too much was being done to help too many people, and instead they should 'stand on their own two feet'. Another way of putting this is to say that only the fittest deserve to survive, and by their own efforts.

This chapter will challenge naturalistic and individualistic explanations such as these, in its exploration of sociopolitical and economic factors which combine to increase the odds of unfavourable pregnancy and childbirth experiences and outcomes for significant numbers of women in contemporary Britain. The analysis will include a focus on two groups of women who are at particular risk during pregnancy because of poverty, namely lone mothers and teenage mothers. Poverty as a concept will be explored, focusing on a number of difficulties with regard to its measurement and definition. The efficacy of politico-economic and health policy responses to the presence of poverty, and the health-damaging effects of poverty in the lives of women and their children, will be evaluated. The chapter will conclude with a discussion of the challenges for midwifery practice that are presented by poverty.

Defining and measuring poverty

Poverty is not an historical relic. It has not been eradicated. Certainly the advent of welfare policies, ushered in by the Liberal Reforms of 1904 and culminating in the Welfare State in 1948, improved the lot of many people in British society although, as will be seen later in the chapter, policy has tended to favour men over women. Most theorists distinguish between *absolute poverty*, in which a person lacks the means necessary to sustain life, and *relative poverty*, in which a person struggles with a standard of living below that of the majority within a given society. Absolute poverty is a grim reality for those living in the so-called 'developing world', where daily suffering and death as a result of malnutrition, diseases contracted through exposure to contaminated water, and conflict, are commonplace.

In contrast, the 'relatively poor' find themselves excluded from participation in ways of life which are taken for granted by others in society, such as having a home of one's own, an inside toilet, a refrigerator, a car, a garden, or sufficient income to afford a 'healthy lifestyle', whether in terms of food or leisure activities. Whether their poverty is classed as 'absolute' or 'relative' possibly matters little to those who are experiencing it. Poverty carries a degree of stigma, which may mean that some poor people are reluctant to take on this identity, thereby also shutting off the possibility of benefits which might help them (Alcock, 1997).

> What is more, people at the bottom of the income distribution in Britain may not see themselves as poor, particularly if they make comparisons with those elsewhere in the world who face starvation and destitution, or even with those elsewhere in Britain who are worse off than themselves – relative judgements of poverty are shared by the poor, too.
>
> (Alcock, 1997: 8–9)

According to a recent report, more than five million people are currently living in *absolute poverty* in the UK (Gordon and Townsend, 2001). The study used a definition of absolute poverty based on a statement by the United Nations in 1995, which identified the lack of basic human needs such as health, sanitation, shelter, safe drinking water and food, together with access to education and benefits, as key characteristics. Gordon and Townsend (2001) found that 17% of households in the UK considered that their income was below the level required to prevent conditions of absolute poverty. This overall statistic includes the 54% of single parents who stated that their income was insufficient to ensure that basic needs could be met.

A significant feature of this study was its use of the participants' own perceptions of their lived experiences as the basis for measuring poverty. Such an approach differs radically from that which is usually adopted, where the emphasis is on external indicators of poverty or wealth (e.g. income level), and enables completely new data to emerge, compared with the more orthodox findings that will be discussed later on in this section. Both objective and subjective perspectives have a significant contribution to make to studies of poverty (Alcock, 1997). Both women and men experience poverty, but significantly more women than men have consistently featured in poverty statistics (Payne, 1991; Doyal, 1998). This is borne out by the data generated by successive governments, examples of which are provided in the tables below. Table 3.1 provides a breakdown of the distribution of poverty within particular groups in society, while Table 3.2 shows the rates, over a span of two decades, of lower than average income for households of different types between 1981 and 2000.

Given that the majority of lone parents are women, and also given the significantly greater representation of women within the 'elderly' population group, it can be seen from the data in Table 3.1 that substantially more women than men can be defined as poor.

The data in Table 3.2 demonstrate that the trend over the last 20 years, in terms of the number of people living in poverty (defined as having an income below 60% of the average), has remained constant. Following a sharp increase in 1991–92, the rate levels off at 18% of the population.

Table 3.1   The bottom line: the number of people living in poverty, according to personal, economic and family status, during the period 1996–97 in the UK

	Total number	Proportion who are poor	Number living in poverty
Adult women	22.2 million	24%	5.3 million
Children	13.0 million	35%	4.5 million
Adult men	21.1 million	20%	4.2 million
Elderly	9.8 million	31%	3.0 million
Lone-parent families	4.3 million	63%	2.9 million
Unemployed	4.6 million	78%	2.3 million
Total		25%	14.1 million

*Poverty is defined as below 50% of average income after deduction of housing costs.
Source: Department of Social Security (1998).

Table 3.2   People living in households with below 60% median income* according to household type in the UK/Great Britain†

	1981	1991–92	1996–97	1998–99	1999–2000
Single people without children	8	18	16	15	16
Single pensioners	15	29	23	23	23
Lone parents	22	46	38	36	35
Couples without children	5	10	10	10	10
Pensioner couples	17	29	20	23	21
Couples with children	15	20	19	18	17
All individuals	13	21	18	18	18

*Equivalised disposable income before deduction of housing costs.
† Data for 1981 and 1991–92 are based on the Family Expenditure Survey, which covers the UK. Data for 1996–97 to 1999–2000 are based on the Family Resources Survey which covers Great Britain only.
Source: Office for National Statistics (2002).

Income has traditionally been used as a primary indicator of poverty and its effects (Payne, 1991; Alcock, 1997). Until recently, this was problematic because of the assumption that in households consisting of a married couple (and children, if any), the female partner would be financially dependent on the male breadwinner's income. A married woman's paid contribution to the family income was thus rendered invisible, and the husband's socio-economic status ('social class') was automatically conferred on his wife. However, in 2001, a new system known as the National Statistics Socio-Economic Classification was introduced by the Government, and this tool, unlike its predecessor, promises to render women more visible in their own right within the data (Macfarlane, 2002). However, the introduction of a new methodology will make it difficult to measure or estimate trends over time, since the data that were collected using the 'old' classification will not be directly comparable with those generated in studies using the new approach, a point which Macfarlane (2002) has highlighted.

The traditional assumption that women are or should be financially dependent on men was linked to the belief that such dependence offered women protection from poverty. However, income within the household is not necessarily equally shared. According to the Scottish Poverty Information Unit (1997), as many as 52% of all women in the UK would be classified as living in poverty, if individual income assessment was to be used instead of assuming equal sharing within married households.

There has been a lack of consensus about the minimum income level below which poverty obtains, which has acted somewhat like a 'smokescreen', arguably extending the debate, but contributing little to definitive action. Oppenheim (1997) is critical of the use made by some politicians of data which indicate that significant numbers of poor individuals have moved up the income ladder, and points out that such movement is often very temporary, given the insecurity of much low-paid work. In general, studies of poverty by UK researchers have made use of 'proxy' measures of poverty, in the form of 'deprivation indexes'. These are designed to account for the complex nature of poverty deprivation by assessing the degree to which a poor individual's ordinary life experiences vary from agreed 'social norms'. The present Government has brought such *social exclusion* effects of poverty and deprivation to the heart of its analysis and policy. Alcock (1997) offers the following comment:

> A full picture of the problem of poverty within a society needs to address these fine grains of the experiences of deprivation, which the simplified definitions and statistical measures necessarily overlook. ... This broader focus on deprivation thus requires the development of an appreciation of what *we do or do not do*. ... Townsend has probably been the most articulate proponent of the notion of relative deprivation. ... He distinguished three different forms of relative deprivation:
>
> • lacking the diet, clothing and other facilities that are customary and approved in society
> • falling below the majority or accepted standard of living
> • falling below what could be the majority standard, given a better redistribution or restructuring of society.
>
> (Alcock, 1997: 85–6)

The lack of an agreed tool for measuring and defining poverty may also be understood as contributing to its perpetuation, although there is something of a 'chicken-and-egg' dilemma here. Have the politics of poverty failed because of 'academic' problems of measurement and definition, or has the acceptance of an agreed definition and a tool for its measurement been constrained by the politics of poverty?

> Poverty is a term which is rarely heard on the lips of policy-makers. ... The debate has been characterised by bland euphemisms – 'low income', 'below average income', 'the bottom 10%' – terms which obscure the reality of deprivation, poverty and hardship.
> (Scottish Poverty Information Unit, 1997: 2)

Human beings do not exist in a vacuum. The individual is situated within a complex system of interrelationships with other people, only some of which are directly experienced as part and parcel of everyday life, but which nevertheless exert an influence. Thus, for example, the decision that is made by a financial business in the City to push up the price of some commodity can result in less food on the table for a lone mother and her children.

Constructing societies and engendering poverty

Arguably, therefore, poverty is not simply a case of 'the roll of the dice', nor is it an inevitable part of the human condition. Sociological analysis demonstrates that the dice may be loaded to start with, because of the existence of inbuilt social inequalities. Health, well-being and illness are profoundly influenced by the ways in which particular societies are structured, and the structure of a society is manufactured from political and economic ideas and decisions. As industrialisation and capitalism have evolved, the 'world of work' (the labour market) has become increasingly diverse and specialised, with concomitant variability and disparity in income. Differences between individuals and groups within a society are thus manufactured by the unequal distribution of wealth and material resources, which in turn have an impact on potential status and power. The data in Table 3.3 illustrate the persistent inequalities in the distribution of wealth within the UK. Table 3.4 shows the income differentials for various types of job.

Gender divisions also form part of social stratification and, together with ethnicity, class, race and age, are supported by ideologies which include political systems of thought. The roles traditionally ascribed to women within evolving UK society have ensured their unequal representation within the social system, whether in terms of restricted access to the labour market and lower rates of pay, or disparities in pensions and welfare benefits (Abbott and Wallace, 1997; Watson and Doyal, 1999; Equal Pay Task Force, 2001). Figures 3.1 and 3.2 illustrate the differentials in income between women and men, using current data, thus providing insight into the contemporary situation within the UK.

Table 3.3 Distribution of wealth* in the UK, expressed as percentage values

Marketable wealth (%) owned by:	1976	1981	1986	1991	1996	1997	1998	1999
Most wealthy 1%	21	18	18	17	20	22	23	23
Most wealthy 5%	38	36	36	35	40	43	43	43
Most wealthy 10%	50	50	50	47	52	54	55	54
Most wealthy 25%	71	73	73	71	74	75	75	74
Most wealthy 50%	92	92	90	92	93	93	94	94
Total marketable wealth (£ billion)	280	565	955	1711	2092	2248	2594	2752

Marketable wealth (less value of dwellings) (%) owned by:	1976	1981	1986	1991	1996	1997	1998	1999
Most wealthy 1%	29	26	25	29	26	30	32	34
Most wealthy 5%	47	45	46	51	49	54	58	58
Most wealthy 10%	57	56	58	64	63	66	70	71
Most wealthy 25%	73	74	75	80	81	83	85	86
Most wealthy 50%	88	87	89	93	94	95	96	97

*Distribution of personal wealth: estimates for individual years should be treated with caution, as they will be affected by sampling error and the particular pattern of deaths that year.
Source: Office for National Statistics (2002).

Table 3.4 Highest and lowest paid occupations in the UK in April 2000

Highest paid	Average gross weekly pay (£)
Treasurers and company financial managers	1059
Medical practitioners	964
Organisation and methods and work study managers	813
Management consultants, business analysts	812
Underwriters, claims assessors, brokers, investment analysts	775
Police officers (at rank of inspector or above)	766
Computer systems and data-processing managers	757
Solicitors	748
Marketing and sales managers	719
Advertising and public relations managers	690

Lowest paid	Average gross weekly pay (£)
Educational assistants	212
Other childcare and related occupations	205
Counterhands, catering assistants	196
Launderers, dry cleaners, pressers	196
Hairdressers, barbers	190
Waiters, waitresses	189
Petrol station forecourt attendants	189
Retail cash-desk and check-out operators	185
Bar staff	184
Kitchen porters, hands	184

Source: Office for National Statistics (2002).

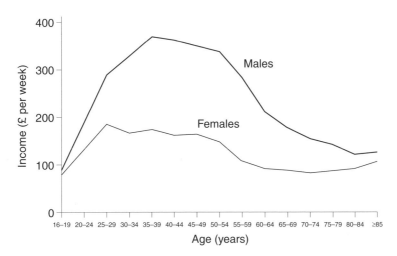

Figure 3.1 Median individual gross income in the UK by gender and age for the period 1999–2000. (Reproduced from Office for National Statistics, 2002.)

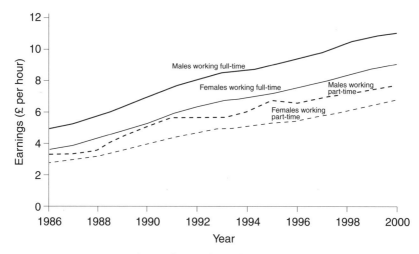

Figure 3.2 Gross earnings in the UK by gender and according to whether working full-time or part-time. (Reproduced from Office for National Statistics, 2002.)

Women have most of the caring and nurturing roles within the home, providing childcare and housework, or caring for a sick or disabled family member (Doyal, 1995; Land, 1999). These responsibilities can impact negatively on women's availability and capacities within the world of paid work. Thus women are disproportionately represented within the lowest-paid jobs, and are also much more likely than men to be in part-time work (Twomey, 2002).

Although issues of gender inequality were addressed in the latter part of the twentieth century, women remain disadvantaged relative to men in terms of their position in the labour market. This is confirmed by data from the spring 2001 Labour Force Survey, published by the Government in the form of a 'special feature' to coincide with Mother's Day 2002 (Twomey, 2002), and in Social Trends (Office for National Statistics, 2002). The data also attest to the fact that there is wide variation among women from different social classes. Those in the lower classes (where social class is defined as occupational grouping) experience a proportionally greater burden of material disadvantage both relative to men belonging to the same social class and relative to women and men belonging to higher social classes.

Women who belong to particular ethnic minority groups may be exposed to yet further disadvantage. The African-Caribbean, Pakistani and Bangladeshi communities are disproportionately represented within the lower social classes, which may reflect exposure to the effects of institutionalised discrimination both within the labour market and within the social system more generally (Nazroo, 1998; Office for National Statistics, 2002). Although not all poor women develop poverty-related illness, or health problems during pregnancy and childbirth, they are at greater risk than are non-poor women, given the now well-established relationship between poverty and health inequalities (Acheson, 1998).

If women are in paid employment outside the home, they tend to have jobs which are part-time and low paid (Abbott and Wallace, 1997; Twomey, 2002). This reflects women's involvement in childcare and other domestic roles. They may choose part-time work to facilitate these additional roles, or they may find themselves denied access to full-time employment, perhaps because of discrimination by employers on the grounds that caring responsibilities are likely to interfere with work performance. Most women who are in paid employment have jobs in the service sector, such as hairdressing retailing, nursing, midwifery and education. These roles mirror the domestic and childcare work which women perform in an unpaid capacity at home, and are considered 'women's work' because of the assumption that such work requires skills which 'come naturally' to women (Doyal, 1995; Crompton, 1997). It is perhaps because of this 'feminisation' that such jobs attract low rates of pay.

Women in jobs that are also held by men tend to occupy the lower strata. Senior positions (especially management roles) are overwhelmingly reserved as 'jobs for men'. There is also evidence that women are denied promotion or career development by employers who take the view that most women will take a break to have children at some point, and that this justifies denying women the same opportunities as their male counterparts (Abbott and Wallace, 1997; Equal Pay Task Force, 2001).

Until very recently, only limited help was available for women who wished to undertake paid work in addition to their childcare roles (Lewis and Piachaud, 1992; Watson, 1999). On the whole, employers have provided neither flexible working patterns nor childcare facilities. The costs of purchasing private care may have the effect of trapping some women, particularly lone mothers, in a cycle of deprivation and unemployment, with all of the associated risks for the health of these women and that of their children.

The politics of poverty

Some political theorists (e.g. Margaret Thatcher) have argued that the State should have a minimal role in ensuring the well-being of its citizens. Others (e.g. Aneurin Bevan, the architect of the Welfare State which was established in Britain in 1948) have argued an equally passionate case for a radical redistribution of wealth, in order to ensure that all members of a society have at least the minimum requisites. Welfare approaches go at least some way towards wealth redistribution. The main political parties in the UK have traditionally espoused fundamentally differing welfare strategies, broadly characterised as either *individualist* or *collectivist*, although more recently the high costs of welfare have resulted in some 'blurring' of the traditional boundaries.

Jordan (1996) put forward a strong case for an approach which acknowledges that any human society will inevitably include individuals who are disadvantaged in terms of competing for work. He cites as examples the very young (children), those who are disabled or sick, those who are old and those who lack skills or qualifications. Doyal and Gough (1991), in suggesting the existence of a number of *universal human needs*, propose that a new approach to social policy is needed if the old inequalities are to be extinguished. Their 'theory of human need' rejects both what might be called *social Darwinism* (briefly discussed earlier), with its emphasis on *individualism*, and *State collectivism*, which emphasises *the social (collective)*

Doyal and Gough (1991) contend that *autonomy* and *health* are fundamental human needs. From their perspective, traditional approaches to welfare policy have compromised autonomy. On the one hand, they have ignored some individuals who, for whatever reason, cannot themselves meet their basic living needs. On the other hand, personal choice and freedom may be limited if policy dictates too strongly how people should live their lives. The problems relating to health inequalities, already referred to above, will be further explored later in this chapter.

The creation of the British Welfare State in 1948 seemed to break new ground. There was an explicit recognition that British society as a whole had a responsibility to each citizen for ensuring that he or she had at least the basic requirements for sustaining life. This included provision for those who were without employment, or whose income was limited. Successive governments after 1948 have restructured the welfare system according to their particular political philosophies. The result has been that a balance between individualism and collectivism, such as would ensure *autonomy*, has arguably never been achieved, and has certainly never been sustained.

There is also evidence to suggest that the very essence of the traditional concept of 'Welfare' was founded on approaches which compounded and even exploited women's disadvantaged structural position within society.

> Because of their part-time and discontinuous employment patterns, women have less access than men to private and occupational pension and sickness schemes. ... The privatisation of 'care' through policies of community care has meant a greater burden of care falling upon 'carers', many of whom fail to qualify for the invalid care allowance ... generally women have had rather 'less to lose' from welfare state restructuring and reductions than men. As has been well documented, the social security system was created with the needs of men rather than those of women in mind.
>
> (Millar, 1997: 106)

Thus women have found themselves denied equitable pension rights because they did not work full-time (housework and mothering being excluded from definitions of work, because 'real' work happens outside the home). There is a paradox here, given that it is largely women who perform 'welfare work', whether in the home or in the labour market. Where welfare work is happening outside the home, women are doing this in addition to their other roles (Lewis and Piachaud, 1992). Formal acknowledgement and valuing of these contributions made by women, in the form of flexible working hours or workplace childcare facilities, have been largely absent from traditional welfare policy (Lewis, 2000; Lister, 2000). Very recently some inroads have been made, with the extension of pension rights and paid sick and holiday leave to part-time workers. However, Watson (1999) wryly offers the following comment on the unfolding welfare reforms:

> Blair's Labour Party was elected to power in the summer of 1997 after nearly 20 years of a Conservative Government which had restructured the welfare state and made swingeing cuts under a rhetoric of, on the one hand, individualism and the end of society, and on the other, a return to traditional gender roles and the patriarchal nuclear family. ... The Blair proposals to restructure the welfare state were to be expected. ... The shock came with the first group to be targeted: single parents' benefit was to be reduced by £10 with a view to encouraging them back into work.
>
> (Watson, 1999: 2)

Women are vulnerable to both poverty and poverty-related illnesses in unique and complex ways, not least of which is the mediation and reproduction of inequalities by welfare approaches that are gendered (Payne, 1991; Glendinning and Millar, 1992; Alcock, 1997; Doyal, 1998; Kent, 2000).

Society, poverty, health and illness: lessons from recent history

Society can either make people sick or it can enable them to flourish and be well. Sociologists have been able to demonstrate that the patterns of illness or wellness which exist in a society such as that of the UK cannot be explained in purely biological terms. They argue that social factors, such as income levels and type and location of housing, have a direct effect in producing biological events which result in illness. This is not a new revelation – it has been known for at least 160 years. Chadwick (1842, cited in Payne, 1991) published a 'Report on the Sanitary Conditions of the Labouring Population of Great Britain' and provided the earliest clear evidence that health varies with social class. Scambler (1997) observed that the work of Chadwick and others demonstrated the 'vicious circle' of poverty and disease, whereby poor people develop diseases which in turn reinforce or compound their poverty.

The evidence that there is a strong relationship between material living conditions and poorer health and earlier death again leads to questions about the structure of human societies. The same health inequalities have persisted over the 160 years since Chadwick's study. Contemporary UK society is thus constructed in ways that ensure inequalities between people. To ignore this fundamental fact, and state that each person as an individual must assume responsibility for his or her own survival and well-being, seems something of a double standard. Social stratification ensures that some people start out with better material resources and access to opportunities than others.

Doyal and Gough (1991) assert that society should be accountable where the social conditions which foster poverty and deprivation, and their consequences for health, are a product of political-economic decisions. Their position therefore seems to echo that of Jordan (1996), whose work was discussed earlier. There have been a succession of studies by social scientists in the UK over the last 22 years, which have sought to present evidence to guide political policy towards a radical response to health inequalities (Townsend and Davidson, 1982; Whitehead, 1987; Townsend et al., 1988; Drever and Whitehead, 1995; Acheson, 1998). However, the problem remains that politicians of differing political persuasions interpret the research in different ways.

Poverty, pregnancy and childbirth

There is evidence that poverty and deprivation play a significant part in the poorer health of women. 'One in twenty mothers in Britain – particularly lone mothers on income support – go without food to meet the needs of their child' (Scottish Poverty Information Unit, 1997: 3).

The findings of a research study conducted 12 years ago resonate closely with those generated by more recent research. Rutter and Quine (1990) demonstrated a relationship between poor housing and higher rates of miscarriage and infant mortality, when housing type and quality were used as indicators of poverty and deprivation. Underlying poverty, with its combination of disadvantages, has a negative impact on the health of women and their children, whether during pregnancy or in the years following birth. Women who are not in full-time paid employment outside the home, or who are only working part-time, spend more time in the home. Thus while both women and men may be living in shared poor housing, women's exposure to these conditions may be greater and may thus render them more vulnerable to the cumulative effects of, for example, inadequate heating, damp, overcrowding, distance from shops, or inoperative lifts in high-rise blocks. Payne (1991) and Benzeval *et al.* (1995) reported similar evidence, and contemporary research in this field is yielding a depressingly familiar picture, which attests to the absence of effective anti-poverty strategies up to the present time.

Lone mothers constitute the majority of lone parents and, as demonstrated in Tables 3.1 and 3.2, they feature significantly in the statistics for households with below average income. Women who are lone mothers are very likely to be poor, and they and their children are therefore at greater risk of ill health. Far from attracting compassionate welfare policy responses, in recent years lone motherhood has become stigmatised. One of the most pervasive stereotypes is that which represents the lone mother as a manipulator who deliberately becomes pregnant in order to secure housing. The evidence presented here tends to give the lie to that view. At present the percentage of lone mothers within the population as a whole remains high, although as can be seen from the data presented in Table 3.5, the rate appears to have levelled out between 1999 and 2001.

There has been a trend towards housing lone mothers in hostel accommodation, which confers additional risks during pregnancy. More than a decade ago, Payne (1991) cited a survey by the London Food Commission, Maternity Alliance and Shelter, which demonstrated that hostel living was associated with a number of negative health effects on women and children. These included a higher than

Table 3.5   Families with dependent children and headed by lone parents* in the UK, expressed as percentage values

	1971	*1981*	*1991*	*1999*	*2001†*
Lone mothers					
Single	1	2	6	8	9
Widowed	2	2	1	1	1
Divorced	2	4	6	6	6
Separated	2	2	4	4	4
Total	7	11	18	20	20
Lone fathers	1	2	1	2	2
All lone parents	8	13	19	22	22

*Lone mothers (by marital status) and lone fathers.
† At spring 2001.
Source: Office for National Statistics (2002).

average incidence of premature births and babies born with low birth weights. Research conducted some years later reinforced the association between poverty, deprivation (including housing type and location) and increased incidence of low-birth-weight babies (Wilcox *et al.*, 1995). Sawtell (2002) reported on the findings of a small-scale study conducted by Maternity Alliance in 2001, in which the experiences and perceptions of women living in temporary accommodation were explored. Almost half of those interviewed were lone mothers, and women from black and minority ethnic groups were disproportionately represented. The conditions in which women (some of whom were pregnant) and their children were living are graphically described by Sawtell:

> Eighteen of the women were living in bed-and-breakfast (B&B) accommodation, six were in hostels and four were in temporary flats. With the exception of those in flats, most were living in one room and sharing amenities such as the kitchen, bathroom and toilet. All three types of accommodation were generally of very poor quality. Overcrowding, sharing of amenities and infestation with mice or cockroaches were common concerns for the women. One woman estimated she was sharing a toilet with 19 others. The accommodation was often in areas of London that the women did not know, where they felt unsafe and where they did not have pre-existing local networks.
>
> (Sawtell, 2002: 518)

These conditions caused the women concern about their own health (including psychological effects) and also that of their children. They had a sense of their deprivation, and were also aware that, at some level, this felt punitive. There has been a great deal of stigmatising political rhetoric about lone mothers during the last two decades, which has underpinned 'hardline' approaches at the level of statutory agencies (e.g. the £10 reduction in benefits as an inducement to seek employment, referred to earlier in the chapter).

Nutrition is of enormous importance during pregnancy and if a mother is breastfeeding. There is evidence that poor nutrition may be causally linked to congenital abnormalities, and there is an increased incidence of poor nutrition among pregnant women who are enduring poverty and deprivation (Acheson,

Table 3.6 Benefit rates for an unemployed single pregnant woman in 2001

Age of single woman (years)	Weekly benefit income	Proportion of income required for adequate diet costing £20.75
≥25	£53.03	39%
18–24	£42.00	49%
16–17*	£31.95	65%

*Pregnant 16- to 17-year-olds are only entitled to benefits (and welfare foods) in the last 11 weeks of their pregnancy. A 16- or 17-year-old may be entitled to the same rate as 18- to 24-year-olds if she can prove that she lives apart from her parents for certain specified reasons. Pregnant teenagers under 16 years of age are not entitled to benefits (or welfare foods) in their own right.
Source: McLeish (2002).

1998). Payne (1991) observed that the state maternity allowance was insufficient to meet the cost of the recommended nutritional intake during pregnancy. As such, it was unlikely to enable women who had to rely on that allowance and other state benefits to afford to eat healthily. More recently, the same dilemma has been noted in relation to 'twenty-first-century poor woman's' experience of pregnancy (Goodman, 1999; McLeish, 2002). The data in Table 3.6 contrast with a national average figure of less than 10% of income being spent on food.

Teenage pregnancies that lead to maternities account for a very small percentage of all pregnancies, the most recent data available (from 1999) showing a rate of 38.6 per 1000, and a declining trend over the last 7 years. The incidence in girls under 16 years of age is 3.9 per 1000 pregnancies, and again it is declining (Office for National Statistics, 2002). Teenage mothers are at particular risk of poverty, given that they are more likely to be unemployed, they are at the very beginning of life as an independent adult, and their pregnancy may have interrupted a nascent career or job development pathway (MacKeith and Phillipson, 1997). Considerable moral opprobrium arguably underpins the political invective surrounding teenage pregnancy, and the rather punitive approach to benefits for this age group (*see* Table 3.6 above) can be interpreted as providing evidence of this. Viewed from this perspective, policy seems to have been directed at the teenage mothers themselves, as a negative sanction.

Perhaps the belief is that an imposed experience of deprivation will discourage further 'irresponsible' behaviour in the future, and that it will also convey a strong message to dissuade other potential teenage mothers. Were the focus to be set on the welfare of the unborn baby, then measures aimed at maximising the mother's health and well-being would be clearly in evidence. McLeish (2002) has commented that neither the present Government nor its predecessor have acted to correct this benefit inequality, despite the availability of evidence and recommendations from a number of studies. Hanna (2001), in documenting the experiences of five teenage mothers in Australia, could be describing the reality of life as a teenage mother in the UK today:

> It was concluded that becoming a sole-supporting mother during the teenage years was a difficult struggle for the young women, because of their youth, their lack of preparation for motherhood and their reliance on welfare supports. In addition, they experienced negative public attitudes directed towards them wherever they went, and this included their visits to community child health centres.
>
> (Hanna, 2001, 456)

In February 2001, the Government announced an initiative as part of its 'Sure Start' strategy, which would give a '£60 million boost' to improve the health of children in low-income families. The aims include the improvement of the health of women and their unborn babies during pregnancy, in order to ensure that babies are born healthier. It remains to be seen how successful this will be in tackling the income-related causes of maternal and infant morbidity. Davies (1997) refers back to a project carried out between 1983 and 1987, in which antenatal midwifery services were 'taken to' women defined as being at high risk because of poverty. The emphasis of the project was on meeting the women in their home environment, with the midwives establishing a local base which made them more accessible and more visible within the community to which their clients belonged. This approach enabled successful health education and support to be provided, as evidenced by the positive evaluation by participants. 'Sure Start' is premised upon similar principles of community involvement, which bodes well for its success.

Salmon and Powell (1998) drew on a wide range of research and policy literature to provide a review of the problems and challenges raised by poverty for mainstream midwifery practice. They echo Payne's analysis of nearly a decade earlier (Payne, 1991) in warning that women who are struggling to meet basic living needs may not be able to make the healthy lifestyle choices which midwives exhort them to during pregnancy. Midwives need to take the facts of poverty fully on board, or they will run the risk of actually increasing the burden of anxiety for poor pregnant women.

What a dreadful paradox it would be if the very substance of antenatal advice produces stress, which in turn may bring about adverse physiological effects that are damaging to the health of both the mother and her unborn child. What about women who are working to a limited budget and perhaps having to juggle the demands of a job and childcare, and who do not live near a large supermarket that offers a range of healthy foods at affordable prices? The reality for many is that they have to rely on what is available locally, and such traders cannot usually afford the mark-down prices of the retail giants.

Thus simply reciting the 'mantras' of health education advice to women, without being empathetically aware of how difficult such advice might be for some women to follow, is arguably at best patronising and at worst dangerous. If it is experienced as moral censure (i.e. it makes a woman feel conflict or guilt), it may possibly so alienate the woman that she does not attend future antenatal appointments. Reisch and Tinsley (1994) found that poverty itself may have a significant effect on the health beliefs of women who are pregnant, influencing their uptake of antenatal services. Armed with such knowledge and insight, midwives are better able to establish a relationship based on respect and empathy with women living in poverty. Getting to know and understand the beliefs which such women may have about how they should behave with regard to health matters during their pregnancy is a prerequisite for introducing any change. The alternative is simply to deal in prejudgements which assume that non-compliance is the result of 'deviance' or ignorance, and as such this constitutes a recipe for failure from the outset.

Crafter (2002) urges midwives to be realistic about the complex processes involved in attitude changes. Expectations about timescales within which change can take place need to be informed by insights from psychological frameworks, and not simply aligned with political target dates. Being able to unravel the 'paradoxical messages' which are part of what might be referred to as 'the current professional rhetoric' from which a midwife is expected to operate is a key skill that she will need to develop if she is to avoid reproducing this in her practice:

> It is important to address this issue of mixed messages because they can create confusion and inconsistency, and undermine the confidence of both women and midwives. ... Furthermore, if midwives do not acknowledge that they may be the agents of giving mixed messages to

women, and women do not understand the paradoxes of what they see and hear, our good relationships may flounder.

(Crafter, 2002: 59)

The image of a woman depriving herself and her unborn baby of adequate nourishment because she is putting her family's needs first in a situation where there is not enough to go round is truly a dreadful one. It is the stuff of which tear-jerking scenes in Dickens novels are made. However, it is also real life for some in contemporary Britain (Salmon and Powell, 1998; McLeish, 2002). The report by Acheson (1998) includes a section on the health and nutrition of women and children, and a focus on health during pregnancy, and makes recommendations for improving these. The emphasis is not just on short-term improvements in the health of pregnant women and their unborn babies. The importance of a 'healthy start in life' for the prevention of illnesses much later in life (e.g. coronary heart disease, mental illness, diabetes) is also strongly argued.

Goodman (1999) contends that midwives need to use these findings as leverage for achieving increased involvement in planning and decision making with regard to health and social policy at both local and national levels. It is possible that the 'Sure Start' initiatives which were introduced in 2001 (referred to earlier in this chapter) came about at least in part as a result of lobbying of the kind that Goodman recommends.

Being poor is not just about physical effects. Self-esteem, which is a core component of well-being, may be reduced by the experience of poverty, particularly in a social climate where being poor is regarded as a 'moral failing'. The relationship between low self-esteem and depression among women living in poverty has been well documented (Brown and Harris, 1978; Graham, 1993). Recent research suggests that postnatal depression may actually start during pregnancy. It is reasonable to assume that poor women are likely to be at greater risk of developing depression during pregnancy, given the limitations and uncertainties which they may have to face. They may be unable to rely on support or material help from family or friends, either because their social support network is limited, or because these people are also poor (Oakley 1992; Millar, 1997).

Conclusion

Midwives can make a difference to the quality of a woman's experience of pregnancy and childbirth, and to the future health and well-being of her baby. If they are to practise effectively, they need to possess sound understanding and knowledge of poverty and its effects. Insights from sociology can inform good midwifery practice by replacing naturalistic and individualistic assumptions about poverty (that were learned in the course of socialisation) with knowledge of its social basis. At the very least such knowledge should enable midwives to avoid simply reinforcing the stigma that is attached to poverty and to engage in non-judgemental ways with women who are poor. At best it may inspire some midwives to challenge those in positions of leadership and influence within midwifery to lobby for social and political change. Meanwhile, the impact of poverty on pregnancy remains an issue of social justice (Hunt, 1999).

- Poverty is an historical and contemporary feature of UK society.
- There are difficulties in defining and measuring poverty.
- An intrinsic relationship exists between social inequalities and poverty which impacts directly on the health and well-being of individuals.
- Women experience poverty in unique ways, particularly in relation to being lone or young mothers, and these experiences can lead to unfavourable outcomes of pregnancy and childbirth.
- Poverty poses a real challenge for midwives.

References

- Abbott P and Wallace C (1997) *An Introduction to Sociology: feminist perspectives* (2e). Routledge, London.
- Acheson D (1998) *Independent Inquiry Into Inequalities in Health Report.* The Stationery Office, London.
- Alcock P (1997) *Understanding Poverty* (2e). Macmillan, Basingstoke.
- Benzeval M *et al.* (1995) *Tackling Inequalities in Health: an agenda for action.* King's Fund, London.
- Brown G and Harris T (1978) *The Social Origins of Depression.* Tavistock, London.
- Crafter H (2002) The practical aspects of health promotion in pregnancy. *MIDIRS Midwif Digest.* **12 (Supplement 1)**: S8–11.
- Crompton R (1997) *Women and Work in Modern Britain.* Oxford University Press, Oxford.
- Davies J (1997) Them and us: poverty, deprivation and maternity care. In: I Karger and R Phillipson (eds) *Challenges in Midwifery Care.* Macmillan, Basingstoke.
- Doyal L (1995) *What Makes Women Sick.* Macmillan, Basingstoke.
- Doyal L (ed.) (1998) *Women and Health Services.* Open University Press, Buckingham.
- Doyal L and Gough I (1991) *A Theory of Human Need.* Macmillan, Basingstoke.
- Drever F and Whitehead M (1995) Mortality in regions and local authority districts in the 1990s. *Popul Trends.* **82**: 19–26.
- Equal Pay Task Force (2001) *Just Pay: a report to the Equal Opportunities Commission.* Equal Opportunities Commission, Manchester.
- Glendinning C and Millar J (eds) (1992) *Women and Poverty in Britain: the 1990s.* Harvester Wheatsheaf, Hemel Hempstead.
- Goodman M (1999) The poor health of poor women. *Pract Midwife.* **2**: 4–5.
- Gordon D and Townsend P (2001) Breadline Europe: the measurement of poverty. In: K Catchside (ed.) *Millions Live in Poverty in the UK;* http//www.Newsvote. bbc.co.uk/hi/english/health/newsid_1207000/1207241.stm (accessed 8 October 2001).
- Graham H (1993) *Hardship and Health in Women's Lives.* Harvester Wheatsheaf, Hemel Hempstead.
- Hanna B (2001) Negotiating motherhood: the struggles of teenage mothers. *J Adv Nurs.* **34**: 456–64.

- Hunt SC (1999) Pregnancy and poverty: an issue of social justice. *RCM Midwives J.* **2**: 36.
- Jordan B (1996) *A Theory of Poverty and Social Exclusion.* Polity Press, Cambridge.
- Kent J (2000) *Social Perspectives on Pregnancy and Childbirth for Midwives, Nurses and the Caring Professions.* Open University Press, Buckingham.
- Land H (1999) The changing world of work and families. In: S Watson and L Doyal (eds) *Engendering Social Policy.* Open University Press, Buckingham.
- Lewis J (2000) Gender and welfare regimes. In: G Lewis, S Gewirtz and J Clarke (eds) *Rethinking Social Policy.* Sage Publications, London.
- Lewis J and Piachaud D (1992) Women and poverty in the twentieth century. In: C Glendinning and J Millar (eds) *Women and Poverty in Britain: the 1990s.* Harvester Wheatsheaf, Hemel Hempstead.
- Lister R (2000) Gender and the analysis of social policy. In: G Lewis, S Gewirtz and J Clarke (eds) *Rethinking Social Policy.* Sage Publications, London.
- Macfarlane A (2002) Measuring health inequalities in pregnancy and its outcome. *MIDIRS Midwif Digest.* **12 (Supplement 1)**: S3–5.
- MacKeith P and Phillipson R (1997) Young mothers. In: I Karger and R Phillipson (eds) *Challenges in Midwifery Care.* Macmillan, Basingstoke.
- McLeish J (2002) All I ate was toast: poverty and diet in pregnancy. *MIDIRS Midwif Digest.* **12 (Supplement 1)**: S6–8.
- Millar J (1997) Dimensions of poverty and social exclusion: gender. In: A Walker and C Walker (eds) *Britain Divided: the growth of social exclusion in the 1980s and 1990s.* Child Poverty Action Group, London.
- Nazroo JY (1998) Genetic, cultural or socio-economic vulnerability? Explaining ethnic inequalities in health. *Sociol Health Illness.* **20**: 710–30.
- Oakley A (1992) *Social Support and Motherhood.* Basil Blackwell, Oxford.
- Office for National Statistics (2002) *Social Trends No. 32.* The Stationery Office, London; http://www.statistics.gov.uk/downloads/theme_social/Social_Trends32/Social_Trends32pdf (accessed 10 March 2002).
- Oppenheim C (1997) The growth of poverty and inequality. In: A Walker and C Walker (eds) *Britain Divided: the growth of social exclusion in the 1980s and 1990s.* Child Poverty Action Group, London.
- Payne S (1991) *Women, Health and Poverty.* Harvester Wheatsheaf, Hemel Hempstead.
- Reisch LM and Tinsley B (1994) Impoverished women's health: locus of control and utilization of prenatal services. *J Reprod Infant Psychol.* **12**: 223–32.
- Rutter DR and Quine L (1990) Inequalities in pregnancy outcome: a review of psychsocial and behavioural mediators. *Soc Sci Med.* **30**: 553–68.
- Salmon D and Powell J (1998) Caring for women in poverty: a critical review. *Br J Midwifery.* **6**: 108–11.
- Sawtell M (2002) Lives on hold: homeless families in temporary accommodation. *MIDIRS Midwif Digest.* **12 (Supplement 1)**: S18–20.
- Scambler G (ed.) (1997) *Sociology as Applied to Medicine* (4e). WB Saunders, London.
- Scottish Poverty Information Unit (1997) *Poverty Debates*; http://www.spiu.gcal.ac.uk/briefing2.html (accessed 1 October 2001)
- Townsend P and Davidson N (1982) *Inequalities in Health: the Black Report.* Penguin, Harmondsworth.

- Townsend P, Phillimore P and Beattie A (1988) *Health and Deprivation: inequality and the north*. Croom Helm, London.
- Twomey B (2002) *Women in the Labour Market: results from the spring 2001 LFS*; http://www.statistics.gov.uk/downloads/theme_labour/LMT_March02pdf #p = 21: (accessed 3 March).
- Watson S (1999) Introduction. In: S Watson and L Doyal (eds) *Engendering Social Policy*. Open University Press, Buckingham.
- Watson S and Doyal L (eds) (1999) *Engendering Social Policy*. Open University Press, Buckingham.
- Whitehead M (1987) *The Health Divide*. Health Education Council, London.
- Wilcox M *et al.* (1995) The effect of social deprivation on birth weight, excluding physiological and pathological effects. *Br J Obstet Gynaecol.* **102**: 918–24.

CHAPTER 4

The family

Val Dunn-Toroosian

In industrialised societies, forms or models of families are changing rapidly, but one form, the nuclear family, is generally portrayed by the media as normative, because it is regarded as well adapted to the demands of modern societies. Family life has become a topic for political debate, and various policies have been devised to try to support families. In this chapter, the diversity of family structures and some of the social and demographic changes that impact on family structure and type are explored. Marriage remains popular in the UK, and is considered together with an examination of the roles of women in this context. Some sociological theories emphasise tensions and conflicts within the family, whereas others view family structure and roles as the product of social consensus. The various sociological approaches with regard to the family are compared, and there is a particular focus on feminist perspectives, with their emphasis on women's experiences of oppression within the family.

Introduction

The idea of the 'family' is an elusive one, as the word is used in a variety of different senses, and it tends to hold different meanings for different people. Families are supposed to signify security and love, and for the majority of individuals they do so. Family and marriage are also viewed as two of the most familiar, fundamental and enduring social institutions in virtually all societies (Giddens, 1997). However, the debate continues as to whether the nuclear two-parent family is a central ideal type, or whether it is essentially a socially constructed concept and as such is influenced by the cultural and historical social practices in which it is situated.

Furthermore, families are unlikely to conform to any stereotypical image. In industrialised and western societies, families are changing rapidly. Modern Britain, for example, is characterised by a range of different family and household structures, but the media always seems to portray a particular type of family. It is therefore hardly surprising that politicians have a traditional view of the family and fail to acknowledge the increasing disparity between family realities and family ideology. This chapter will explore the diversity of family structures and some of the social and demographic changes that impact on family structure and type. The various roles and responsibilities and the gendered division of household tasks will also be discussed with reference to the various theoretical perspectives.

First, the terms 'family' and 'social institution' require clarification.

The family

Families may be regarded as dynamic sets of social relationships, where each individual makes a unique contribution that combines with others to form the whole family unit. Giddens defines the family as 'a group of persons directly linked by kin connections, the adult members of which assume responsibility for caring for children' (Giddens, 1997: 140).

Family members can be interrelated by biological, legal or functional relationships, which means that they are essentially a crucial support system, both structurally and emotionally, and they can be nuclear, inter-generational or extended in configuration (Kristjanson, 1992). The United Nations definition of the family unit is based on 'the conjugal family concept', which is a traditional and unrealistic perspective of modern family life, as it assumes that most families are based on marriage and it therefore excludes a huge number of families which do not necessarily fit within this narrow definition. According to 1987 recommendations:

> the family should be defined in the narrow sense of a family nucleus — that is, the persons within a private or institutional household who are related as husband and wife or as parent and never-married child by blood or adoption. Thus a family nucleus comprises a married couple without children or a married couple with one or more never-married children of any age or one parent with one or more never-married children of any age.
>
> (Hantrais and Letablier, 1996: 8)

It must also be acknowledged that every family functions within and is uniquely influenced by its cultural and social context. Different demographic structures, cultural traditions and economic characteristics of various ethnic groups will necessarily influence family composition. Thus lifestyle differences may be due to ethnicity, social class or religious beliefs, and families will differ not only across cultures but also within a given culture. For example, all indigenous white British families do not function in the same way. There will be variations in household type, family structure and the division of domestic labour.

Social institution

A social institution is a way of referring to particular social groupings that are common to the majority of people in a society. They are often viewed in terms of the social need or function that they serve. According to Giddens: 'Social institutions are the "cement" of social life. They provide the basic living arrangements that human beings work out in their interactions with one another and by means of which continuity is achieved across the generations' (Giddens, 1995: 387).

This definition of a social institution seems to aptly describe a view of the family, which is recognised as the most complex but also the most familiar of the social institutions. It is the primary socialising agency, responsible for transmitting the values of a society and fostering the growth of children into competent adulthood. It is also the main context within which children receive care and protection. Furthermore, *the family*, where common residence, marriage and parenthood are frequently seen as central features, represents the first experience of social life, and for many individuals it will be the most enduring social group to which they will belong (Murdoch, 1949, cited in Hantrais and Letablier, 1996). Most people have some experience of family life, and irrespective of whether it was good or bad the experience will undoubtedly influence what they think a real family should be. These personal experiences can result in judgemental attitudes which are detrimental to effective client care.

Family models

Because of the great diversity of family types and structures which exists within a given society, Gittins (1993) suggests that the use of the term 'families' rather than 'the family' is more appropriate, as it demonstrates cognisance of this reality. However, despite the many variations, there are underlying similarities in cultural perceptions of family life. The evidence suggests that, for most people, family is regarded as a kin relationship (biological, legal or functional), and links are maintained by frequent telephone calls, correspondence and visits. The family provides mutual structural and emotional support (Hantrais and Letablier, 1996). 'Kinship' is a term often employed by sociologists and anthropologists when exploring what constitutes 'families', and it is defined as the ties that exist between individuals. 'Ties' can be described as a special social relationship that creates the social and/or biological attachment between individuals. In some cases, friendship ties can provide much more social support than biological ties with brothers, sisters and other family members.

A broad distinction can be made between what sociologists and anthropologists refer to as the *nuclear family* and the *extended family*. These are the two main types of family. Most other family structures, namely lone-parent families, reconstituted families, mono-gender families, symmetrical families, cohabitation and matrifocal or matriarchal families, can fit within these two distinctions.

Box 4.1 Family structures

- Extended family
- Nuclear family
- Symmetrical family
- Mono-gender family
- Lone-parent family
- Matrifocal family
- Reconstituted family
- Cohabitation family

Nuclear families

Nuclear families consist of two adults, namely mother and father, and dependent children (biological or adopted) living together in a household (Giddens, 1997). Two-parent nuclear families predominate in western and industrialised societies.

According to Jones (1994), this model is considered to be the typical and ideal family unit in UK culture, and this view is reinforced by current political ideology. Despite acknowledging the significant changes that the family has undergone in recent decades, the Government still asserts that the traditional patriarchal family (within a marriage) provides the most reliable framework for raising children (Home Office, 1998). However, it is clear that the 'cereal-box' family, as it is sometimes referred to, is not the norm for a large number of children, and reinforcing the traditional family as the ideal can have detrimental consequences for children who are being raised in non-traditional families. The reality is that household composition has undergone significant transformation in recent decades. The percentage of two-parent family households with dependent children has fallen, while the proportion of lone-parent households with dependent children has increased. Although divorced lone mothers have traditionally been the most numerous category, the last decade has seen a sharp increase in the incidence of births outside marriage. However, despite recent social and demographic changes, illustrated by the Office for National Statistics, the traditional two-parent nuclear family with dependent children remains the commonest type of family in the UK, representing 79% of family households (Office for National Statistics, 2002).

Table 4.1 Percentage of dependent children living in different family types in the UK (General Household Survey and Labour Force Survey, Office for National Statistics)

Family type	1972	1981	1991–92	2001*
Two-parent families				
1 child (%)	16	18	17	18
2 children (%)	35	41	37	37
3 or more children (%)	41	29	28	24
Lone-mother families				
1 child (%)	2	3	5	6
2 children (%)	2	4	7	7
3 or more children (%)	2	3	6	5
Lone-father families				
1 child (%)	–	1	–	1
2 or more children (%)	1	1	1	1
All dependent children (%)†	100	100	100	100

*In spring 2001.
† In spring 2001, including cases where the dependent child is a family unit (e.g. a foster child).

Extended families

The extended family, which is a multi-generational unit, includes three generations or more living in the same household or in close proximity, or having continuous contact. It may include grandparents, brothers and sisters and their partners, aunts, uncles, nieces or nephews. Extended families predominate in most non-industrialised parts of the world. They are also more likely to conform to the traditional model of family life, with a male breadwinner who is the head of the household. They are often patriarchal units characterised by a dominant male and (usually) subordinate female and children, with unequal distribution of power and status. Female heads of households are less common except where the women are single, divorced or widowed and there are no other adult members present (Haralambos and Holborn, 2000).

Symmetrical families

Young and Willmott (1973) believe that there has been a growth in the symmetrical family, which is characterised by more egalitarian role sharing. The symmetrical nuclear family is said to be home-centred, self-reliant and self-contained. Women take up paid employment and their partner participates in the household chores and childrearing. Free time is spent around the house sharing chores. However, contemporary sociological evidence suggests otherwise. There certainly is a trend for more women to be in employment, but often it is either part-time or flexible working hours in order to enable them to fulfil their childcare and household responsibilities. They therefore carry the double burden of labour in the home and in the waged economy (Jones, 1994). Women undertake the bulk of household chores, and only a very small minority of men participate in domestic work on an equal basis. This finding holds regardless of whether wives or partners work outside the home or are full-time homeworkers. Women's share of total waged employment increased throughout the European Union (EU) during the 1980s, and in the UK women are now almost outnumbering men in the labour market, albeit in part-time and low-paid jobs. Despite these changes, men's level of participation in the home and family life has not changed significantly (Mintel Report, 1994; Office for National Statistics, 2001). This evidence dispels the myth of the 'new man'.

Lone-parent families

Another significant demographic change is the increasing number of single-parent families, which may be headed by either the male or female parent. However, the vast majority of single-parent families are headed by a lone mother. Approximately 19% of dependent children are raised by their mother, while lone fathers account for just 2% of all families with dependent children (*see* Figure 4.1). The majority of lone-parent families result from separation or divorce, but they may also be the result of bereavement or individual choice. Statistics show a rise in the number of births outside marriage and an increase in the number of divorces following the implementation of the Divorce Reform Act in 1971 (Office for National Statistics, 2001). The UK is estimated to have the highest proportion of lone-parent families in the EU (Jones and Millar, 1996). However, there appears to be an ethnic difference here. Nearly 50% of black families are lone-parent families, compared with only 8% of Indian families (Office for National Statistics, 2002).

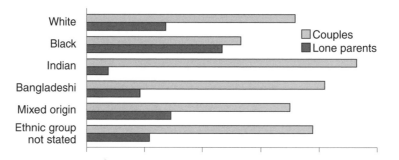

Figure 4.1 Families with dependent children in the UK, by ethnic group, in autumn 2000. Percentage values are shown. (These families may also include non-dependent children.)

Matrifocal families

Matrifocal families (female-headed families or matriarchal families) often consist of a woman with her dependent children, and sometimes their grandmother. Such families are common in low-income black communities in New World societies, and in the USA 29% of all black families are headed by women (Haralambos and Holborn, 2000). In the UK, 49% of black families are lone-parent (generally mother-headed) families (Office for National Statistics, 2002). According to Haralambos and Holborn (2000), female-headed families are more common in black communities for the following reasons.

- Historically in West Africa 'polygyny' (a form of extended family consisting of one husband and two or more wives) was practised. Perhaps this continues to influence black family structures.
- Economic deprivation may lead to desertion by the husband or partner because he cannot fulfil the responsibilities of paying the bills, being head of the household and being the main breadwinner.
- Poverty is the primary cause of matrifocal families, and they have become the subculture of poverty.

Patrick Augustus' autobiographical novel *Baby Father*, which was serialised by the BBC, explores the lives of young black men who have children with more than one woman and boast about it. Darcus Howe once said 'We are black men; that means we make babies all the time' (Alibhai-Brown, 2000). This is one of the worst stereotypes of black men. It portrays them as extremely irresponsible, but there are a number of complex reasons why young men behave in this way. Some men never agreed to be fathers (which is not a valid excuse), and are therefore resentful and feel no responsibility towards either their child or the mother of the child. The women involved are referred to as 'Baby Mothers' in the above-mentioned novel.

However, despite the statistics, matrifocal families are neither the norm nor the ideal within black communities. They are usually the result of the breakup of a nuclear family. This would suggest that many matrifocal families are the products of both culture and poverty. It is well documented that financial stressors are a significant factor in family breakup.

Stepfamilies

Households which are composed of one biological parent and a step-parent living with dependent children from more than one marriage or a non-marital relationship are referred to as stepfamilies, reconstituted, multiparental families or reordered families. Children whose biological families have not broken up, but who live with both parents and their stepbrothers or stepsisters, also belong to a re-ordered family (Hantrais and Letablier, 1996). The evidence indicates that the number of stepfamilies or reconstituted families in the UK is increasing for a variety of reasons, and the rising divorce rate is but one of these. There is also an increase in the number of children being born premaritally (Office for National Statistics, 2001). However, lone-parent status is often a temporary state, as most individuals still marry or remarry. Studies indicate that 50% of divorced or separated men will remarry within 2 years, and that 50% of divorced or separated women will do so within 5 years (De'ath, 1992). This evidence suggests that stepfamilies or reconstituted families are also on the increase. According to the National Children's Bureau, 2.5 million out of 12.5 million dependent children are in stepfamilies, and 300 000 children are born into stepfamilies (Foley *et al.*, 2001). These figures are still an underestimate, as they do not take into account cohabiting couples with stepchildren, who do not have to register their union or their separation in the UK.

According to the General Household Survey in 1998–99, stepfamilies (married and cohabiting) in which the head of the family was under 60 years of age accounted for about 6% of all families with dependent children. It is socially expected that children will remain with their mother if a partnership breaks up, and the statistics indicate that almost nine in ten stepfamilies consist of a couple with at least one child from the *female* partner's previous relationship (Office for National Statistics, 2002).

Stepfamilies are far more complex than biological families, and all family members have to make huge adjustments in order to make them work. The average stepchild will spend time in at least two homes and have four adults trying to

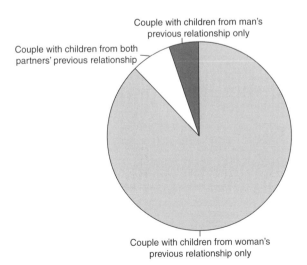

Couple with children from man's
previous relationship only

Couple with children from both
partners' previous relationship

Couple with children from woman's
previous relationship only

Figure 4.2   Stepfamilies with dependent children by family type, for the period 1998–99, in the UK. Families with one or more children, and with head of family aged 16–59 years, are included.

parent them. In families where grandparents are involved the numbers increase and the dynamics become even more complex. Thus there are sometimes three sets of parents and three sets of rules to observe and accommodate. Carers/parents often have very different rules, standards and goals for effective childrearing, which can sometimes cause confusion or conflict for the children, especially with regard to the issues of behaviour and discipline. Sibling rivalry may be exaggerated, and children may be concerned that the parents love their brothers or sisters more than them. For some families there may be a need to appear like an 'ordinary' family, thus underplaying or denying the complexities of their family arrangement (De'ath, 1992).

Gay families

Gay families may consist of two adult females or two adult males who are caring either for their own children from a previous heterosexual relationship, or for adopted children. New reproductive technologies or surrogate motherhood may have been utilised (Haralambos and Holborn, 2000). There is still much controversy about gay families arising from the belief that homosexuality is undesirable and therefore not the ideal environment in which to raise children. There is concern that children may be stigmatised, taunted or bullied by intolerant peers, and therefore it is suggested that gay families must be discouraged (King and Pattison, 1991). Of course there is no real evidence to show that children in such households are worse off. The quality of the relationship between the children and their carers is the major outcome determinant, not the carer's sexuality.

It is also known that because the current laws discriminate against gay couples as adoptive parents, most children of gay couples are from a previous heterosexual relationship. Therefore relationships between children and their parents, good or otherwise, are already established. Children more often remain with their mother in a marital breakup, and consequently lesbian mothers living with dependent children are more common than gay fathers living with dependent children (Haralambos and Holborn, 2000). The evidence also suggests that homosexual fathers very rarely gain sole custody of their children, partly because few of them apply to do so, but also because those who do are usually denied. Lawyers are hesitant to advise clients to apply for custody, because if a heterosexual family is available that option is likely to be favoured (King and Pattison, 1991). Social disapproval of and prejudice against gay fathers raising children is much more acute than for gay mothers, and this attitude seems to be reinforced by the courts.

In most western societies gay couples are not allowed to marry, and they are not considered to be 'proper' families by some. In the UK, Section 28 of the Local Government Act 1988 explicitly states that a local authority shall not 'promote the teaching in any maintained school of the acceptability of homosexuality as a "pretended" family relationship' (Secretary of State for Environment and Transport, 1988).

Parents and Friends of Lesbians and Gays (PFLAG),[4.1] which is a national organisation in the USA that offers support and understanding to these families,

---

[4.1] Parents and Friends of Lesbians and Gays (PFLAG) *Family Values*; http://www.pflag.org/about/family.html

points out that same-sex families should be given the same recognition and support which is afforded to traditional families. These families are often under huge emotional strain, and they need support from society for the family unit. They see the family as:

> two or more persons who share resources, share responsibility for decisions, share values and goals, and share commitments to one another over a period of time. The family is that climate that one comes home to; and it is that network of sharing and commitments that most accurately describes the family unit, regardless of blood, legalities, adoption or marriage.
>
> (PFLAG; http://www.pflag.org/about/family.html)

The past Vice President Gore made clear his support for gay families, especially in adoption cases, where he promised to eliminate discrimination. He stated that the only factors which ought to be considered in adoption are what is in the best interests of the child (Barillas, 1998). In British Columbia, Canada, the Government has recognised homosexual relationships as being 'on a par' with heterosexual relationships with regard to child support, custody and access. These changes to the Family Relations Act gave same-sex couples the same rights as heterosexual couples. However, some areas, such as Toronto and Alberta, are not nearly so inclusive (Lundie, 1998). These changes and the general trend for more inclusive legislation are further affirmed by Callahan, who argues that:

> gay or lesbian households that consist of intimate communities of mutual support and that display permanent shared commitments to inter-generational nurturing share the kinship bonding we observe and name as family.
>
> (Callahan, 1997, cited in Haralambos and Holborn, 2000: 507)

In the UK, Section 28, a law that prevents local councils from promoting or encouraging homosexuality through publications or campaigns or in schools, was brought in by Margaret Thatcher in 1988. The present New Labour Government promised to repeal the law in England and Wales as a measure against intolerance, and so that teachers would not be prevented from tackling homophobic bullying in schools (Stonewall Survey, 1996), to which Section 28 has contributed significantly. This met with strong opposition from the Conservatives, and was voted down in February 2000. However, in Scotland Section 28 has been repealed and education authorities are free to discuss alternative lifestyles. In May 1996, South Africa became the first country in the world to enshrine equality, regardless of sexual orientation, in the constitution (Achmat, 1998).

According to Giddens (1999) in the Reith Lectures, up to the beginning of the twentieth century, due to the absence of effective contraception, sexuality in the traditional family was dominated by reproduction. With the advent of the pill, sexuality was separated from reproduction, and was no longer defined in relation to marriage and legitimacy. This being the case, the increasing acceptance of homosexuality may become evident. As Giddens (1999) says, 'sexuality which has no content is by definition no longer dominated by heterosexuality'.

Functions of the family

Sociologists are in general agreement that the family has several core functions which may be seen as essential to the reproduction and maintenance of society. These functions also play a significant part in ordering society and in determining individual life chances. Within the family, children learn discipline, acceptable ideas about right and wrong and the limits of tolerated behaviour. Fletcher (1988) divided these into essential and non-essential functions, the essential functions being reproduction, sexual activity and the provision of a home. Each family also takes responsibility for childcare, primary socialisation, informal healthcare, economic provision and maintaining the household. Traditionally, the family fulfilled many of the functions which are today provided by State-sponsored institutions, and the family is expected to utilise these services. Some examples include healthcare, education and the health surveillance role of health visitors.

The functions of the family have changed over time. The modern family is now seen more as a unit of consumption, whereas the pre-industrial family was regarded as a unit of production. Some writers assert that the role of the family is being eroded, and they bewail the breakdown of the traditional family. However, Fletcher (1988) suggests that the family has retained its central roles and that these have actually increased and intensified. Significantly, political leaders in the UK also urge the return to earlier family values (focusing specifically on the assumed evils of single parenthood), since an adequately functioning family is believed to contribute to the orderly maintenance of an industrial society. The Government has pledged to support families and children because they believe that a secure family life gives a child a good start in life and the best chance of succeeding (Home Office, 1998).

The 'deviant' or 'problem' family is defined by the powerful as one that is a burden on society, either because it relies on welfare support or because such families are perceived as being unable to 'control' their children, thus failing in their responsibility for socialisation. Again, mothers in particular bear the brunt of the criticisms. The case of a mother who was jailed for failing to prevent her children from playing truant made the media headlines recently (Staff and Agencies, 2002).

An increase in industrialisation demanded a more mobile workforce, and this contributed to a change in family structures and role relationships, such as an increase in the number of symmetrical nuclear families (Young and Willmott, 1973) and a reduction in the number of extended families. These changes are of interest to the State because there is a reduced role for grandparents in supporting young working families with dependent children, and this in turn creates a need for the State to provide adequate childcare facilities, as well as care for the elderly and dependent.

The notion of the family is reinforced by social policy, which is based on the assumption that everyone is in a traditional family. The family ideology in state policy asserts that:

- men are primarily breadwinners
- women are their dependents
- a woman's primary role is that of housewife and mother.

There is a dichotomy here. Conservative politicians in particular would prefer mothers not to work, as they need to be at home to care for and protect their children. On the other hand, they do not want single mothers to be claiming income support.

Marriage

Marriage, according to Giddens, is 'a socially acknowledged and approved sexual union between two adult individuals' (Giddens, 1997: 140). This is a predominantly western definition, as there are some cultures in which individuals marry before adulthood. Of course this calls into question the way in which the terms 'adult' and 'child' are defined. Although falling in love is the most obvious reason for marrying in western societies, marriage is also of great social significance, in that it is an effective way of ensuring societal continuity through reproduction and socialisation.

Most European Union (EU) member states recognise the family as an important social institution and are committed to its protection, focusing in particular on the 'legitimate' family sanctioned by marriage. Where there is a strong Roman Catholic belief or where marriage is a defining feature of family life, divorce reform has been difficult to institute. For instance, Ireland had not legalised divorce by the early 1990s (Hantrais and Letablier, 1996). The Family Law (Divorce) Act of 1996 legalised divorce.

Women are socialised at an early age that their main role is to be a mother, and that men must first have a career and secondly be a father. Women are therefore likely to leave work in order to bear and raise children. Once she is married, a woman's career is less important than that of her husband. Perrone (2001) has examined the sacrifices that both men and women are forced to make when attempting to juggle career and family life. She notes that in the USA men are becoming more active in parenting and homemaking as more women pursue full-time careers. However, women are more likely than men to describe sacrifices made with regard to promotion or pay in order to enable them to lead a more balanced life. It seems irrelevant that today most mothers are in paid employment out of necessity. They have to juggle both of their roles, and therefore they are disproportionately represented in low-paid jobs and in social class five (Abbott and Wallace, 1992, 1997; Crittenden, 2001). Their choice of hours and employment is governed by domestic and childcare responsibilities (Abbott and Wallace, 1997). Furthermore, 'duty' is a sentiment that is often expressed within marriage, and women are made to feel guilty or deviant if they put their career before their family. It is also a reality that women can be poor even within an affluent household, because men generally control the finances and women receive a relatively small share of the household resources. They may also make sacrifices for their children, and are then left with even less to spend on themselves. This economic dependence reinforces the inequality between men and women (Abbott and Wallace, 1997).

Once they are married, women are expected to undertake the housework and childcare. Ann Oakley, in her classic study, *The Sociology of Housework*, concluded that housewives worked up to 72 hours a week, and were not rewarded by a wage or even status (Oakley, 1974). Household labour, which is classified as non-market work, is deemed to be insignificant by male economists, even though studies show that non-market work contributes around 40–60% of production in many countries (Crittenden, 2001).

Until the 1960s, the rights of mothers were legally subordinated to those of the partner and/or father. However, legislation is adapting in recognition of the fact that the male partner is often not the sole or even main breadwinner, and therefore he is not the undisputed head of the family in economic terms. Men and women are jointly responsible for managing family affairs, and legal subordination of women and children has been removed in most EU states. For example, the concept of parental authority was introduced to replace paternal authority. In the UK, the 1989 Children Act introduced the concept of parental responsibility, which could be shared with another person − for example, the father. After separation or divorce and in consensual unions, when unions are dissolved, the mother is presumed to be more capable of caring for the child than the father (Hantrais and Letablier, 1996). This fact goes some way towards explaining why there are more lone mothers than lone fathers.

Social practices such as the wife and children using the father's surname after the couple are married confirm male dominance within the family. However, the sharing of parental authority and responsibility, division of property and the right of women to retain their maiden name after marriage and to choose their children's surname are some factors which symbolise a trend towards greater gender equality in some countries. In the UK, the father's surname generally takes precedence, but parents can give their child either the father's or the mother's name.

Marriages are legally registered and confer certain rights and responsibilities on spouses. However, English law does not automatically give cohabitees the same recognition, and when these consensual unions break up, if property was jointly owned, property disputes have to be established through property law. Most EU member states have now formally recognised the rights of cohabiting couples, and heterosexual consensual unions can be registered. Case law has made provision for issues with regard to inheritance, division of jointly acquired property and parental authority on separation. However, some countries (e.g. Greece, Luxembourg and Ireland) have still not formally accepted consensual unions, and this places cohabitees, especially women, in a very vulnerable position (Hantrais and Letablier, 1996).

Only a few countries have extended their legislation on heterosexual cohabitees to homosexual couples. Sweden has done so, and in The Netherlands same-sex partners can draw up cohabitation contracts to cover property rights and taxation, just like unmarried heterosexual partners (Collins, 1992).

The terms 'legitimate' and 'illegitimate' are used to indicate whether a child was born in or out of wedlock. These are old-fashioned, value-laden terms and reflect society's attitude to marriage and childbearing. Furthermore, they reinforce the New Right view and the Conservative pro-family movement, derived from Christian morality, that the traditional family (with wives economically dependent on their husbands) is the ideal, and that marriage binds the family together. However, it is encouraging to note that discrimination between children born in wedlock or extramaritally is now being abolished by most governments, so that where paternity is recognised, regulations governing care, maintenance and inheritance are the same for both. This arrangement may, though, inadvertently disadvantage the resident married partner. The UK, Germany and Sweden have acknowledged the rights of children born extramaritally since 1969 (Hantrais and Letablier, 1996).

Because of the nature of role division in families, with women taking the greater role in childcare and housework, they are disadvantaged in the labour market. Due to the fact that they interrupt their careers to raise children and because of family commitments, women may also have relatively less education, training and work experience and so be forced to take low-paid, low-status jobs. Feminists have repeatedly called for mothers to be paid, thus giving them some economic independence and raising their status. In the UK, women's average gross income was £119 a week, compared with £247 for men (Office for National Statistics, 2001), and in the USA women earn 75% of what men earn (Crittenden, 2001). Motherhood is considered by Crittenden (2001) to be the greatest obstacle to economic equality for women. On the whole, women draw the short straw in marriage in all respects. They are disadvantaged even with regard to their morbidity and mortality. It is well documented that women have a higher morbidity rate than men (Acheson, 1998; McDonough and Walters, 2001), although this may be accounted for by sex-role socialisation and structural disadvantage, but married women have a still higher morbidity rate than their unmarried counterparts, especially with regard to mental health (Abbott and Wallace, 1997).

Sociological perspectives

Families are said to be the building blocks of society, and they remain the basic unit for the protection and rearing of young children. They provide emotional and financial support for both adults and children and have several core functions, which are important in terms of the reproduction and ordering of society. Thus it is important to explore their roles and functions from different sociological perspectives.

Interpretive sociology studies the meaning that is given to everyday life by those involved in its construction. The cultures in which people live have a profound effect on what is perceived as 'common sense' or 'reality', and this is just as true for family life. The definitions that are used for family life are the product of shared meaning. Goffman (1969, cited in Steel and Kidd, 2001) states that people are actors and that they act out their social roles as public performances. Each role has a script, which includes cues to expect from others with whom one interacts. Some roles are *ascribed* (that is, given at birth) (e.g. female), whereas others are *achieved* (that is, gained through life experiences) (e.g. parent). According to interpretive sociology, these roles and corresponding scripts give meaning to social life (Steel and Kidd, 2001).

The functionalists and the New Right adopt a *consensus* perspective, which means that they uphold consensus-based family values. Feminism and Marxism are *conflict* perspectives, which view 'family values' as part of the problem in relation to power, control, status and inequality.

From a *functionalist* perspective, social roles are culturally determined and adopting these roles contributes to the smooth running of society. The importance of integration and harmony between the various parts of society which are *functionally* related is emphasised. In general, functionalists define the family by the 'needs' it fulfils in society. Functionalists believe that roles give people their place in society and thus ensure 'normal' functioning of family and society. Families have an important role in the primary socialisation of children, who will conform to the norms and values of society. A distinction is made between male and female roles with regard to the division of domestic labour. Roles are segregated along traditional gender lines. Functionalists talk of a female expressive role, which implies that females are more suited to caring, nurturing and providing emotional support.

The male instrumental role provides financial support and is the breadwinner. A gendered division of labour is perceived as best serving the needs of industrial society (Abbott and Wallace, 1997).

The anthropologist George Murdoch (1949) regards biological differences as the basis of sexual division of labour in all societies, since this is the most efficient way of organising society. Woman's biological function of childbearing confines them to the home, and their physique limits them to less strenuous tasks. Men can wander further from home and perform heavier tasks. These were studies of 'primitive' family units, but one can still draw parallels in today's families (Haralambos and Holborn, 2000).

Parson (1951, cited in Haralambos and Holborn, 2000) viewed the family as serving universal (biological) human and social needs, and emphasised the necessity for a gendered division of labour so that care and nurturing (expressive role) and material resources (instrumental role) can be provided.

The *New Right* takes a similar perspective to the functionalists. They are clear that men's role is as head of the family and economic provider. The woman is the homemaker and responsible for childcare (Abbott and Wallace, 1992). However, many couples today rebel at the notion of traditional marital roles.

The New Right and Conservative administrations since the 1970s have emphasised support for the stable patriarchal nuclear family with a dependent female and a dominant male. The Conservative Family Campaign was established in 1986 to restore the traditional patriarchal family and revive fundamental Christian values. Moral decline and family breakdown are considered to be the cause of economic and military decline in the UK. Conservative members of parliament have in public speeches blamed a variety of social ills, namely delinquency, vandalism, juvenile crime and a decline in educational standards, on the weakened position of parents. In a 1988 speech, Margaret Thatcher famously said that 'family breakdown … strikes at the very heart of our society'. A major problem, as they see it, is poor single-parent (single-mother) families (Abbott and Wallace, 1992; Jones and Millar, 1996). This was an era of 'lone-parent' bashing, and even though New Labour has played this down, their rhetoric continues to idealise nuclear families and marriage.

Feminists believe that functionalists support patriarchy by claiming that men and women are biologically suited to different roles in the family, and that therefore their ideology is problematic. Feminist sociologists argue that the family is the main means by which women are oppressed in modern Britain, and they have looked primarily at the gender roles within families. For them the unequal division of domestic labour is a matter of real concern. The heavy burden of housework and childcare leads to the 'captivity' of women in traditional gender roles. The stereotypical view of the family has assisted the subordination and exploitation of women and other dependants, and perpetuates the domination of men (Abbott and Wallace, 1997). Feminism has also emphasised the heavy emotional and financial price that is paid by women in families with traditional gender roles where they have little autonomy or emotional support and are responsible for most domestic labour (Finch and Groves, 1983). The majority of men take on a minor share of childcare and household chores, but on the other hand may work long hours with much overtime. These expectations make it difficult for women to compete on equal terms with men in the labour market. Their occupational choices are constrained by family roles and responsibilities. As mentioned earlier, most working married women take employment and hours that are governed by the need to juggle domestic and childcare responsibilities and work. Oakley (1974) also emphasised the extent to which housework is built into the feminine role. Women are disproportionately represented in part-time, low-paid jobs and in social class 5, living in poverty with dependent children (Oakley, 1974; Abbott and Wallace, 1992; Office for National Statistics, 2001).

Feminists view domestic labour as real and physically demanding work, and as such they consider that it should be paid. Oakley (1974) also points out that housework is unrecognised and under-rated, and radical feminists consider that men benefit from women's unpaid work, so they have an interest in maintaining the status quo. Marxist feminists, on the other hand, emphasise that women's exploitation in the family serves the interests of capitalism. Marxist analysis tends to concentrate on the way in which families encourage and reproduce hierarchical and inegalitarian relationships. They maintain the status quo by providing tomorrow's labour force, and by offering a secure place for relaxation and rest. Through socialisation and day-to-day relationships, rebellious spirits are quelled. Therefore the family is seen as detrimental to the development both of the individual (woman) and of society. Feminists and Marxists are in agreement that the family oppresses women (Abbott and Wallace, 1997). Capitalism also oppresses women by excluding them or making it difficult for them to participate in the public sphere of waged labour, and by exploiting their labour in the domestic sphere. However, women's oppression pre-dates capitalism. It is argued that it is the patriarchal social system, with all of its structural constraints, that oppresses women.

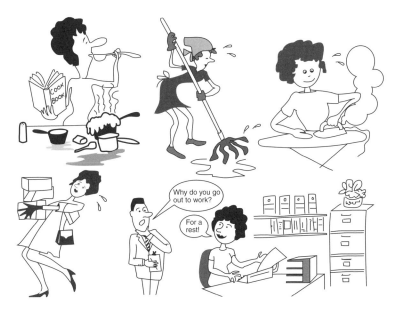

Figure 4.3   Women at work. (Reproduced with permission from Moore S (1987) *Sociology Alive!* Stanley Thornes Publishers Ltd, London.)

The ideology of 'familism' supports this position, and Dalley (1988) states the following:

> The ideology of familism is based on the assumption that the family, and particularly the nuclear family, with breadwinner male and dependent female and children, is the normal and natural unit for nurturing and caring. It is the standard against which all forms are measured and, importantly, judged. Accordingly, non-family forms are deemed to be deviant and/or subversive.
>
> (Dalley, 1988, cited in Jones, 1994: 93)

Postmodernism suggests that the world is shaped by pluralism, religious freedom, consumerism, mobility and increasing access to news and entertainment. The postmodern is inclusive, and dismisses the existence of an absolute reality. It acknowledges that there are multiple realities. By definition, therefore, the postmodern family is less uniform and includes a variety of family forms, as described earlier. Furthermore, the purpose and function of families have changed and are more diverse. Shorter may have been the first to describe the emerging postmodern family. He noted the following three important characteristics:

> Adolescent indifference to the family's identity; instability in the lives of couples, accompanied by rapidly increasing divorce rates; and destruction of the 'nest' notion of nuclear family life with the liberation of women.
>
> (Shorter, 1975)

According to Elkind (1995), the postmodern family values autonomy, and is parent-centred, basing decisions on the needs and aspirations of both parents. 'Maternal love' is believed to be a social construction that can be expanded to include 'paternal love', and shared parenting replaces the 'universal' construction of mother as sole carer. These trends are often seen as the breakdown of the family (O'Neill and Pittman, 2001).

All industrialised countries have seen a change in families from the predominantly extended institutional family to the small self-contained modern or postmodern family. For many postmodern children there is dual socialisation by family and childminder or nursery. This can create new problems, because while some children thrive, others are unable to adjust to the demands of a daily transition from one environment to the other.

Functionalists tend to ignore the harmful effects of family life and the inequalities of domestic life, while feminists question common-sense and conventional sociological assumptions of the family. Thorne (1982) states that feminists argue against the view that any specific family form is natural. Family forms are socially constructed around assumptions about people's roles, and there is no biological reason for the gendered division of labour. Families have 'power relationships that can and do result in conflict, violence and the inequitable distribution of work and resources' (Abbott and Wallace, 1997: 140). Family crime, a term that is used to define violence and abuse in domestic life, is seen as less serious than 'real crime', even though domestic violence accounts for 25% of all violent crime (Saraga and Muncie, 2001) (*see* Table 4.2 for a summary of sociological perspectives on the family).

Roles and relationships within the family are not becoming more democratic and symmetrical, and equality remains an illusory goal. The Omnibus Survey

Table 4.2 Summary of sociological perspectives on the family

Sociological perspectives	Description (view)	Division of labour	Functions	Paid employment (earnings, dependence)
Consensus perspectives Functionalists	Traditional, patriarchal nuclear family with dominant man and dependent woman and children seen as the ideal. Other family forms are undesirable	Gendered division of domestic labour is taken for granted. Male breadwinner, female housewife who cares for children and breadwinner. Female has expressive role and male has instrumental role	Seen as a necessary institution in society. Emphasis is on the benefits of families, namely procreation, socialisation, economic and emotional support. Traditional nuclear family is most suited to the needs of industrialised society	Men need a family wage, as their prime responsibility is earning to support the family. Women do not need a family wage. They work for non-essentials, their prime responsibility is as a homemaker, and therefore they usually have low-paid or part-time jobs
New Right	Similar to functionalist. They take a moralist view and they emphasise heterosexual marriage as central to a family unit	Social/gender roles are prescribed and have biblical origins	Women should be at home caring for the children and pampering the male breadwinner. All social ills are blamed on the woman rebelling against her traditional role	New Right feel that women should not take up paid employment
Conflict perspectives Feminists	Feminists argue against the view that any specific family form is 'natural' or 'normal'. They focus attention on the diversity of families, and they draw on anthropological evidence to demonstrate a wide variety of kinship systems across the world	Women have the major responsibility for domestic labour (the essential repetitive tasks), while men 'help out'. Even when in full-time employment, women bear the double burden because domestic labour is not viewed as 'real' work	The family is the main means of oppression and subordination of women and children. It reinforces and perpetuates women's subordinate roles, while men exploit women's unpaid domestic labour	Motherhood, domestic responsibilities and childcare restrict the choice of jobs. Therefore women are predominantly in low-paid, part-time work. Restricted work opportunities mean that economic and political power lies with men
Marxists	Similar to feminists. They question the assumption that the traditional nuclear family is best for the individual	The unequal division of domestic labour oppresses women, and women's traditional role within the family helps to maintain the status quo – and provides a healthy, happy workforce	Families meet the needs of a capitalist society at the expense of the individual (female). Capitalists exploit women's unpaid labour as carers and homemakers. Marxists view the family, where socially acceptable behaviour and social responsibility are learned, as an agent of social control	Capitalism makes it difficult for women to compete with men in the workplace

(Office for National Statistics, 1999) clearly illustrated that the family is still essentially patriarchal. In the UK, the average male spends more time eating out, watching television and gardening than his female partner, and does less than a quarter of the cooking and routine housework, even though he is less likely to be the sole or even main breadwinner. The proportion of women in employment increased during the latter half of the twentieth century, while for men the proportion has declined. However, men do spend more time on gardening, caring for pets and home improvements, and on average they work longer hours than women in waged labour (Office for National Statistics, 2001).

Conclusion

This chapter has explored the diversity of family forms, noting the various demographic changes and cultural influences on families, and considering some sociological perspectives. Roles within the family have also been explored, especially the division of domestic labour.

Family structures have become more diverse and complex during the last decade but, despite these changes, families will continue to play a very important role in people's lives. The family will survive in a plurality of family forms, and does not have a static, fixed definition. A postmodern family perspective will become more common. Cohabitation is a popular prelude to marriage, and this trend will continue as social attitudes become increasingly tolerant, but evidence suggests that it will not replace marriage. Dual-earner families, stepfamilies and single-parent families are also on the increase. Homosexual families and families using new advances in reproductive technology create another set of issues, and introduce debates about biological versus social definitions of kinship.

There are some advantages to traditional families. Two-parent families are less vulnerable to socio-economic deprivation and health problems than lone-parent families. This does not mean that they are necessarily better than alternative family structures, which even in today's climate tend to be devalued. There is greater social acceptance that children can and indeed do flourish in non-traditional family environments, even though Government policy and ideology continue to promote the idea of a traditional nuclear heterosexual two-parent family as the ideal. However, it should not be forgotten that the traditional family is essentially patriarchal, with subordinate women and children, and domestic violence towards women and children is a consequence of unequal power relationships and male authority.

- There is a great diversity of family structure and family types in society in the UK.
- Ideologies of the family, such as familism, patriarchy and the gendered division of domestic labour, impact on women's lives.
- Families play an important role in ordering society.
- Marriage remains a popular social institution.

References

- Abbott P and Wallace C (1992) *The Family and the New Right.* Pluto Press, London.
- Abbott P and Wallace C (1997) *An Introduction to Sociology: feminist perspectives* (2e). Routledge, London.
- Acheson D (1998) *Independent Inquiry Into Inequalities in Health.* The Stationery Office, London.
- Achmat Z (1998) *World: Africa gay rights win in South Africa*; http://news.bbc.co.uk/hi/english/world/africa/newsid_190000/190268.stm
- Alibhai-Brown Y (2000) We are black men. That means we make babies. *Guardian.* **13 April**: 8.
- Barillas C (ed.) (1998) *VP Gore Promises to Protect Gay Families*; http://www.datalounge.com/datalounge/news/record.html
- Collins H (1992) *The Equal Opportunities Handbook. A guide to law and best practice in Europe.* Blackwell, Oxford.
- Crittenden A (2001) *The Price of Motherhood: why the most important job in the world is still the least valued.* Henry Holt and Company, New York.
- Dalley G (1988) *Ideologies of Caring: rethinking community and collectivism.* Macmillan, Basingstoke.
- De'ath E (1992) Stepping into family life. *Health Visitor.* **65**: 15–17.
- Ekind D (1995) School and family in the postmodern world. *Phi Delta Kappan.* **77**: 8–14.
- Finch J and Groves D (1983) *A Labour of Love: women, work and caring.* Routledge and Kegan Paul, London.
- Fletcher R (1988) *The Shaking of the Foundations. Family and society.* Routledge, London.
- Foley P, Roche J and Tucker S (eds) (2001) *Children in Society: contemporary theory, policy and practice.* Palgrave, Basingstoke in association with Open University Press, Buckingham.
- Giddens A (1995) *Sociology* (2e). Polity Press, Cambridge.
- Giddens A (1997) *Sociology* (3e). Polity Press, Cambridge.
- Giddens A (1999) *Family. BBC Reith Lectures 1999*; www.lse.ac.uk/Giddens/reith_99/week4
- Gittins D (1993) *The Family in Question* (2e). Macmillan, Basingstoke.
- Hantrais L and Letablier M-T (1996) *Families and Family Policies in Europe.* Longman, London.
- Haralambos M and Holborn M (2000) *Sociology Themes and Perspectives* (5e). Harper Collins, London.
- Home Office (1998) *Supporting Families. A consultative document.* The Stationery Office, London.
- Jones H and Millar J (eds) (1996) *The Politics of the Family.* Avebury, Aldershot.
- Jones L (1994) *The Social Context of Health and Health Work.* Macmillan, Basingstoke.
- King MB and Pattison P (1991) Homosexuality and parenthood. *BMJ.* **303**: 295–7.
- Kristjanson LJ (1992) Conceptual issues related to measurement in family research. *Can J Nurs Res.* **24**: 37–52.

- Lundie L (1998) B.C. gives gay families equality in the eyes of the law. In: *The Peak: Simon Fraser University's Student Newspaper*; http://www.peak.sfu.ca/the-peak/98–1/issue5/family.html
- McDonough P and Walters V (2001) Gender and health: reassessing patterns and explanations. *Soc Sci Med.* **52**: 547–59.
- Mintel Report (1994) *Men 2000.* Lifestyle Report, London.
- Murdoch GP (1949) *Social Structure.* Macmillan, New York.
- Oakley A (1974) *The Sociology of Housework.* Martin Robertson, Oxford.
- Office for National Statistics (1999) *National Statistics Omnibus Survey.* The Stationery Office, London.
- Office for National Statistics (2001) *Social Trends No. 31.* The Stationery Office, London.
- Office for National Statistics (2002) *Social Trends No. 32.* The Stationery Office, London.
- O'Neill L and Pittman K (2001) *Mapping the Modern–Postmodern Divide. Volume 4*; http://www.ascd.org/readingroom/classlead/0012/1dec00.html
- Perrone K (2001) Learning to balance career and family increases lifetime satisfaction. In: *BSU Alumnus Magazine: Ball State University's Alumni Publication*; www.bsu.edu/alumni/alumnus/may2001/faculty.html
- Saraga E and Muncie J (2001) Family Crime. In: E McLaughlin and J Muncie (eds) *The Sage Dictionary of Criminology.* Sage Publications, London.
- Secretary of State for Environment and Transport (1988) *Local Government Act 1988.* HMSO, London; www.hmso.gov.uk/acts/acts19/Ukpga_19880009_en_5.htm
- Shorter E (1975) *The Making of the Modern Family.* Basic Books, New York.
- Staff and Agencies (2002) No place for a mother. Truancy is bad: prison won't solve it. *Guardian.* **15 May**: 17.
- Steel L and Kidd W (2001) *The Family.* Palgrave, Basingstoke.
- Stonewall Survey (1996) 'Queer bashing'. In: *Citizen 21 – together for equality*; http://www.c21project.org.uk/information_h3_1.htm
- Thorne B (1982) *Feminist Rethinking of the Family: an overview.* Longman, New York.
- Young M and Willmott P (1973) *The Symmetrical Family.* Penguin, Harmondsworth.

CHAPTER 5

'Race' and ethnicity

Dave Sookhoo

Pregnancy and childbirth are unique life events. They cannot be reduced to primarily biological events, since the social and cultural context is central to the subjective and collective experiences of women. Personal factors such as the woman's age, ethnicity, social class, religion and culture may influence her experiences of pregnancy and childbirth. This chapter explores the concepts of 'race', ethnicity and culture in relation to pregnancy and childbirth. The issues of access to maternity services, stereotyping and racism are explored within the context of midwifery service provision and practice. The challenge of caring for someone whose cultural beliefs and practices are not similar to one's own raises questions about the cultural competence of healthcare professionals, particularly the midwife.

Introduction

In health sciences, as elsewhere, the definition and meanings of terms such as 'race', 'ethnicity' and 'culture' have been extensively debated. The mosaic or maze approach does not clarify the situation. The use of these terms, sometimes without any clarification of the context or the perspective being adopted, does little to eliminate the confusion that can arise, particularly when the terms are used synonymously or assumed to be implicit in their sense. The common-sense approach does not help either, because sometimes these terms have been used to advance particular political and economic viewpoints, with ideological values bound up in the process of illuminating issues that are assumed to be of significance. The values that are implied may be real and may enhance or impede understanding. In the health sciences and health service provision, the gulf between intellectual argument and real-life encounters can be overwhelming. The need to address more fundamental and sensitive issues that are of practical value becomes a professional imperative in order to influence differences in the care of women and the newborn.

This chapter examines the definitions and terms, sets them in the context of the evolutionary framework, and attempts to illustrate their usefulness or otherwise with evidence from the literature. Much of the discussion will be conceptually based and applied to midwifery to inform practice. As we become increasingly multicultural in our communities, or as the *Parekh Report* (Runnymede Trust, 2000) puts it, a 'community of communities', the pluralism that we embrace becomes self-evident even in the air that we breathe – invisible, yet life itself. Defining the terms is difficult and not without pitfalls and risks of over-simplifying complex issues.

'Race'

Any discourse about ethnicity today requires that we also engage with 'race' from an historical perspective, in order to bring clarity to the context within which these terms are used. The complex use of the term 'race' can be traced back to the nineteenth century, when it was employed to express the 'interweaving of biology, culture and language' (Tonkin *et al.*, 1996). Today it is generally accepted that 'race' as a concept is a social construct. The use of the word 'race' in quotation marks has come to emphasise this acceptance of its use in debates about races and racial groups, with the understanding that race does not exist (Sarup, 1996; van Dijk *et al.*, 1997). The evidence suggests that genetically there is no such thing as race (McKenzie and Crowcroft, 1994; Bhopal, 1998b). However, among certain populations the biological component tends to assume significant importance with regard to diseases that are genetically transmitted, such as sickle-cell anaemia and thalassaemias. In the context of the appropriateness of healthcare services provision, such racialisation of diseases impacts both on the political ideologies and sensibilities of resource allocation, and on cultural competence in care and genetic counselling.

Ahmad (1993) has argued that an ideological stance has permeated the use of the term 'race', thus projecting a racialisation of health and illness within health research. The use of 'racial' or 'ethnic' groups as primary categories, and reliance upon these categories in an attempt to present robust explanatory models, play down the role of inequalities that are based on stratification by class, income, education, occupation and employment. When this happens, 'issues of institutional and individual racism as determinants of health status or healthcare become peripheral' (Ahmad, 1993: 19).

Although there is a much more critical appreciation of the anomalies associated with the use of the term 'race', the sometimes negative, attitudinal and behavioural values that it may convey cannot be ignored, nor can it be said that there is any lack of evidence for such precedence. Events within the UK in recent decades have suggested and serve as reminders that racism and institutionalised racism are real challenges to all of us as citizens and healthcare professionals.

Racism

Everyday experiences of racism reported by individuals from minority ethnic groups vary according to gender, age and social class (Virdee, 1995). Racism is the attitude of racists and 'not an inevitable feature of the ethnic minority' (Bradby, 1995: 413).

The acknowledgement of the existence of racism suggests that healthcare professionals themselves are contextualised within a frame in which racism affects everyday lives (Beishon *et al.*, 1995). As far as patients are concerned, the services are bound to reflect some of the wider societal issues in relation to racism and the fact that there are local and regional variations in the way in which the services are perceived. The understanding of others and their cultural values and beliefs are often misunderstood simply because the overt behavioural acts are judged on sight, without analysis of the underlying motives and intent. However, institutional racism has been a fact of everyday life for many non-white people from minority ethnic groups (Macpherson, 1999). It is recognised that planned, concerted and outcome-oriented action is urgently required to address racism in the NHS (NHS Executive, 1998).

Thus although this is not often recognised as such by professionals and service providers, to service users the concerns and experiences of 'racism', behavioural and attitudinal dispositions and actions are real and demeaning (Bassett, 1994). Therefore in health and social care services, racism is a real concern for people who are accessing these services, and the eradication of racism is high on the agenda for action. Midwifery care is one such area of practice for action on tackling racism (Hunt and Richens, 1999).

Ethnicity

Ethnicity is a multi-dimensional concept (Christian *et al.*, 1976; Nazroo, 1997; Culley, 2000). Ethnic identity is not a fixed entity. It is socially constructed and is given particular emphasis in diverse contexts. 'Ethnicity' is a term that is used more often in place of 'race'. However, this has not escaped the attention of those who regard it as being as problematic as the former. It is a difficult term to define and pin down, as the ethnicity of individuals is not fixed, but rather it is fluid and situational as described by Senior and Bhopal (1994). Ethnicity is generally taken to mean 'shared origins' in terms of geographical regions, shared and distinct culture and traditions that are maintained over generations, and common language or religion, which all give a person a distinct sense of identity and group affiliation (Brass, 1996; Nash, 1996).

In a similar way to the use of 'race' as a category, which is meaningless but may be dangerous, the use of ethnicity as a category has been criticised both for its vagueness and, more importantly, for the misinformation or distortion that it presents. Even with ethnicity, it appears that the conception is about 'them' and 'their ethnicity', thus failing to acknowledge both that we all have ethnic groups to which we belong, and that we all have an 'ethnicity'. In the white European context, white ethnic groups are often 'invisible' (McAuley *et al.*, 1996). Further problems arise when terms are used synonymously with nationality, and the picture is complicated still more if religion and geographical regions are introduced when defining the ethnic groups.

The use of ethnicity as a variable in health data is problematic (Sheldon and Parker, 1992; Ahmad, 1993; Senior and Bhopal, 1994; Bradby, 1995). De Bono (1996) has argued that there is an equally pressing need to describe accurately the ethnicity of 'white' populations. As mentioned above, the use of ethnicity as a variable has major flaws and disadvantages because of its imprecise and fluid nature. As Ahmad (1994), Smaje (1995) and Nazroo (1997) have argued, ethnicity-related data tend to camouflage the real materialist inequalities and outcomes of discrimination.

Ethnic monitoring and health needs assessment

The needs of the population whom we serve at local level and the demographics are essentially what generate the planning for care. The issues involved in needs assessment of minority ethnic groups are well established in the literature (Rawaf and Bahl, 1998).

In general, there is concern about the accuracy and completeness of data collection at local levels in maternity units (Kenney and Macfarlane, 1999). Incomplete information certainly seems to raise concern with regard to effective management of the systems of care. As a reflection of data about the health needs of the community and minority ethnic women, this represents a gap. The audit of the accuracy of data and their availability needs to be improved (Kenney and Macfarlane, 1999). The limitations of ethnic statistics lie in the accuracy with which the categories are filled, how and from whom the information is obtained, and the completeness of the data. The implementation of the Race Relations (Amendment) Act 2000 in April 2001 heralded a new era in tackling indirect discrimination. This Act removes exceptions to indirect discrimination by institutions and agencies, including the NHS and higher education (Home Office, 2001). Thus health and social care services will be required to demonstrate legally acceptable standards for information and workforce planning. However, the relevance of any data lies in their interpretation and their influence on the context of local services provision.

The concept of ethnicity as being fixed or static, and referring to a stable set of cultural traits or attributes, is misleading and may be instrumental in leading to stereotyping. Therefore it is useful and less restricted to think of ethnic and cultural identities of individuals as transitions through social and cultural adaptation and acculturation. The conceptualisation of ethnicity may benefit from a broader perspective through analysis first of the multidimensional and dynamic nature of ethnic identity, and secondly of the transitions that ethnic identities undergo over time. This may be exemplified by what Bhachu (1991) has tried to demonstrate with regard to Punjabi Sikh women. She has emphasised the self-determinative role of Punjabi women. This is in contrast to the view which is often erroneously held, and generalised, that women with a South Asian background are oppressed and have little or no opportunity for self-determination.

Inter-generational differences in the beliefs and practices of women with regard to care during pregnancy, childbirth and following delivery have been reported by Katbamna (2000). She illustrates these differences with the interview data from her study of Bangladeshi (Muslim) and Gujarati (Hindu) women. The differences were greater among women who had lived in the UK for longer and who had become acculturated with regard to the norms of the ways of life in the UK. Although there are similarities, Katbamna (2000) suggests that the differences between Bangladeshi and Gujarati women were also due to socio-economic factors, family structure and religious beliefs.

Stereotypes and cultural relativism

The ethnocentric attitudes that are held by healthcare professionals may prevent them from establishing relationships with their patients or clients unless those relationships are based on equality and mutual respect. Generalised beliefs that are held about others may or may not be true. Stereotypic thinking and behaviours may serve many functions, such as bolstering the person's self-esteem in what might be considered to be situations of threat (e.g. being in the presence of others who are not of the same group) (Hilton and von Hippel, 1996). However, stereotypes reflect misguided or ill-informed beliefs about people of different ethnic origin with regard to their traits, attitudes and behaviours. They tend to be negative or to arouse negative images about non-group members, and are perpetuated by various means. The media in particular, having access to large sections of the population, the institutions and social networks, may be influential in promoting stereotypes. It has been observed that racist views are common in the media (van Dijk *et al.*, 1997). Stereotypic beliefs that are held by midwives, such as those reported by Bowler (1993), demonstrate the need for education and greater understanding of the values and beliefs of others in our care. Bowler (1993) reported four themes that emerged from a qualitative study of midwifery care of women of South Asian descent:

1 difficulty in communication
2 women's lack of compliance with care, and abuse of services
3 a tendency to 'make a fuss about nothing'
4 lack of maternal instinct.

Earlier research by Larbie (1985) had shown that women with an African-Caribbean background had also experienced similar stereotyping and discrimination. It becomes apparent from these studies that racism may take the form of *cultural racism*, which is associated with the belief that the cultural values, beliefs and practices of others are inferior to one's own. Such racism, which is based on cultural and religious discrimination, is prevalent throughout the health services (Weller *et al.*, 2001).

Cultural relativism

Cultural relativism maintains that cultures are unique, that they must be evaluated according to their own values and standards, that specific cultural practices are exempt from criticism from outsiders, and that such judgement by outsiders is primarily based on ethnocentric standards (Haviland, 1993; Baker, 1997). Cultural relativism emerged as an approach to confronting racism and ethnocentric views and promoting respect and tolerance for the other. However, as Brannigan (2000) has argued, ethical issues arise from adopting positions of cultural relativism, not least as a consequence of an uncritical acceptance of the cultural practice of others. Therefore it is important that a critical understanding of the explanations of cultural practices, and their impact on the perceptions and experiences of women during pregnancy and childbirth, is generated through dialogue and reflection. However, there are ethical problems with this stance.

Suspending any judgement about others is not easy, and it involves deeper cognitive processes and attitudinal integration. In the context of a system of care, it is easy to forget some of the perspectives that govern professional practice. From the consumer's perspective, not knowing the acceptability or otherwise of certain practices is unacceptable not just in a cultural, moral context, but also more seriously in the legal context of professional practice. Values and beliefs can be challenged, otherwise the relativistic position leads to a cul-de-sac (Baker, 1997).

Women's experiences

The cultural perspectives of birth cannot be ignored (Thomson, 1997). Kitzinger (2000) has illustrated the ways in which birth is perceived in different cultures. The experiences of women with regard to pregnancy, childbirth and motherhood vary according to their perceptions of their pregnancy and how they feel and negotiate their relationships with others during these transitions. The experiences of women suggest that there is a large divide between the professional and lay perceptions. MacVicar (1990) recognised that the information provided and the expectations of women during pregnancy and the antenatal visits were at odds, simply because the women and the midwives were not the same.

When confronted with people who have different ethnic and sociocultural backgrounds to our own, 'difference' seems to be the most common aspect in the discourse about ethnic groups (van Dijk *et al.*, 1997). The experiences of women from minority ethnic backgrounds suggest that assumptions are made about them on the basis of skin colour, presentation, traditional dress, language spoken and their apparent willingness to respond to requests or their perceived lack of co-operation.

The maternity services have been criticised for not being flexible enough in the past (Larbie, 1985; James, 1997). The problem seems to lie in the resistance to change and the lack of empowerment and choice that is extended to women in general, not just women from minority ethnic backgrounds. The medical model and the ethnocentric views of pregnancy and childbirth promote conformity. When conformity is not perceived, then the pattern of behaviours or attitudes is interpreted as deviation from the accepted norms. There is no doubt that various stereotypes may characterise women with disability and lead to stigmatisation of some women (Thomas, 1997). Bowes and Domokos (1996) have suggested that the participation of women in decision making is limited, and that expressions of emotion and pain are frowned upon, giving the distinct impression that the voices of Pakistani women are muted during labour. Thus in the spirit of emancipation and empowerment of women, the raising of muted voices represents an even greater social challenge for women themselves, their advocates and care providers.

The Audit Commission report highlighted postnatal maternity services as an area about which service users expressed dissatisfaction (Audit Commission, 1997). It is contended that what often underpins dissatisfaction with postnatal services is the balance between an unfair overemphasis on the women's characteristics and a less than critical evaluation of the appropriateness of many aspects of the maternity services (Phoenix, 1990: Parsons *et al.*, 1993). For example, access to maternity services remains problematic for some women from minority ethnic groups (Hayes, 1995). It is not as simple as it is claimed to be. In many instances, access involves structural barriers that disadvantaged women have to overcome. Explanatory models may include not only ethnicity but also the interactions between many other factors such as educational and socio-economic status.

In general, the services fail women on several counts. Language appears to have been a major problem for a long time. The Bangladeshi women in Katbamna's study frequently referred to language as a barrier to communication with healthcare professionals (Katbamna, 2000). Inadequate interpreter services often mean that patients have to rely on relatives to act as interpreters. Brooks *et al.* (2000) reported that of a sample of 277 Asian patients, 31% did not speak or understand English, and about a third of the patients in the sample were not aware of the interpreter services provided. This may reflect local variations where the minority ethnic population is highly represented. One would expect that the use of interpreters and advocates would be widespread in maternity services. Where interpreter services are provided, women should be informed of their availability and usefulness. Service providers need to address those issues that are well known and documented, and to ensure that ineffective communication does not remain a recurrent major problem with a less than acceptable level of care provision.

Antenatal classes and screening

Narang and Murphy (1994) showed that only about 50% of the women in their study had any understanding and knowledge of the tests and screening procedures, and only a few women knew the reasons for the tests being performed. This lack of knowledge was indicative of the lack of information and poor decision making during the management of these women's pregnancies.

Atkin *et al.* (1998) concluded that ethnic and racial stereotypes adversely influence policy decision making in the provision of antenatal screening for the haemoglobinopathies, with the result that choice is often limited, and there appears to be an inability to provide culturally sensitive care. They also found that there tended to be ad hoc referral to screening services, with poor understanding among healthcare professionals about the value and purpose of genetic screening.

An understanding of the sociocultural aspects of minority ethnic women's sexuality and associated taboos may provide some explanation for any perceived lack of responses with regard to the uptake of antenatal examinations and procedures. Assumptions about what is expected from a professional viewpoint may underestimate elements of embarrassment, anxiety and fear that are perceived by women. The person whose integral self feels threatened in the environment of risk discourse may not be attuned to the 'medicalised bodies' that are so much a part of professional attitudes. However, as Crawford has argued, 'Cultural meanings are not only shared or given, they are fragmented and contested' (Crawford, 1984: 95). This requires that assumptions are always critically appraised in each case. Women's feeling of loss of control with regard to their pregnancy and childbirth is a serious issue for the self-esteem of women. Lack of self-esteem, traumatic experiences and a sense of disempowerment may lead to depression (Kitzinger, 2000).

Men's involvement

The part played by men in the transitions of women through pregnancy, childbirth and parenthood is a welcome one, and there is evidence to suggest that more men from various ethnic groups are now taking part in antenatal classes and are present at the birth of their children. However, beliefs and cultural issues surrounding the presence of men during what, in traditional cultures, is very much a women's event

(Kitzinger, 2000) may influence whether or not the husband or partner chooses to attend during labour.

Husbands and partners are encouraged to attend the birth, and if the father does not wish to attend the birth, this is often attributed to lack of interest or concern. However, such negative stereotypes of men are unwarranted. In some cases such attitudes and behaviour may be explained in terms of the legitimate wishes of women in the social context of gender relationships. Somali women's experiences in hospital in Sweden suggest that there are some women who, due to the cultural and socially differentiated roles during pregnancy and childbirth, are not comfortable about the presence of their husbands or partners at the birth (Wiklund *et al.*, 2000). Cultural influences on body modesty may be a critical issue, as well as the deeper issues of the self, disclosure, and the ethics of the social and medicalised body.

Technology and interventions

The medical model and its emphasis on risk management and surveillance sometimes fails to give enough credence and attention to the psychological and social needs of women (Oakley, 1984). The NHS environment of childbirth may be alien to many women who were not born in the UK. Indeed, it can be overwhelming even to those who are familiar with the services. The system of care and the specialised approach to maternity care, with technological interventions and screening procedures, may reinforce the feeling of loss of control, particularly if language is a barrier to the accessibility of services. As Sandelowski (1999) has suggested, technological systems maintain the knowledge and power differentials between patients and professionals, and serve the process by 'muting' the voices of women.

Lack of support is another aspect that is not taken into account. For those women who have extended families and friends, the experience may be very different to those who do not have such support. Many assumptions about support and its availability prevail both with regard to immigrant communities (Choudhry, 2001) and in relation to support during pregnancy and postnatal care (Katbamna, 2000). Due to these assumptions there is often a lack of understanding of women's care needs.

Management of labour

Bowler (1993) described how midwives perceived pain in women of South Asian descent in labour in a stereotypical manner, and did not respond by providing more analgesia when it was required. This was partly due to their apportioning blame on the women or being punitive. The stance of the midwives was very much that it was the women's fault for not attending antenatal classes where they would have been taught 'how to breathe', and since they did not attend these classes, they suffered pain. Needless to say, such an approach to the management of pain is unacceptable. The lack of analgesia is a recurrent theme in the literature (Bowler, 1993; Cheung, 1994). However, in some circumstances the woman herself may regard pain during childbirth as natural and acceptable. Zaidi (1994) suggests that Muslim women may accept pain during childbirth as part of the will of Allah (God).

Postpartum care

It is common practice to place the newborn on the mother's abdomen immediately after birth. However, in some cultures and according to some religious beliefs, placing the newborn on the mother's abdomen without first washing it is regarded as unacceptable because blood is viewed as 'contamination'. This may partly explain the observation that some women from Indian, Pakistani and Bangladeshi backgrounds do not or are reluctant to hold their babies immediately after birth (Midwives Information and Resource Service, 1998). Breastfeeding is another area of care that may reveal differences in beliefs and practices. Littler (1997) has reported how the perceptions and beliefs that are held by women about colostrum influence their breastfeeding behaviour. This may be observed in particular in Bengali women. What is pertinent about Littler's findings is that a lack of knowledge on the part of midwives about the cultural and religious beliefs of Bangladeshi women perpetuates the stereotypes that are held by midwives. Zaidi (1994) has provided a brief but useful guide to the care of Muslim women.

Rest and recovery

There is a common belief that after labour and childbirth, women need much rest and care. A long period of rest is traditionally expected, and this has been reported among Asian and Chinese women (Cheung, 1997; Gervais and Jovchelovitch, 1998; Katbamna, 2000; Davis, 2001). This may well be misinterpreted as the woman being 'lazy' (Bowler, 1993). However, if a culture-specific approach is adopted, this is seen as giving time for recovery and balancing the body (Davis, 2001).

Some socio-cultural issues
Stillbirth and infant mortality

Stillbirth and infant mortality rates among mothers from certain ethnic groups tend to be higher than the average for mothers born in the UK (Balarajan and Raleigh, 1993). The rates are highest among Pakistani women, followed by Bangladeshi, African-Caribbean and Indian women. In *Social Inequalities* (Drever *et al.*, 2000), it is reported that five out of every 1000 babies who are born to mothers who were themselves born in the UK, will die during the first year of life. For mothers who were born outside the UK, this figure rises to six in 1000 babies, and for those mothers who were born in Pakistan or the Caribbean, it rises to 10 in 1000 babies. Health inequalities are well-known by-products of poverty and social deprivation, and materialist explanations shed light on the rates of infant death among different ethnic groups (Andrews and Jewson, 1993). Among ethnic groups, the socio-economic status of Pakistani and Bangladeshi communities tends to be the lowest (Berthoud, 1997; Chandola, 2001). Distinctions should be made between the diverse groups that are subsumed under the label 'Asian'. In relation to health, the Indian group is better off than the 'Pakistani' or the 'Bangladeshi' groups, and the 'Bangladeshi' group is worst off (Nazroo, 1997). This may well be a direct reflection of settlement patterns and time of arrival, combined with education and occupational opportunities. Other ethnic groups such as Somalis, Vietnamese, Ethiopians and Albanians may show similar trends. Poverty has long been one of the major critical factors in health inequalities among the population in general as well as various ethnic groups (Haines, 1997; Nazroo, 1998).

Family size and family structures

Family size varies, and it would appear that the Pakistani and Bangladeshi ethnic groups on average have larger family sizes than others (Nazroo, 1997; Katbamna, 2000). This is partly explained by attitudes towards family planning and having or not having children, as well as religious beliefs.

The family structures in different ethnic groups vary, and the localities that people inhabit tend to be associated with proximity to kin. The joint family system emphasises the collectivist approach, which poses problems for the individualist oriented, especially in the context of one-to-one interactions (Laungani, 1999). The role of women within certain family structures influences the perceptions of motherhood itself. Traditional views about pregnancy and childbirth may become superimposed on the role expectations of the pregnant woman with regard to other family members. As is illustrated by Katbamna (2000), there is a need to be alert both to familial influences on the woman and to her attitudes and responses in relation to the role and expectations of the extended family. There is always a risk of stereotyping, and it is important to be aware that cultural norms are not fixed with regard to social mobility, personal biography, values and beliefs.

Religion

Religion plays an important part in the everyday lives of many individuals. People from the Indian subcontinent have diverse origins, with regional variations in language, diet, religious beliefs and practices, and social structure (Bhopal, 1998a). Indeed, one of the major criticisms of the 1991 Census was that 'the strong differentiation of the South Asian groups by religion was not captured' (Aspinall, 2000: 586). To Hilton (1996) it is inconceivable to think of ethnicity without giving equal consideration to religion. The Indian category conceals individuals of religious faiths such as Muslims, Sikhs, Hindus, Christians and Jains. With regard to regional variations, people may view themselves as Gujeratis or Punjabis. The pattern of migration from East Africa also adds to the subtle differences that may exist within the categories (Bhachu, 1991).

Bhopal (1998a) reported differences between single and married women with regard to their affiliation to religious beliefs and practices in South Asian communities. Married women were more likely to adhere to religious practices than single women, and Muslim women identified themselves by reference to Islam. These findings have implications both for continuity of identity formation and for identities in the context of place of birth. The Parekh Report (Runnymede Trust, 2000) further showed that religion is helping to redefine cultural identities among communities.

However, although it may not be immediately perceived as such, the religious beliefs and practices of people from non-European backgrounds appear to govern their lives to a much greater extent by comparison. If professionals are not familiar with the diversity of religious beliefs and practices, this may give rise to misunderstandings and lack of sensitivity to women.

Research and anti-racist perspectives

A number of issues involved in researching minority ethnic groups present difficulties, including access, participation rates and response rates. It is well documented that the response rate and participation rate in research are low among individuals from minority ethnic groups (Bowler, 1997). Part of the problem lies in the perceptions of what research is and what it is not. Bowler (1997) gives examples of how initial willingness to take part in research later turned into refusal because of the potential respondents' lack of understanding about why their views were being sought and the importance of their views in informing service delivery. When conducting research one has to be cognisant of the cultural factors that may influence the respondent's decision to participate. Bowes and Domokos (1996) regard their approach as meeting the principles of anti-racist, sensitive research. It becomes critical to the process of research to ask the women what they perceive to be problems, rather than having predetermined ideas about what those problems may be. Gerrish (2000) has described useful ways of understanding ethnic categories and practical issues when conducting research among ethnically diverse populations.

Cultural competence

Effective communication and an understanding of the expectations and practices of women from diverse sociocultural and religious backgrounds influence the degree of advocacy and empowerment that may be achieved. It is therefore important that when caring for women the midwife shows a level of cultural competence that builds on her role in advocacy and empowerment. In order to become culturally competent, the midwife has to embrace skills and knowledge that will enable one-to-one communication based on an understanding of the social, cultural and religious needs of these women.

Although culturalist analysis has come under criticism, the value of understanding cultures should not be underestimated. It is only through an understanding of the culture in its context that one can begin to make sense of the comparative (Jahoda, 1984; Alasuutari, 1995). In ways that are not immediately apparent, the stereotyping of women appears to go hand in hand with the perpetuation of certain myths, and in the context of woman-to-woman interactions, the management of pregnancy and childbirth becomes a series of negotiations within an arena of power positions, mutual respect and rights.

The individualistic and collectivist perspectives

An understanding of the orientation of the individual or ethnic group may be helpful when differentiating the needs of the individual and the family. The notion that the individualistic perspective prevails, no matter what meanings are attached to the event, mitigates against care that is appropriate for those women who may well come from cultural groups that have a collectivist orientation towards life and life events. Policies that are drawn up may not necessarily sit comfortably with the goal of providing culturally competent care, be it at the individual level with the practitioner or at the collective level with the institution, unless a cultural assessment of women's needs is made.

Conclusion

This chapter has attempted to explore the issue of the terminologies that are used in the literature and everyday practice with regard to the experiences of childbirth of women and men from diverse ethnic backgrounds. The women's experiences are unique, and unlike different diseases and their outcomes, pregnancy and childbirth have different moments for women, these transitions being defined by the experiences themselves. 'Race', ethnicity and culture are concepts that are frequently used in the discourse of pregnancy and childbirth. However, they should not be used without some critical analysis, as argued by those who suggest that advancing any explanatory model based on these concepts simply detracts from addressing the socio-economic inequalities that reflect inequalities in health (Andrews and Jewson, 1993).

Although various explanations have been proposed for the experiences of women from different ethnic groups with regard to pregnancy, childbirth and the associated mortality, no single explanation can be assumed to be conclusive, as each has its merits and limitations. The explanations of service providers and the experiences of women suggest that there is much to consider in relation to the appropriateness of and satisfaction with the care that women report receiving from the maternity services. The disadvantage that is associated with ethnicity and social positions may be partly based on social inequalities that cut across ethnic and cultural divides.

However, the experiences of women and the responses of healthcare professionals to the perceived needs of women should be a matter of serious concern for the professionals who come into contact with these women. Only through an understanding of the factors that contribute to the women's experiences – not only their biological condition but also their psychosocial and cultural needs – can the healthcare professional begin to offer care in an equal partnership. The development of anti-racist anti-discriminatory practice and cultural competence in caring for a woman through her pregnancy, childbirth and the postpartum period is essential for professional education and training in the pursuit of excellence in maternity care. The culture of midwifery itself requires further exploration and action to be taken for the empowerment of midwives (Kirkham, 1999).

- Midwives need to understand the personal subjective experiences of women during pregnancy and childbirth.
- Midwives need to explore the influences of ethnicity and culture on women both as individuals and as recipients of services.
- Midwives need to explore their own beliefs, attitudes and practice with regard to respecting and valuing diversity.

- Midwives should be cognisant of inadvertent or direct racism and discrimination that women may experience when accessing and using maternity services.
- Midwives should develop an understanding of the social and cultural needs of women from all ethnic backgrounds, with regard to similarities and differences.
- Midwives need to demonstrate anti-discriminatory and culturally competent care.

References

- Ahmad WIU (1993) Making black people sick: 'race', ideology and health research. In: WIU Ahmad (ed.) *'Race' and Health in Contemporary Britain*. Open University Press, Buckingham.
- Alasuutari P (1995) *Researching Culture. Qualitative method and cultural studies.* Sage Publications, London.
- Andrews A and Jewson N (1993) Ethnicity and infant deaths: the implications of recent statistical evidence for material explanations. *Sociol Health Illness.* **15**: 137–56.
- Aspinall PJ (2000) Should a question on 'religion' be asked in the 2001 British census? A public policy case in favour. *Soc Policy Admin.* **34**: 584–600.
- Atkin K, Ahmad WUI and Anionwu EN (1998) Screening and counselling for sickle-cell disorders and thalassaemia: the experiences of parents and health professionals. *Soc Sci Med.* **47**: 1639–51.
- Audit Commission (1997) *First-Class Delivery: improving maternity services in England and Wales.* Audit Commission Publications, Abingdon.
- Baker C (1997) Cultural diversity and cultural relativism: implications for nursing practice. *Adv Nurs Sci.* **20**: 3–11.
- Balarajan R and Raleigh VS (1993) *Ethnicity and Health: a guide for the NHS.* Department of Health, London.
- Bassett C (1994) Not just a black-and-white issue. *J Commun Nurs.* **6**: 12–14.
- Beishon S, Virdee S and Hagell A (1995) *Nursing in a Multiethnic NHS.* Policy Studies Institute, London.
- Berthoud R (1997) Income and standards of living. In: T Modood, R Berthoud, J Lakey *et al.* (eds) *Ethnic Minorities in Britain.* Policy Studies Institute, London.
- Bhachu P (1991) Culture, ethnicity and class among Punjabi Sikh women in 1990s Britain. *New Community.* **17**: 401–12.
- Bhopal K (1998a) South Asian women in East London: religious experience and diversity. *J Gender Studies.* **7**: 143–56.
- Bhopal R (1998b) Spectre of racism in health and health care: lessons from history and the United States. *BMJ.* **316**: 1970–3.
- Bowes AM and Domokos TM (1996) Pakistani women and maternity care: raising muted voices. *Sociol Health Illness.* **18**: 45–65.
- Bowler I (1993) 'They're not the same as us': midwives' stereotypes of South Asian descent maternity patients. *Sociol Health Illness.* **15**: 157–78.
- Bowler I (1997) Problems with interviewing: experiences with service providers and clients. In: G Miller and R Dingwall (eds) *Context and Method in Qualitative Research.* Sage Publications, London.

- Bradby H (1995) Ethnicity: not a black-and-white issue. A research note. *Sociol Health Illness.* **17**: 405–17.
- Brannigan M (2000) Cultural diversity and the case against ethical relativism. *Health Care Anal.* **8**: 321–7.
- Brass PR (1996) Ethnic groups and ethnic identity formation. In: J Hutchinson and AD Smith (eds) *Ethnicity.* Oxford University Press, Oxford.
- Brooks N, Magee P, Bhatti G *et al.* (2000) Asian patients' perspective on communication facilities provided in a large inner-city hospital. *J Clin Nurs.* **9**: 706–12.
- Chandola T (2001) Ethnic and class differences in health in relation to British South Asians: using the new National Statistics Socio-Economic Classification. *Soc Sci Med.* **52**: 1285–96.
- Cheung N (1994) Pain in normal labour: a comparison of experiences in southern China and Scotland. *Midwives Chronicle.* **107**: 212–16.
- Cheung NF (1997) Chinese *zuo yuezi* (sitting in for the first month of the postnatal period) in Scotland. *Midwifery.* **13**: 55–65.
- Choudhry UK (2001) Uprooting and resettlement experiences of South Asian immigrant women. *West J Nurs Res.* **23**: 376–93.
- Christian J, Gadfield NJ, Giles H and Taylor DM (1976) The multidimensional and dynamic nature of ethnic identity. *Int J Psychol.* **11**: 281–91.
- Crawford (1984) A cultural account of health, control, release and the social body. In: JB McKinlay (ed.) *Issues in the Political Economy of Health.* Tavistock, London.
- Culley L (2000) Working with diversity: beyond the factfile. In: C Davies, L Finlay and A Bullman (eds) *Changing Practice in Health and Social Care.* Open University Press, Buckingham and Sage Publications, London.
- Davis R (2001) The postpartum experience for Southeast Asian women in the United States. *MCN Am Matern/Child Nurs.* **26**: 208–13.
- De Bono D (1996) Describing race, ethnicity and culture in medical research: 'white' populations also need to be accurately described. *BMJ.* **313**: 425.
- Drever F, Fisher K, Brown J and Clark J (2000) *Social Inequalities. 2000 edition.* The Stationery Office, London.
- Gerrish K (2000) Researching ethnic diversity in the British NHS: methodological and practical concerns. *J Adv Nurs.* **31**: 918–25.
- Gervais M-C and Jovchelovitch S (1998) *The Health Beliefs of the Chinese Community in England.* Health Education Authority, London.
- Haines A (1997) Working together to reduce poverty's damage. *BMJ.* **314**: 529–30.
- Haviland WA (1993) *Cultural Anthropology* (7e). Harcourt Brace Jovanovich, Orlando, FL.
- Hayes L (1995) Unequal access to midwifery care: a continuing problem? *J Adv Nurs.* **21**: 702–7.
- Hilton C (1996) For debate: collecting ethnic group data for inpatients: is it useful? *BMJ.* **313**: 923–5.
- Hilton J and von Hippel W (1996) Stereotypes. *Ann Rev Psychol.* **47**: 237–71.
- Home Office (2001) *The Race Relations (Amendment) Act 2000. New laws for a successful multi-racial Britain: proposals for implementation.* The Stationery Office, London.
- Hunt S and Richens Y (1999) Unwitting racism and midwifery care. *Br J Midwifery.* **7**: 358.

- Jahoda G (1984) Do we need a concept of culture? *J Cross-Cult Psychol.* **15**: 139–51.
- James D (1997) Maternity services: the Audit Commission reports. Listen to women, especially after delivery. *BMJ.* **314**: 844.
- Katbamna S (2000) *'Race' and Childbirth.* Open University Press, Buckingham.
- Kenney N and Macfarlane A (1999) Identifying problems with data collection at local level: survey of NHS maternity units in England. *BMJ.* **319**: 619–22.
- Kirkham M (1999) The culture of midwifery in the National Health Service in England. *J Adv Nurs.* **30**: 732–9.
- Kitzinger S (2000) Some cultural perspectives on birth. *Br J Midwifery.* **8**: 746–50.
- Larbie J (1985) *Black Women and Maternity Services. A survey of 30 young Afro-Caribbean women's experiences and perceptions of pregnancy and childbirth.* Health Education Council and National Extension College for Training in Health and Race, London.
- Laungani P (1999) Client-centred or culture-centred counselling? In: S Palmer and P Laungani (eds) *Counselling in a Multicultural Society.* Sage Publications, London.
- Littler C (1997) Beliefs about colostrum among women from Bangladesh and their reasons for not giving it to the newborn. *Midwives.* **110**: 3–7.
- McAuley J, De Souza L, Sharma V, Robinson I, Main CJ and Frank AO (1996) Describing race, ethnicity and culture in medical research: self-defined ethnicity is unhelpful. *BMJ.* **313**: 425–6.
- Macpherson W (1999) *The Stephen Lawrence Inquiry. Report of an inquiry.* Home Office, London.
- MacVicar J (1990) Obstetrics. In: BR McAvoy and LJ Donaldson (eds) *Health Care for Asians.* Oxford University Press, Oxford.
- McKenzie KJ and Crowcroft NS (1994) Race, ethnicity, culture and science. *BMJ.* **309**: 286–7.
- Midwives Information and Resource Service (1998) Infant feeding in Asian families. *MIDIRS Midwif Digest.* **8**: 358–61.
- Narang I and Murphy S (1994) Assessment of antenatal care for Asian women. *Br J Midwifery.* **2**: 169–73.
- Nash M (1996) The core elements of ethnicity. In: J Hutchinson and AD Smith (eds) *Ethnicity.* Oxford University Press, Oxford.
- Nazroo JY (1997) *The Health of Britain's Ethnic Minorities.* Policy Studies Institute, London.
- Nazroo JY (1998) Genetic, cultural or socio-economic vulnerability? Explaining ethnic inequalities in health. *Sociol Health Illness.* **20**: 710–30.
- NHS Executive (1998) *Tackling Racial Harassment in the NHS. A plan for action.* Department of Health, London.
- Oakley A (1984) *The Captured Womb: a history of the medical care of pregnant women.* Basil Blackwell, Oxford.
- Parsons L, Macfarlane A and Golding J (1993) Pregnancy, birth and maternity care. In: WIU Ahmad (ed.) *'Race' and Health in Contemporary Britain.* Open University Press, Buckingham.
- Phoenix A (1990) Black women and the maternity services. In: J Garcia, R Kilpatrick and M Richards (eds) *The Politics of Maternity Care.* Clarendon Press, Oxford.
- Rawaf S and Bahl V (1998) *Assessing Health Needs of People from Minority Ethnic Groups.* Royal College of Physicians, London.

- Runnymede Trust (2000) *The Future of Multi-Ethnic Britain. The Parekh Report.* Profile Books, London.
- Sandelowski M (1999) Culture, conceptive technology and nursing. *Int J Nurs Stud.* **36**: 13–20.
- Sarup M (1996) *Identity, Culture and the Postmodern World.* Edinburgh University Press, Edinburgh.
- Senior P and Bhopal R (1994) Ethnicity as a variable in epidemiological research. *BMJ.* **309**: 327–30.
- Sheldon T and Parker H (1992) Race and ethnicity in health research. *J Pub Health Med.* **14**: 104–10.
- Smaje C (1995) *Health, 'Race' and Ethnicity. Making sense of the evidence.* King's Fund, London.
- Thomas C (1997) The baby and the bath water: disabled women and motherhood in social context. *Sociol Health Illness.* **9**: 622–43.
- Thomson A (1997) The importance of culture in the provision of midwifery care. *Midwifery.* **13**: 53–4.
- Tonkin E, McDonald M and Chapman M (1996) History and ethnicity. In: J Hutchison and AD Smith (eds) *Ethnicity.* Oxford University Press, Oxford.
- van Dijk TA, Ting-Toomey S, Smitherman G and Troutman D (1997) Discourse, ethnicity, culture and racism. In: TA van Dijk (ed.) *Discourse as Social Interaction.* Sage Publications, London.
- Virdee S (1995) *Racial Violence and Harassment.* Policy Studies Institute, London.
- Weller P, Feldman A and Purdam K (2001) *Religious Discrimination in England and Wales.* Home Office Research Study 220. Home Office, London.
- Wiklund H, Aden AS, Högberg U, Wikman M and Dahlgren L (2000) Somalis giving birth in Sweden: a challenge to culture- and gender-specific values and behaviours. *Midwifery.* **16**: 105–15.
- Zaidi F (1994) The maternity care of Muslim women. *Prof Midwife.* **4**: 8–10.

CHAPTER 6

Refugee women

Jo James

In the UK, refugee women face overwhelming obstacles to their health and well-being. Many have been through traumatic events and experiences, and exile and loss (both cultural and material) will add to their suffering when they are here. The refugee experience in the UK is not a comfortable one. These women face bigotry, ignorance, disinterest, hostility and poverty. Pregnancy and childbirth represent a dangerous time for these individuals, who can be particularly vulnerable. In order to provide the support and care that a refugee woman needs, the healthcare professional must understand who she is, what she has been through and the challenges that she faces when bearing a child in her country of exile.

Introduction

Refugee women are among the most marginalised and misunderstood groups in the world today. They face the stigma of being refugees as well as gender persecution, and they often suffer in a culture of silence because of their sex. Women and their dependent children represent 'the overwhelming majority of refugee caseloads in almost every country' (Marshall, 2000). Many will find their way to the UK, either through cross-border flight or after languishing in a neighbouring country's refugee camp, sometimes for years. Although these women are survivors who will have shown remarkable fortitude and resourcefulness to get here at all, they are also vulnerable and often severely traumatised by their experiences. A high percentage of them will be pregnant – some when they arrive, and others soon afterwards. This in itself may seem odd. Why should women want to give birth at a time of such hardship and uncertainty? First, they may not be pregnant through choice. The great majority (approximately 80%) of refugee women are Moslem and come from a culture of short birth spacing (Wali, 1995). Secondly, they may be pregnant due to lack of available contraception, or as a result of rape. Finally, women who are already in their host country may choose to become pregnant. Possibly, as one doctor who cares for refugees has suggested, this has to do with a reaffirmation of life and an attempt to move towards normality by entering into a life experience which encompasses both ritual and tradition, as well as a new beginning. Once they are in the UK, refugees experience deteriorating health, poor housing and poverty (Directorate of Public Health, 1999). They are the subjects of resentment and sometimes violence. The policy of dispersal of refugees throughout the UK has led to problems with existing communities, an issue that was tragically illustrated by the murder of an asylum-seeker in Glasgow in 2001.

Refugees are a diverse group, coming from extremely varied social and cultural backgrounds. They will all have had different experiences, and may or may not be coping in their host country. However, there are certain common issues of which those caring for them need to be aware. It is vital to be able to understand and contextualise these experiences in terms of the pregnant woman if she is to receive the care that she needs. Van der Veer (1998) suggests that refugees are subject to trauma which is similar to that experienced by immigrants, disaster victims and war veterans, but which is a unique amalgamation of all three.

One of the most important factors which contributes to an understanding of these women is a knowledge of the different statuses of refugees in the UK, as their living conditions and concerns will be significantly different. The asylum-seeker does not have access to benefits, has no long-term security and faces the possibility of forced repatriation. She may still be preoccupied with survival, and could be heavily involved with asylum applications or appeals. The refugee, on the other hand, will have access to all of the benefits available to a UK citizen, and she will know that she can live and raise her child in the UK, and she will be adjusting to her new life and dealing with the loss of her homeland.

The term 'refugee' means:

- a person who has been granted refugee status – that is, full access to all of the facilities and benefits available to UK nationals
- a person who is in the process of applying for refugee status. Asylum-seekers have rights to NHS services, no income support, and receive vouchers worth £36.54 per week plus £10 cash. They have no rights to other services, and are not allowed to work for 6 months
- a person who has been granted exceptional leave to remain/enter (ELR/ELE). Designed for situations of war, this gives full access to all facilities, but the refugee is expected to return to their homeland when the conflict has been resolved
- family and dependants of the above

The aim of this chapter is to consider these women in terms of who they are, how they came to seek asylum, and how the experiences of persecution, war, loss, flight and exile may have affected them physically and psychologically. In addition, strategies will be discussed which will help professionals to care for these women and to ensure that the journey through pregnancy and childbirth does not traumatise them further.

Who becomes a refugee?

Member states of the United Nations are obliged to offer refuge to any person who steps on to their soil and requests asylum. It is then incumbent on that state to decide whether the person concerned will or will not be granted refugee status. The guide that is used to decide this is the 1951 United Nations Refugee Convention, which defines the refugee as follows:

(any person who) owing to a well-founded fear of being persecuted for reasons of race, religion, nationality, membership of a particular social group or political opinion, is outside the country of his nationality and is unable or, owing to such fear, is unwilling to avail himself of the protection of that country ... is unable or, owing to such fear, is unwilling to return to it.

(United Nations, 1951, cited in United Nations
High Commission for Refugees, 1998)

The UK has had a recognition rate of 34.9% over the last 10 years. Overall, only approximately 20% of asylum-seekers in the European Union will achieve full refugee status (United Nations High Commission for Refugees, 2000). The convention is made more notable by its lack of reference to gender as a reason for persecution. Women still have a low status in the world, and are often subjected to maltreatment, sexual abuse and domestic violence by their husbands or families. The practice of female genital mutilation also abounds in many countries. As governments came under greater pressure from refugee numbers in the late twentieth century, the convention was interpreted in an increasingly narrow fashion, culminating in the assumption that a refugee, by definition, could only be someone who had been persecuted by government forces. For the thousands of women fleeing persecution by their families and husbands, this meant being sent back to appalling living conditions. However, in 1985 the problem of vulnerable women was finally recognised, and it was agreed that women who faced harsh or inhuman treatment and received no help from their government could become refugees under the convention. Despite this, the majority of host countries are still reluctant to grant asylum on these grounds (United Nations High Commission for Refugees, 2000).

It is important for professionals caring for refugees to be aware that there is an assumption that every refugee is an escapee from war or civil unrest, and that they will be missing their home and desperate for the company of their own race. The woman who has sought refuge from gender-based persecution may be reluctant to engage with anyone from her own country. She may also be living in fear of being returned, or of being found by a UK-based branch of her family.

However, most of these women will be fleeing from situations of war. This is because in modern warfare the civilian population is deliberately targeted. On average, civilians represented approximately 90% of casualties in late twentieth-century wars (Chinkin, 1993). Women bear the brunt of this, as they continue to be particularly vulnerable in times of war or civil unrest. Nikolic-Ristanovic (2000) suggests that this vulnerability stems from a combination of the following factors.

1   Women are usually unarmed and do not have access to weapons. Most of them do not know how to use a weapon.
2   They are less mobile. For example, they may be pregnant, or caring for small children or elderly relatives.
3   They are usually reluctant to leave their homes, as their role is to look after the home in the absence of men.
4   They need to provide for their families, which may lead to dangerous expeditions for basic necessities such as food and also to prostitution.

5   Women are often objectified as the property of their men. Attacking them is therefore often seen as a direct assault on the man concerned and on the honour of his family.

Women will often stay in their homes until the last minute, when a final traumatic event, such as an attack, a rape or a threat to their children, causes them to flee. Many do this reluctantly, torn between their children and their husband, and experiencing guilt about leaving their home and husband, who may return after the war. The account of Olivera, a Serb refugee, clearly illustrates this:

> I can't forgive myself for leaving with the children. You know, I was taught to be always by my husband's side. I thought 'What would happen if he has to go to fight and then gets killed? Would my children tell me that I had left and let him manage everything alone and get killed?'
>
> (Nikolic-Ristanovic, 2000)

Common experiences

Although, as a rule, generalisations are dangerous and should be avoided, they have a use in the refugee situation, if only to act as a paradigm in which to explore the many factors which will affect the pregnant refugee. As mentioned earlier, the refugee woman will have had a unique series of experiences which will have affected her prior to her encounter with the healthcare professional. Many of these women will be suffering from psychological trauma. Kielson, 1979 (cited by Van der Veer, 1998) suggests that the process of traumatisation of the refugee is a slow one and generally takes years. He divides it into three periods, namely the increasing political repression at home, the traumatic events that culminated in flight, and exile itself. This is a useful observation, as it shows how the woman has been moving towards becoming a refugee over a long period of time and will already be showing signs of long-term traumatisation. Seligman (1975) suggests that passivity is often observed as a result of trauma, and this view is supported by Gielis (1982), who introduced a concept of 'learned helplessness' caused by trauma. This has the following features:

1   reduced motivation to react, including passive slow reactions, sluggish thinking, low expectations and no belief in the possibility of an improvement in the situation
2   reduced capacity to learn that actions can lead to desired results
3   negative feelings such as fear, depression, emptiness, and absence of desires
4   self-reproach and low self-esteem.

This is particularly relevant with regard to the pregnant refugee, who could thus appear passive and uninterested in the outcome of her pregnancy as a result of this long-term trauma. So what factors lead to this level of trauma in the woman? Van der Veer (1998) has identified eight types of experience that the majority of refugees will undergo. Although no list could encompass the entirety of every individual refugee's experience, this is useful as a framework for exploring the effects of becoming a refugee on a pregnant woman.

1 Increasing political repression.
2 Detention.
3 Torture and rape.
4 Other types of violence.

5 Disappearance of relatives.
6 Separation and loss.
7 Hardship.
8 Exile.

Increasing political repression

Wars do not start suddenly and refugees are not made instantaneously. There is frequently a slow political shift towards an opposing ethnic or political group. Many individuals experience the loss of privileges first, with increasing restrictions being placed on their lives and work. They will see their own and their children's future slowly becoming less hopeful, and they may begin to be the subjects of abuse in the press and when they go out of the home. As the repression increases, there is a build-up of tension within the family, leading to an increase in domestic violence, and women will be under enormous stress as they work to keep their family safe in this environment. Living in a constant state of fear is both depressing and damaging to health, and there may also be a loss of faith and trust in others as neighbours and friends turn against them. Many refugees will find it difficult to trust anyone again. For the pregnant refugee in the UK, this loss of trust can be very difficult, as she will not automatically trust her care team, and she may require more time and understanding before she has confidence in them. Some women will also be very nervous in the presence of interpreters whom they do not know, as they often suspect them of being spies or members of opposing parties. It is vital for them to develop a rapport with an interpreter and remain with that person if possible. A high turnover of medical and midwifery staff will also worry the woman, as she has come from a world of disappearances and will wonder why different people are present at each appointment.

Detention

Many women will have been detained for a period of time prior to their flight. This may have been a sudden arrest or an expected event. However, the mother will have been separated from her family, and she may have missed important family events or ceremonies. She will be unable to fulfil her role of mother, and this will lead to feelings of guilt and self-reproach, particularly if the arrest is due to any actions on her part (e.g. handing out leaflets). Detention also signifies the loss of hope of any improvement in the political situation, and it is often the catalyst which makes a woman flee.

Torture and rape

Torture is common in repressive regimes. It frequently occurs during detention, and women are tortured as often as men. It would be impossible to determine how many refugee women have been tortured, as there is great stigma attached to it and many would never speak of their experiences, even to loved ones. However, United Nations High Commission for Refugees (UNHCR) figures have suggested that up to 80% of refugees have been tortured either in their own country or during flight.

One of the main aims of the torturer is to silence dissent by using techniques which take away the voice of the victim. These will involve physical violence in all of its forms, psychological violence (e.g. sensory deprivation), threats to the woman and her loved ones, particularly her children, the assault of loved ones in front of her, and sexual torture, including rape, mutilation of genitals and the administration of electric shocks to organs. Sadly, the list of ways that torturers have found to hurt their victims could go on for ever. However, this chapter will concentrate on some of the effects on the woman and her life afterwards. Rape will be discussed as a separate issue.

The physical sequelae of torture include scarring, chronic headaches, shoulder pain, back pain and haemorrhoids. Many women will suffer from chest complaints, after having been imprisoned in damp cells. Some will complain of problems eating, possibly due to the forced ingestion of taboo substances such as faeces, oil and semen (Douglas, 1966) during torture. These women will often have somatised complaints, which can be described as the physical manifestation of psychological pain. Hinshelwood (1996: 195) suggests that 'the body's language to communicate and live with the unspeakable is much more primitive and simple than the spoken word'. Survivors of torture often have difficulty sleeping and are plagued by nightmares and flashbacks.

Women who are pregnant at the time of torture frequently miscarry afterwards. The torturers will often convince them that they will never again bear healthy children because of the torture, and this is one of the most powerful long-term effects of torture for women. The following quote illustrates this clearly: 'Women who have been tortured feel the torture is inside them and that their insides are spoiled and, most particularly, their creative reproductive capacity' (Hinshelwood, 1996: 195).

This sense of internal spoiling is not unusual, and it represents a major psychological stumbling block for the pregnant woman. Consider, for example, the moving story of Sylvia, who begged for a termination because of her belief that anything which came from inside her could only be evil and deformed (Agger and Jenson, 1993). Hinshelwood (1996: 195) also writes of her client who believed 'her body to still be filled with blood and torturer's semen and dead foetus'. There are numerous descriptions of women asking for the removal of something evil which they felt was inside them and tangible. Hinshelwood (1996) suggests that a sensitive gynaecological examination can help to provide reassurance in these situations. Perhaps an ultrasound scan would also serve the same function if it was approached with this purpose in mind. Meeting medical staff and undergoing procedures can be particularly traumatic for the survivor of torture, because much torture is medicalised. Some of the instruments that are used for torture will look 'medical', and rooms will be given ironic, euphemistic names, such as 'intensive care' and 'operating theatres', by the torturers (Morris, 2000).

This leads us on to the subject of rape and the devastating consequences of this for refugee women. In war situations, the incidence of rape increases dramatically (Seifert, 1993), a fact that was most clearly demonstrated by the recent Balkan conflict. Before the war, rape was very rare, but during the war an estimated 20–50 000 women were known to have been raped (it is believed that the true figure is higher). Brownmiller (1993) suggests that this is because women's bodies have become an extension of the battlefield and therefore war is waged on them. Rape is also used with the intention of destabilising society and forcing citizens into exile. For example, many women in the Balkans were kept in rape camps until they became pregnant in order to interfere with the gene pool. Finally, there is a serious problem of rape in refugee camps, where women are unprotected and the incidence of rape is very high. Research has shown that rape during conflict is more brutal, often repeated and involves more than one rapist (Nikolic-Ristanovic, 2000).

Although the refugee woman will not necessarily be pregnant as a result of rape, the fact of the pregnancy is likely to generate very ambivalent feelings within her. Many women never speak of their ordeals because it is so unacceptable to do so (some languages do not even have a word for rape, as they believe that a woman cannot be penetrated unless she is willing, and others punish rape victims as adulterers). On arrival in the UK, there may be pressure from the woman's family to have a baby and she will be unable to explain why this may be a problem for her. Some women who have previously become pregnant as a result of rape may have had a late termination or they may have had the baby and given it away. Nikolic-Ristanovic (2000) describes the conflict of knowing that one is carrying one's rapist's child which is also one's own child as one of the cruellest forms of torture. The children born of these unions are viewed as 'monstrous ' and 'evil'. For these women, pregnancy will be a major memory trigger, and together with the concerns about internal spoiling it may result in significant traumatisation. Labour will inevitably bring back the memories of the previous experience. Zelina, a 13-year-old refugee who had been raped, had given birth to a child and had given it away, described her greatest fear as follows: 'that she would never be able to physically enjoy a man's company or love a baby' (Hinshelwood, 1996: 195).

Therefore for these women, having a baby will be a pivotal moment in their lives which may be a new beginning, but which will also be a painful reminder of what has happened. They will have fears about the baby and whether it will be deformed or evil because their internal reproductive organs have become a bad and unsafe place. Finally, many of these women will be terrified that they bear some kind of visible sign of their experiences, which will be discovered during an examination. To end this section, a vignette is taken from a speech by Gill Hinshelwood. We can assess torture, rape and torment in cool clinical language, but the cost to an individual can only be quantified in humane terms. Asha's story brings to life the suffering and shame that are experienced by these women after being abused.

> Asha arrived in England in 1994 when she was 18 years old. She knew no one. Once in England, she was sent to a bed-and-breakfast hostel, where she stayed in her room, locked away from noise and danger, and only emerged to find help when she could not control her vomiting. She was pregnant. She had an abortion and went back to her miserable room. When she was referred to me some seven months later, her presenting symptom was a carrier bag of medicines with some of which she had tried to take an overdose. Asha had 22 different medicines in her bag for complaints of aches and pains ranging from head to foot. She sat strained and rigid, her face never lightening and never making eye contact. ... The past history that Asha slowly allowed us to hear was one of violence and brutality, beginning with threats and abuse directed at those entering the Kingdom Hall, abuse hurled at her in the

street, and culminating in brutal rape by five policemen in a cell leaving her unconscious, bleeding and, as it later turned out, pregnant. She had been a virgin. Asha had very few words at her disposal to describe what had happened. Many of the words we use are felt to defile the person by the very utterance of them. ... She had coped over the last seven months by her disconnectedness, by being a backache, a sore throat, a painful knee. This consultation with me was the first exposure she had allowed since that day when her clothes were torn off, a rag was stuffed into her mouth and five policemen took over her body, penetrated her, cursed her. ... Asha was a walking picture of shame.

(Hinshelwood, 1997)

Other types of violence

Most refugees are subjected to terror prior to flight. Awareness of the destabilisation of a regime and the increased unpopularity of one's ethnic group will be frightening. During these periods, stories of rape and torture abound, and there will be much agonising over the decision as to whether to leave. The ongoing threat of violence will be present. There will also be terror of being returned. As only 20–25% of applications are upheld, the great majority of refugees will be sent back home.

Disappearance of relatives

This can be extremely painful for the woman. Her relatives may have disappeared years previously, but the lack of closure will keep the pain fresh. Allodi and Rojas (1985) suggest that there is a higher incidence of mental health problems among refugees who have experienced the disappearance of a family member.

Separation and loss

All refugees will experience separation and loss. The woman will have been forcibly separated from her home, and she will have lost her belongings and status. She will no longer have a social structure around her that will help her through her pregnancy. She will also have lost all of the frames of reference that contextualised her as a person, both internally and externally. Afkhami (1999: 214) described this as a 'loss of who I was.'

Coehlo (1982) describes this loss as a form of culture shock, which is particularly pertinent with regard to the pregnant woman, as childbirth is an event imbued with cultural and traditional meanings which will not be relevant in the new social culture. The woman may have lost members of her immediate family, and she will also have lost her social group who would have welcomed the baby into the world. Eisenbruch (1984) suggested that these losses are a form of cultural bereavement, and that they require adaptation which could result in denial, anger and finally depression.

Many women will also have been bereaved in the literal sense, having lost husband, relatives, friends and children in the conflict. They may be recently bereaved, and they could be experiencing feelings of guilt both about surviving and about having a new baby.

There is also loss of the woman's cultural life, and there is little interest in or respect for a refugee's homeland in the host nation. This lack of knowledge and desire to learn is profoundly depressing and deeply insulting for many refugees (Van der Veer, 1998). There will be cultural confusion, particularly in relation to gender, and the woman will often feel isolated and cut off from the female support networks in her own society. The rules which governed her in her homeland may not exist in a western society where there are few limitations for women, and this can result in a loss of stability and balance in the woman's family relationships. Groenenburg (1992) has noted that this leads to conflict and ultimately a higher divorce rate within these families.

Hardship

Mrvic-Petrovic and Stevanovic (2000) stated that there is a widespread impoverishment of women refugees. This impoverishment often begins before the woman becomes a refugee, within her home country. Living in a repressive regime or an area of conflict inevitably leads to hardship of various kinds. There are frequently food and power shortages, and if the refugee is from a minority group, there could be poverty and hunger imposed by the regime itself.

During flight, refugees often experience the most gruelling physical hardship – they may walk through storms, over mountains or through deserts to escape. Some will bribe their way into lorries run by criminals, paying a terrible price to escape, as these criminals often force the women to have sex with them, rape them, rob them, and often do not give them food or water for days at a time. At the borders, guards exact a price as well, often in the form of the belongings of and sexual intercourse with the women.

A huge number of refugees will begin exile in a refugee camp. These again are places of immense poverty and hardship. There are frequently food shortages, and women receive the smallest share of what is available (Marshall, 2000). As aid agencies struggle to manage the vast needs created by these camps, many residents are left without heating, water or shelter for long periods of time.

Finally, having arrived in the UK, these women will again face hardship. The life of the asylum-seeker is not an easy one. They are often housed in the least desirable properties in the least desirable areas, and are forced to live below the poverty line with no access to money, paying for goods with vouchers. Single women are placed in hostels, which are often mixed and which charge fees that use up all of the asylum-seeker's allowance. Asylum-seeking mothers do not even have the right to free milk and vitamins for their babies.

In times of extreme hardship, the woman will be more concerned about survival than anything else. The pregnant asylum-seeker will be likely to have this mind set. She may seem more preoccupied and concerned about housing or her application for refugee status than she is about the baby and attending antenatal clinics at the right time. This is not an indication of lack of interest, but rather it is simply her way of coping with the enormous hurdles that lie in front of her. She will need flexibility and understanding from the midwives, and even help with organising her time so that she can attend her appointments and receive the support that she needs.

Exile

All refugees, for whatever reason, have been exiled. They have been exiled from the smell, the feel and the sights of home, and this sense of not belonging often remains with refugees for the rest of their lives. Many of them will be concerned with events at home, and will be disturbed if there is news coverage of a particular event. The pregnant woman will be adapting simultaneously to her new social setting and her pregnant state. She will be aware that her child will be born into exile and may never know its country of origin. She will also be coming to terms with the fact that she has become a refugee and her child will be born with this identity and denied his or her birthright. This can cause overwhelming feelings of guilt and sadness. In exile, the woman may also have a great deal more responsibility than she had before. She may suddenly be the head of the household and be faced with decision making for the first time in her life.

Remembering

People who have been through significant trauma will have a different way of remembering events. In fact, it is probably misleading to use the term 'memory' in this context, as it implies a sense of an event being viewed in the past, whereas for the traumatised refugee quite the opposite will be the case. Langer (1991) identified a concept of durational memory in Holocaust victims. This is a form of remembering which does not age or fade with time. Durational memories are fresh and are described as being 'like yesterday'. They are also physical or sensory, involving smell, sensations and emotions rather than details and overviews. This means that the woman can be remarkably vague (to the point of being difficult to believe) about details, but will nevertheless remember and feel the event as if it were yesterday. Seifert and Hoffnung (1987) suggest that this is due to an overload of information in the long-term memory causing spillage into the short-term memory, which results in flashbacks and nightmares. They also suggest that the short-term memory is then filled up inappropriately, resulting in problems with regard to memory and concentration.

This is a crucial factor to consider when caring for the refugee woman. Her pregnancy, the examinations and the birth may all trigger durational memories which could be very damaging and frightening. She needs to be treated as if her experiences had happened yesterday, as chronological time has no relevance in this situation. She should not be expected to remember things easily, so information that is given to her should be repeated and written down.

Conclusions

Faced with this list of appalling experiences and tragedy, it seems difficult to envisage that anything other than understanding can be offered to the refugee woman who is facing childbirth in the UK. However, this is not the case, as with resourcefulness and knowledge healthcare professionals can adapt their approach to the needs of the woman and greatly improve her care.

One of the most difficult problems for these women is lack of knowledge – of who they are, where they are from, what they have been through and what is important in their lives. In the busy world of the NHS these issues are rarely addressed, but they are vital to the person who has lost most of this knowledge. We need to be able to show interest, learn a little about the countries they come from and acquaint ourselves with some of the major cultural features (particularly birthing rituals) of our refugee patients. The ability to discuss refugee topics with these women will be a step towards reducing the stigma attached to their position. It is also vital for the carer to understand the importance of survival issues to the refugee. It is pointless to assume that they are safe now and therefore there is no longer a problem. They will not feel safe – they will fear strangers, fellow nationals, people in uniform, and of course the Home Office who may send them back to their homeland. Instead of fighting this, and the healthcare professional trying to impose their own set of values on these women, it would be more productive to help them work through the survival issues or to direct them towards someone who can do this.

Bearing a child in the UK can represent a loss of control over one's body, particularly in the hospital setting. This can be very challenging for the refugee patient, who has seen all control removed from her life in previous years. In particular, victims of torture need to have control over their bodies, as they have been subject to a total loss of autonomy during the torture. The loss of control over one's body, associated with pain such as labour, may trigger durational memories, flashbacks and terror. Because of this, the healthcare professional should ensure that any decision – even simply touching the woman – is made by the woman herself without pressure or coercion. Any refusal of an examination or treatment must be regarded as an informed choice. For example, some survivors of torture have said that they would prefer to die rather than undergo a procedure which triggered a flashback (Matthews, 1997).

This chapter has provided a snapshot of the refugee woman and her life. We can see that the effects of experiences such as rape and torture are overt and numerous. Basic functions such as eating and sleeping are disrupted, as are mechanisms for communication, due to fear and lack of language. The woman's body has acquired a new set of meanings through her experiences, and these make it a dangerous place for her. We can also see how the violation of boundaries during rape and torture leads to a sense of social pollution. It is hardly surprising that many women refugees struggle to come to terms with their lives in the UK. There is a high rate of suicide and depression among refugees in this country (Directorate of Public Health, 1999). However, most refugees will carry on, despite feelings of desperation and severe traumatisation. They are survivors and that is what they do, often at immense personal cost. Importantly, Amen (1985) suggests that refugees often cope well until they are faced with something unexpected, or until physical illness undermines their ability to cope, and then they collapse. This is why pregnancy and childbirth represent such a dangerous time for the refugee woman, as it is a time of emotional significance and great vulnerability, when the woman will miss her home, her family and her loved ones more than ever and require greater support than before. Mrvic-Petrovic (2000) supports this view, stating that women refugees are especially vulnerable to new stressors when pregnant.

This chapter has focused on what *makes* refugee women more than on what *happens* to them in the UK, because if we are to understand the context of their

- Refugee women are stigmatised, and experience poverty and hardship in their host country.
- Women seek asylum for a variety of different reasons.
- They will be diverse and have had widely different experiences, but certain common factors will be present.
- Many will have endured physical and mental abuse which they will be reluctant to discuss. This could have profound psychological effects.
- Apparent lack of interest and apathy may be misleading and require the carer to consider the possible causes, such as trauma and a preoccupation with survival.
- The rape and torture of refugee women is common.
- Traumatic memories remain recent and painful.
- Pregnant refugees are particularly vulnerable and require special care and consideration. The midwife needs to understand and anticipate the difficulties which may arise.

lives, it is necessary to look back to the start of the fear and repression and how the process of becoming a refugee has affected these women. During pregnancy and childbirth they require knowledge, sensitivity and understanding. The midwife should be alert to signs of trauma and aware of the complex issues in the refugee woman's life.

Useful addresses

Medical Foundation for the Care of Victims of Torture
96–98 Grafton Rd
London NW5 3EJ
Tel: 0208 813 7777
Provides medical consultations and treatment, medical documentation of torture, practical help and advice, marital, family and child therapies, and a range of complementary therapies.

Refugee Council
3 Bondway
London SW8 1SJ
Tel: 0208 820 3000
Campaigns for refugee rights, provides direct services such as day care, housing advice, etc., and produces information on refugee issues.

Liberty
21 Tabard Street
London SE1 1LA
Tel: 0207 403 3888/0207 374 8659 (advice)
Offers legal advice and assistance on all areas that affect asylum-seekers and refugees.

Refugee Women's Network
c/o Refugee Council
3 Bondway
London SW8 1SJ
Tel: 0207 820 3000
Networking of refugee women to provide support and motivation, and campaigning for women's rights.

References

- Afkhami M (1999) A woman in exile. In: M Agosin (ed.) *A Map of Hope.* Penguin Books, Harmondsworth.
- Agger I and Jenson S (1993) The psychosexual trauma of torture. In: J Wilson and B Raphael (eds) *International Handbook of Trauma Stress Syndromes.* Plenum Press, New York.
- Allodi F and Rojas A (1985) The health and adaptation of victims of political violence in Latin America. In: P Pichot (ed.) *Psychiatry: the state of the art.* Plenum Press, New York.
- Amen DG (1985) Post-Vietnam stress disorder: a metaphor for current and past life events. *Am J Psychiatry.* **39**: 580–86.
- Brownmiller S (1993) Making female bodies the battlefield. In: A Stiglmayer (ed.) *Mass Rape: the war against women in Bosnia-Herzegovina.* University of Nebraska Press, Lincoln, NE.
- Chinkin CM (1993) Peace and force in international law. In: DG Dallmeyer (ed.) *Reality, Women and International Law.* Asil, New York.
- Coehlo GV (1982) The foreign student's sojourn as a high-risk situation: the culture-shock phenomenon re-examined. In: RC Nann (ed.) *Uprooting and Surviving.* D Reidel Publishing Company, Dordrecht.
- Directorate of Public Health (1999) *East London and City Health Authority Health of Londoners Report. Refugee health in London. Key issues for public health.* King's Fund, London.
- Douglas M (1966) *Purity and Danger.* Routledge, London.
- Eisenbruch M (1984) Cross-cultural aspects of bereavement: a conceptual framework for comparative analysis. *Culture Med Psychiatry.* **8**: 283–309.
- Gielis A (1982) Geleerde hulpeloosheid all depressiemodel, Een literatuurstudie. *Gedragstherapie.* **15**: 3–31.
- Groenenburg M (1992) Female victims. In: G Van der Veer (ed.) *Counselling and Therapy with Refugees.* John Wiley & Sons, New York.
- Hinshelwood G (1996) Women, children and the family. In: D Forrest (ed.) *A Glimpse of Hell.* Cassell, London.
- Hinshelwood G (1997) *Gender-Based Persecution.* Transcript of unpublished paper given to United Nations Medical Foundation Library, London.
- Langer L (1991) *Holocaust Testimonies.* Yale University Press, New Haven, CT.
- Marshall R (2000) Refugee women. *Refugees Magazine.* **Issue 100**: 78–89.
- Matthews J (1997) *After the Pain: the body of the torture survivor.* Unpublished research paper. Brunel University, Brunel.
- Morris T (2000) Disguise and deny. *New Internationalist.* **327**: 28.

- Mrvic-Petrovic N (ed.) (2000) Social acceptance and the difficulty adapting to a new environment. In: V Nikolic-Ristanovic (ed.) *Women, Violence and War: wartime victimization of refugees in the Balkans.* Central European Press, Budapest.
- Mrvic-Petrovic N and Stevanovic I (2000) Life in refuge – changes in socio-economic and familial status. In: V Nikolic-Ristanovic (ed.) *Women, Violence and War: wartime victimization of refugees in the Balkans.* Central European Press, Budapest.
- Nikolic-Ristanovic V (ed.) (2000) *Women, Violence and War: wartime victimization of refugees in the Balkans.* Central European Press, Budapest.
- Seifert K and Hoffnung RJ (1987) *Child and Adolescent Development.* Houghton Mifflin, Boston, MA.
- Seifert R (1991) War and rape – a preliminary analysis. In: A Stiglmayer (ed.) *Mass Rape: the war against women in Bosnia-Herzegovina.* University of Nebraska Press, Lincoln, NE.
- Seligman M (1975) *Helplessness: on depression, development and death.* Freeman, San Francisco, CA.
- United Nations High Commission for Refugees (1998) *Basic Obligations: refugee rights and the State.* Unpublished guidance document.
- United Nations High Commission for Refugees (2000) *The State of the World's Refugees.* Oxford University Press, Oxford.
- Van der Veer G (1998) *Counselling and Therapy with Refugees and Victims of Trauma.* John Wiley & Sons, Chichester.
- Wali S (1995) Muslim refugee, returnee and displaced women: challenges and dilemmas. In: M Afkhami (ed.) *Faith and Freedom.* Syracuse University Press, Syracuse.

CHAPTER 7

Domestic violence

Sally Price

This chapter discusses domestic violence experienced by women in pregnancy. It explores the social context of domestic violence in the UK from both historical and present-day perspectives, as well as the effects that it has on women and their experience of pregnancy. The impact that health professionals and the maternity services can have on women's experience is also discussed, with some suggestions on how health professionals can help to ensure that women who experience violence receive appropriate support.

Introduction

Domestic violence in pregnancy is a major public health issue with serious consequences for both maternal and infant health. It is a primary cause of gender-specific health inequalities, which should be of concern not only to health professionals but also to society as a whole (Baird 2002). Violent behaviour displayed towards one person by another should not be a justifiable form of human behaviour. However, male domination of women is still regarded as normal and natural within patriarchal societies. This in turn allows the perpetuation of domestic violence as an acceptable method of controlling women.

Definition

Domestic violence can be defined as 'any violent or abusive behaviour, whether physical, sexual, psychological, emotional, verbal or financial, which is used by one person to control and dominate another with whom they have or have had a relationship' (Hester *et al.*, 1998). It may include various forms of coercion and intimidation, such as degradation, humiliation, deprivation, systematic criticism and belittling (Home Office, 1995).

It is widely accepted that the vast majority of violence in a domestic relationship is perpetrated by men against women and their children, although it is acknowledged that abuse may occur in same-sex relationships or may be committed by women against men (Department of Health, 2000a). However, it is also important to acknowledge that the issue of domestic violence perpetrated against women by their male partners is not the same violence that is displayed towards children or older people. Failure to acknowledge this would be to ignore or minimise the gender implications that are central to this issue.

The language that is used to describe domestic violence and the women who experience it can be problematic. Terms such as 'victim' and 'battered wife' are frequently applied to women who experience domestic violence, implying weakness and passivity. This denies women's resistance and coping strategies, and encourages a culture of victim blaming (Hester *et al.*, 1996). A more appropriate descriptor might be 'survivor' to emphasise the determination, action and bravery shown by women (Dobash and Dobash, 1992) and to reflect the complexity of responses to the experience of domestic violence.

Who experiences domestic violence?

Domestic violence is often secret, hidden and undisclosed. Only one in three incidents that result in injury are reported to the police (Home Office, 1996). However, a self-report questionnaire which was used in the British Crime Survey indicates that domestic violence is a common experience, with nearly one in four women being assaulted by their partner at some point in their lives, and one in eight being repeatedly assaulted in this way (Mirrlees-Black, 1996). Domestic violence is rarely an isolated incident, but rather involves an escalating spiral of abuse, sometimes resulting in death. The criminal statistics for England and Wales in 1997 demonstrate that almost 50% of all female murder victims are killed by a present or former partner. Indeed, one woman dies every three days in the UK as a result of domestic violence (Home Office, 1999).

Women of all ages, classes and ethnic groups are known to experience abuse in the home (Radford, 1987), although recently some age-related differences have been noted, with young women aged 16–24 years being most at risk (Mirrlees-Black, 1996). However, there appears to be a common view that violence is more prevalent or somehow different among individuals from the lower socio-economic groups. This is exemplified by the writings of Frances Cobbe, who described domestic violence as:

> The blow or two delivered occasionally in the gentlemen's drawing room, through thrashings with a fist in London, to its climax in the overcrowded centres of manufacturing, trade and mining in the north, where tramplings and purrings with hobnailed boots are common.
> (Cobbe, 1878, cited in Stark and Flitcraft, 1996)

The majority of the research into domestic violence has been conducted among the lower socio-economic groups, thereby contributing to the myth that it is a disorder of the poor. It is also true that the highest level of reporting of domestic violence occurs in this group. However, no differences have been found in the actual incidence of domestic abuse within different social groups in the UK. It could be suggested that middle-class women might be more able to deal with the challenges of addressing domestic violence. They are more likely to be financially able to leave, and to receive respect and be taken seriously by professional support services. However, if they are married to middle-class men, it may be more difficult to enlist the support of agencies such as the police, due to stereotypical assumptions that middle-class men do not beat their wives (Hester *et al.*, 1996).

Pregnancy – a time when women are making physical, emotional and social preparations for motherhood – may offer no protection from abuse. For some women, pregnancy is a result of their male partner's violence towards them, conception having occurred through rape. During pregnancy, the abuse may simply be 'business as usual', but for some women the pregnancy may act as the trigger for domestic violence, with male jealousy or anger being directed towards the unborn baby (Campbell *et al.*, 1993). For almost 30% of women who experience domestic violence during their lifetime, the first incident occurs during pregnancy (Helton *et al.*, 1987). Others experience an increase in the extent and nature of violence, with injuries to the breasts, abdomen and genital area being more common (Hillard, 1985). As part of a cycle of escalating violence, pregnant women may also be murdered by their male partner or relative. Eight such cases were reported in the *Confidential Enquiries into Maternal Deaths in the United Kingdom* (Lewis, 2001). Pregnancy may also offer some women a respite from abuse, often resulting in repeated pregnancies within a short space of time to afford some self-protection (Mezey and Bewley, 1997). However, other research has demonstrated that postnatal women are most at risk for moderate to severe injury (Hedin, 2000).

Historical perspective

For many centuries women have experienced violence at the hands of men with whom they are intimately involved. The abusive nature of this relationship has been well documented since Roman times, the patriarchal society being considered to be the root cause of male violence towards women. There seems no doubt that the origins and perpetuation of domestic violence lie within male authority and control and the associated subordination of women. For example, in the eighteenth century, a married woman was subject to whatever violence her husband felt was reasonably required to correct her (Blackstone, 1765, cited in Dobash and Dobash (1979)). This 'domestic chastisement' was thought to be necessary because husbands were legally answerable for their wives' misbehaviour, although there was no legal recourse for women whose chastisement was excessive or unreasonable.

Throughout the nineteenth century, various Acts of Parliament were passed that made small improvements to the position of women as wives, and through the Matrimonial Causes Act (1878) women were finally afforded the same protection against beatings and ill treatment that animals already had. However, these improvements had little impact on the daily lives of women in abusive relationships. The private institution of the family – upheld by the church and the state as sacred – maintained and promoted the subordinated position of women and their economic dependence on their male partners. Every 20 years or so during the twentieth century a surge of protests about the issue of domestic violence has occurred, perhaps most notably during the 1970s with the emergence of the women's movement against domestic violence. National Women's Aid organisations, working to end violence against women and children, have been a powerful force for social change, supporting individual women, providing accommodation in shelters and generally raising the profile of domestic violence and ensuring its place on the national agenda. Their work and that of others has led to a huge increase in social and political awareness of domestic violence, the experience of women who live in abusive relationships and the impact that this has on their health.

By the end of the twentieth century, Government policy had begun to take a strong line, promoting an inter-agency approach to tackling domestic violence, and guiding the police to take a proactive approach in the enforcement of relevant legislation. Having previously viewed domestic violence as being within the private domain of the family, the police moved from a position of largely ignoring the problem to taking a more positive stance (e.g. setting up domestic violence units within each locality). However, within any institution that is inherently patriarchal, such as the police force, it is difficult not to be critical of their approach. It would seem that police discretion in dealing with the abuse of women allows an enormous number of domestic violence crimes against women to be ignored (Wright, 1995). It is small wonder then that women are reluctant to involve the police, on average being assaulted 35 times before reporting domestic violence (Bewley *et al.*, 1997).

The context of domestic violence

In understanding the context of domestic violence, it is important first to comprehend the context of the lives of men and women within society and to accept the roles that they play in order to fulfil society's expectations. Hoff (1990) asserts that violence against women occurs in a climate of socially structured inequalities for women, exemplified not only by the concept of patriarchy, but also by sexism. In a social system in which women's subordination to men is regarded as natural, violence continues to be viewed as a necessary and acceptable means of controlling women. Alternatively, women may be regarded as willing participants who are thriving on and enjoying an abusive relationship. Frequently heard comments include 'If it is so bad, why doesn't she leave?'. This approach typifies the ideology of women as victims, putting the onus for ending the violence on them, rather than with the perpetrator who is actually responsible. It also fails to take into account how domestic violence can create such low self-esteem in women that they are unable to imagine being able to survive outside their abusive relationship.

Dobash and Dobash (1979, 1998) and Dobash *et al.* (1996) have demonstrated how violence can be regarded as the result of a conflict of interests within a domestic relationship, based on the status and position of men in a patriarchal society. Four themes have been identified that exemplify conflict leading to domestic violence:

- men's possessiveness and jealousy
- disagreements and expectations with regard to domestic work and resources
- men's sense of their right to punish 'their' women for perceived wrongdoing
- the importance to men of maintaining or exercising their power and authority.

This research has highlighted the specific issues that may be a source of conflict and act as a trigger for violence to occur (*see* Box 7.1).

Pregnancy and the birth of a baby could also be regarded as an additional source of conflict, exacerbating those highlighted in this model. Consider the impact of

---

Box 7.1   Sources of conflict (Dobash and Dobash, 1998)

- Domestic work
- Money
- Children
- Alcohol
- Possessiveness and jealousy
- Isolation and restriction of mobility and social life
- Sex

---

pregnancy on women's domestic work. Household chores such as cleaning, washing, ironing, shopping and food preparation are essentially the responsibility of women. During early pregnancy, many women experience extreme tiredness and nausea and vomiting, combined with paid employment outside the home and care of other children. In the later stages of pregnancy, backache and tiredness are commonplace. During the early postnatal period women will need personal time to establish breastfeeding and recover from the physical effects of labour and birth. It is likely that domestic responsibilities will be low on their list of priorities, although the same demands as ever will be present or even increased. Combine this with a male partner's expectation that his needs for food, clothing and a clean house will be met, and it is not difficult to see how this could be an increased source of conflict.

Gelles (1975) investigated the reasons why pregnant women might be abused, and suggested that the normal behaviour of pregnant women, such as a reduction in libido as well as mood swings resulting from normal physiological changes, were credible reasons for male violence towards pregnant women. Thus pregnancy can be viewed as interfering with the woman's ability to perform the roles and duties that the male partner regards as necessary, and this failure as provoking or justifying a violent response. Cultural beliefs about domestic violence reinforce the notion that women are somehow deserving of abuse. However, it is only within the context of a society that perpetuates women's subordination to men that this view could be adopted.

Domestic violence as a women's issue may also be denied on cultural grounds. In discussions of domestic violence one commonly hears of women who perpetrate violence against their male partners. With regard to the crime of domestic violence against women, people instinctively leap to the defence of the perpetrator (Horley, 1991). One of the easiest ways of avoiding the realities of domestic violence is to turn the situation around, and insist that it is a two-sided issue with women being viewed equally as abusers and as the abused. However, there is no doubt that the overwhelming majority of adults who experience domestic violence are women, and that the extent of the injuries and trauma which they experience is far in excess of anything experienced by men (Dobash *et al.*, 1995). With regard to cases of extreme domestic violence that result in death, the number of female victims far outweighs the number of male victims, and there is a significant difference in the way in which the violence is perpetrated. Women who kill their male partners typically do so as a single act of violence after many years of experiencing abuse themselves, in contrast to men who kill their female partners as a final act after a long series of attacks (Lloyd, 1995). However, within the male-dominated criminal justice system, violence against women is too often viewed as justified, provoked or deserved, with women who kill their partners after experiencing years of abuse being discriminated against, and often receiving harsher sentences than men who commit similar or lesser crimes.

Effects of domestic violence

The effects on women of living with violence are wide and varied, ranging from physical injury to poor mental health, social isolation and overuse of drugs for comfort. The abuse may be manifested in a variety of ways, such as bruises, bites, cuts and grazes, broken bones, depression, suicide attempts, loneliness, alcoholism and drug abuse, or there may be no obvious outward signs.

Consistent with the secret, covert nature of the perpetration of the abuse, women may become skilled at hiding the signs and symptoms of violence. This may be due to shame, embarrassment, or fear of retribution if anyone outside the family becomes aware of the abusive relationship. Women who are living with violence may also have a sense of personal responsibility for their partner's actions. Guilt may be a significant factor in women's silence, the experience of violence being interpreted as a signal that the woman has somehow failed, and public knowledge being associated with social stigma (Dobash and Dobash, 1998). If other people do become aware of the abuse, the woman may minimise or deny violent incidents. However, when a woman says that 'nothing really happened', perhaps what she is really implying is how much worse it could have been (Hester *et al.*, 1996).

Specific effects of domestic violence on pregnancy

Pregnant women may experience domestic violence in the same ways as women who are not pregnant. However, the effects may also include some that are specific to pregnancy, including miscarriage, placental abruption, antepartum haemorrhage, premature labour, stillbirth and low-birth-weight babies (Hillard, 1985; Salzman, 1990; McWilliams and McKeirnan, 1993; Mooney, 1993). *In-utero* injuries have also been found, with abdominal trauma to the mother resulting in fractures to the fetus (Mezey and Bewley, 1997). These effects are often not attributed to domestic violence by health professionals, and may partially account for the frequency with which many negative outcomes of pregnancy and birth remain unexplained.

For women who experience 'moderate to severe' violence during pregnancy, the risk of preterm labour has been found to be up to four times higher than in women who experience no abuse (Shumway *et al.*, 1999). A high incidence of miscarriage has also been found. A survey of women living in refuges in Northern Ireland found that 60% had experienced violence during a pregnancy, with 13% having subsequent miscarriages (McWilliams and McKiernan, 1993). Within the health services, considerable emphasis is placed on physiological causes of miscarriage and preterm labour. Women may be diagnosed with an 'incompetent cervix' and offered cervical cerclage, or undergo repeated trans-vaginal ultrasound scans to alert the medical profession to changes in the cervix that may result in preterm delivery. Huge resources are poured into offering these services, yet little is directed to the exploration of social causes such as domestic violence.

Research has shown that 'mildly and moderately' abused women are more frequently admitted to hospital during their pregnancy (Webster *et al.*, 1996). However, it is likely that for many of these women the true cause of their need for admission is never identified. It is apparent to anyone working within the maternity services in the UK today that a considerable number of antenatal admissions are for symptoms that are never adequately diagnosed or explained by traditional medical approaches to care. A woman who has vague abdominal pain at 24 weeks with no specific diagnosis made, or frequent admissions for reduced fetal movements, may simply be seeking a place of refuge from an abusive relationship for a few hours or days. In other cases a woman's physical illness caused by domestic abuse (e.g. a urinary tract infection) is physiologically investigated, diagnosed and treated. If the infection is severe, recurrent or resistant to treatment, a range of further investigative tests may be performed. However, it is unlikely that anyone will stop to consider whether the actual cause of the symptoms, or the reason for the woman's self-referral, could be related to an abusive relationship.

Abused women are more likely to use a range of coping strategies that have associated health risks both for themselves and for the fetus. An increased incidence of over-consumption of alcohol, prescribed and illegal drug abuse and cigarette smoking is evident (Martin *et al.*, 1996; Curry, 1998; Grimstad *et al.*, 1998), with an associated impact on birth weight (McFarlane *et al.*, 1996). Strategies to support smoking cessation are becoming widespread in order to meet the Government's recently set target of significantly reducing the incidence of smoking during pregnancy (Department of Health, 2000b). However, in seeking to promote smoking cessation, it is uncommon for health professionals to address the social causes of women's smoking behaviour, such as domestic violence. In failing to do this, not only are health professionals facing a monumental challenge in meeting this target, but also they are failing women who experience violence in their lives, and who use cigarettes as a means of support that is easily available to them.

Violence directed at the unborn child may be apparent, with abdominal injuries being more common during pregnancy (Hillard, 1985). One-third of domestic violence in pregnancy is thought to be associated with jealousy of or anger directed toward the unborn child (Campbell, 1989, 1998). The welfare of children in households that are affected by domestic violence is also a cause for concern, with children being known to be at great risk of physical harm themselves if their mother is abused (Mullender and Debbonaire, 2000).

Social isolation may be an intrinsic aspect of domestic abuse, as part of the male strategy to control and dominate the female partner (Stark and Flitcraft, 1996). Women may be emotionally unable to or physically prevented from accessing support, either from family and friends or from statutory and voluntary agencies. During pregnancy, abused women may be late bookers and unable to attend for antenatal care, missing planned appointments. They may be labelled by health professionals as a nuisance, deviant or uncaring about the outcome of their pregnancy, with little insight into the difficulties that they face in engaging in normal social interactions.

Not surprisingly, women who experience domestic violence are also known to experience mental health problems. Depression, anxiety and suicide (actual or considered) have been reported (Helton *et al.*, 1987). However, domestic violence as a cause of perinatal mental illness is still largely unrecognised. In recent years, considerable emphasis has been placed on the risks and impact of postnatal depression on new mothers, and it has been proposed that hormonal changes are the main determinant (Dalton and Holton, 2001). This physiological approach denies the social context of birth, offering medical explanations and solutions for depressive illnesses that may in fact have their roots in relationship conflict and domestic violence. Post-traumatic stress disorder has also been found among women who experience domestic violence (British Medical Association, 1998), and parallels between the effects of domestic violence on women and the impact of torture and imprisonment on hostages have been described (Graham *et al.*, 1988). These effects include low self-esteem, dependence on the perpetrator, and feelings of hopelessness and despair (Kirkwood, 1993).

Women are at a high risk of 'moderate to severe' violence during the postnatal period (Hedin, 2000). The birth of a baby and the transition to parenthood is a time of major upheaval, stress and lifestyle changes. An increase in social status for the woman as mother is also evident, with a need for the male partner to redefine his role as father, and to assert his associated power and authority. If violence already exists within a relationship, this period of social role adjustment may be a time when it flourishes. The early postnatal period may be a time of particular vulnerability. It is not difficult to empathise with the postnatal woman who has a painful swollen perineum following an episiotomy. She takes regular analgesia and frequent baths to alleviate her pain. She moves awkwardly, easing herself slowly from standing to sitting position or vice versa, using every possible means to minimise her discomfort. It might be surprising therefore to learn that some midwives have found women who have had their perineal sutures removed by their partner (Hunt and Martin 2001; M Steene, personal communication, 3 May 2001). Imagine the power, coercion or force that must be involved, and the physical and psychological trauma that the woman experiences, for the partner to asssert his conjugal rights. Yet although this is spoken about within professional circles, no documentary evidence existed until recently.

What can health professionals do?

The NHS has until recently largely ignored the problem of domestic violence. Given the incidence of the latter, the level of identification of women who access health services for injuries caused by domestic violence seems staggeringly low. A women may attend for care on many occasions before her injuries are viewed as anything other than accidental. The Department of Health supports a 'joined up' approach of inter-agency working, and has issued clear guidance for health professionals on their role and responsibilities, proposing the following:

> It is essential that public agencies take every opportunity to identify those who may be subject to violence, and by offering practical and emotional support, help prevent the situation deteriorating.
>
> (Department of Health, 2000a)

It is no longer considered acceptable simply to treat the consequential injuries of domestic violence. Health professionals are now expected to work with the

Box 7.2 Possible indicators of domestic violence in pregnancy

- A history of recurrent miscarriage, termination of pregnancy, stillbirth or low-birth-weight babies
- Late self-referral to antenatal care
- Infrequent attendance for antenatal care
- Frequent attendance for antenatal care for minor ailments or for symptoms with no apparent physiological cause
- A history of unexplained or inappropriately explained physical injuries
- A history of unexplained hospital admissions
- Current physical injuries with a delay in seeking medical assistance
- A history of or existing mental health problems, including depression, anxiety, panic attacks or stress-related illness
- Substance abuse (including cigarettes, alcohol, and prescription and illegal drugs)
- A partner who always accompanies the woman, and answers questions on her behalf

survivors of abuse, providing support, advice and appropriate referrals to other agencies, and empowering women to retake control of their lives. To do this, professionals must first acknowledge domestic violence as a women's health issue and then identify those individuals who are experiencing abuse, by screening for possible indicators (*see* Box 7.2).

These indicators may give health professionals some insight into individuals who are experiencing domestic abuse, although the most important factor appears to be a relationship that is under social or financial strain. Key signs include marital separation, young children, financial pressures, drug/alcohol abuse, and disability and ill health (Mirrlees-Black, 1996). Great caution should be exercised before midwives, health visitors, general practitioners and others commence a 'search-and-rescue' mission to save these apparently helpless vulnerable women (Dobash and Dobash, 1998). Hunt and Martin (2001) have highlighted the anger that midwives may feel when confronted with women who are experiencing violence during pregnancy, which may lead to a directive approach and strongly worded advice to leave the perpetrator. However, this merely serves to reinforce the notion that women who experience domestic violence are weak and in need of direction and control. By exercising professional power in this way, although it is rooted in the caring aspects of the role, health professionals may perpetuate the disempowerment of women with regard to controlling their own lives and experiences.

Screening for indicators of abuse may not be particularly fruitful, due to the covert nature of domestic violence. An alternative approach would be for health professionals to ask appropriate and timely questions of all women with whom they come into contact. The form that these questions may take must depend on the individual practitioner, the woman concerned and the circumstances in which they find themselves. However, it is recommended that general questions such as 'How are things at home?' should be followed up with more specific questions related to abuse (Royal College of Midwives, 1997). Fears that women will be offended by health professionals' questions are largely unfounded, as research has demonstrated that the vast majority of women have no objections to being asked about domestic violence (Bradley *et al.*, 2002). No differences in levels of acceptability have been found between those who experience violence and those who do not (Stenson *et al.*, 2001). What appears to be central to the acceptability of screening to women is that it is conducted in a safe, confidential environment, by a trained health professional who is empathetic and non-judgemental (Bacchus *et al.*, 2002).

Alternatively, some women may voluntarily choose to disclose their experience of violence to a health professional, although this may be fraught with difficulties, not least finding a suitable opportunity. Mezey and Bewley (1997) have highlighted the paradox that now faces pregnant women. In the move to empower women, promote informed choice and make birth a social experience, the maternity services have opened previously closed doors to men, and have welcomed them with open arms. Gone is the antenatal clinic or delivery room as a sacred female-only domain. Men are positively encouraged to attend every antenatal clinic appointment with their partner, to participate in birth preparation or 'parentcraft' classes, and to stand vigil while their partner is in labour, soothing, massaging and whispering words of encouragement. A man who is not present at his baby's birth is often regarded as somehow slightly deviant in today's post-*Changing Childbirth* (Department of Health, 1993) era. As a consequence of this, for pregnant women who live with domestic violence there is no longer a place of safety, a respite from the abuse, or a confidential space in which to disclose their experience. Health professionals may be reluctant to ask a woman about the cause of her injuries or symptoms, out of fear of offending or upsetting her partner. Concerns about their own and the woman's subsequent safety may also discourage active questioning.

It is vital that when women do disclose an experience of domestic violence, health professionals respond sensitively, providing ongoing support and information about other services that are available to assist women who are experiencing violence. Encouraging or cajoling a woman into leaving her abuser may not necessarily have the desired effect of protecting her from further violence. The time of highest risk for violence, particularly death, is when a woman leaves or attempts to leave the perpetrator (Binney *et al.*, 1988; Daly and Wilson, 1988). What is essential is that women are supported in making their own decisions, and that if they choose to leave, they are well informed about support services which they can use, such as a refuge or local authority accommodation to ensure their safety. If they choose not to leave, health professionals can help by offering an open door to provide ongoing support and appropriate information. This is not because women are helpless victims, but because an individual's personal coping mechanisms may not on their own be sufficient to counteract the social structure, cultural values and actions of perpetrators that combine to create and perpetuate the domestic abuse of women.

If health professionals are to be effective in identifying and supporting women who experience violence in pregnancy, a 'joined up' approach is required that has adequate resources and the support of health service managers. Close inter-agency liaison is required, with health professionals who are not afraid to challenge historical working practices, and who are willing to work across traditional boundaries. To promote this, staff development programmes should include training in domestic violence issues, and support mechanisms for health professionals who are themselves survivors of abuse. Particular attention should be paid to attitudes and beliefs about abuse that occurs within the private domain of the family, for if health professionals are to be effective they must acknowledge domestic violence as an issue that is everyone's business.

Conclusion

Although much has changed with regard to society's attitudes towards domestic violence, and there is recognition of the need for a coherent strategy to address this issue, there is still a considerable way to go before every woman who is living with violence receives the support and assistance that she requires. For many women who live with abuse in the home, little has changed. Male violence continues to be perpetuated within a patriarchal society as a means of controlling women so that men can assume their socially ascribed place in the natural order. It is vital that health professionals recognise domestic violence as an issue that potentially affects all of the women whom they encounter, regardless of age, social class or ethnic background. Pregnancy may be a particularly vulnerable time, when violence has serious consequences for both maternal and fetal health. It is therefore essential that health professionals provide sensitive and timely advice and support that empower women to survive domestic violence.

- Domestic violence is a common experience, with nearly one in four women being assaulted by their partner at some point in their life, and one in eight being repeatedly assaulted.
- The origins and perpetuation of domestic violence lie within a culture of male authority and control. In a social system where women's subordination to men is defined as natural, violence may be regarded as a necessary and acceptable means of controlling women.
- Domestic violence may be the result of a conflict of interests within a domestic relationship. The most important factor appears to be a relationship that is under social or financial strain. Key signs include marital separation, young children, financial pressures, drug and/or alcohol abuse, and disability and ill health.
- Pregnancy may offer no protection from abuse. For many women the first incident of domestic violence may occur during pregnancy, although postnatal women are most at risk for moderate to severe injury.
- The physical and psychological effects of abuse are often not attributed by health professionals to domestic violence, and may partially account for the frequency with which many negative outcomes of pregnancy and birth remain unexplained.
- It is vital that when women do disclose an experience of domestic violence, health professionals respond sensitively, providing ongoing support and information about other services that are available to assist women who are experiencing abuse at home.

Useful address

Women's Aid Federation of England
PO Box 391
Bristol BS99 7WS
Women's Aid National Domestic Violence Helpline
Tel: 0845 702 3468
Website: www.womensaid.org.uk

References

- Bacchus L, Mezey G and Bewley S (2002) Women's perceptions of routine enquiry for domestic violence in a maternity service. *Br J Obstetr Gynaecol.* **109**: 9–16.
- Baird K (2002) Domestic violence in pregnancy: a public health concern. *MIDIRS Midwifery Digest.* **12 (Supplement 1)**: S12–15.
- Bewley S, Friend J and Mezey G (eds) (1997) *Violence Against Women.* Royal College of Obstetricians and Gynaecologists, London.
- Binney V, Harknell G and Nixon J (1988) *Leaving Violent Men. A study of refuges and housing for battered women.* Women's Aid Federation of England, London.
- Bradley F, Smith M, Long J and O'Dowd T (2002) Reported frequency of domestic violence: cross-sectional survey of women attending general practice. *BMJ.* **324**: 271–4.
- British Medical Association (1998) *Domestic Violence: a health care issue?* British Medical Association, London.
- Campbell J (1989) A test of two explanatory models of women's responses to battering. *Nurs Res.* **38**: 18–24.
- Campbell J (1998) *Empowering Survivors of Abuse: health care for battered women and their children.* Sage, London.
- Campbell J, Oliver C and Bullock L (1993) Why battering during pregnancy? *Clin Issues Perinat Women's Health Nurs.* **4**: 343–9.
- Curry M (1998) The interrelationships between abuse, substance use and psychosocial stress during pregnancy. *J Obstet Gynaecol Neonat Nurs.* **27**: 692–9.
- Dalton K and Holton W (2001) *Depression after Childbirth: how to recognise, treat and prevent postnatal depression.* Oxford University Press, Oxford.
- Daly M and Wilson M (1988) *Homicide.* Aldine de Gruyter, New York.
- Department of Health (1993) *Changing Childbirth.* HMSO, London.
- Department of Health (2000a) *Domestic Violence: a resource manual for health care professionals.* Department of Health, London.
- Department of Health (2000b) *The National Plan for the New NHS: the need for change.* Department of Health, London and NHS Executive, Leeds; www.nhs.uk/nationalplan/
- Dobash RE and Dobash RP (1979) *Violence Against Wives. A case against patriarchy.* Free Press, New York.
- Dobash RE and Dobash RP (1992) *Women, Violence and Social Change.* Routledge, London.

- Dobash RE and Dobash RP (eds) (1998) *Rethinking Violence Against Women.* Sage, London.
- Dobash RE, Dobash RP and Noaks L (eds) (1995) *Gender and Crime.* University of Wales Press, Cardiff.
- Dobash RE, Dobash RP, Cavanagh K and Lewis R (1996) *Research Evaluation of Programmes for Violent Men.* Scottish Office Central Research Unit, Edinburgh.
- Gelles R (1975) Violence and pregnancy. A note on the extent of the problem and needed services. *Family Co-ordinator.* **24**: 81–6.
- Graham P, Rawlings E and Rimini W (1988) Survivors of terror: battered women, hostages and the Stockholm syndrome. In: K Yllo and M Bograd (eds) *Feminist Perspectives on Wife Abuse.* Sage, London.
- Grimstad H, Backe B, Jacobsen G *et al.* (1998) Abuse history and health risk behaviours in pregnancy. *Acta Obstet Gynecol Scand.* **77**: 893–7.
- Hedin L (2000) Postpartum, also a risk period for domestic violence. *Eur J Obstet Gynaecol Reprod Biol.* **89**: 41–5.
- Helton A, McFarlane J and Anderson E (1987) Battered and pregnant: a prevalence study. *Am J Pub Health.* **77**: 1337–9.
- Hester M, Kelly L and Radford J (eds) (1996) *Women, Violence and Male Power.* Open University Press, Buckingham.
- Hester M, Pearson C and Harwin N (1998) *Making an Impact: children and domestic violence.* Department of Health, School for Policy Studies, University of Bristol, Bristol.
- Hillard P (1985) Physical abuse in pregnancy. *Obstet Gynaecol.* **66**: 185–90.
- Hoff L (1990) *Battered Women as Survivors.* Routledge, London.
- Home Office (1995) *Interagency Circular.* Home Office, London.
- Home Office (1996) *British Crime Survey.* Home Office, London.
- Home Office (1999) *The Home Office Agenda on Violence Against Women;* www.homeoffice.gov.uk/domesticviolence/hoagen.htm
- Horley S (1991) *The Charm Syndrome: why charming men can make dangerous lovers.* PaperMac, London.
- Hunt S and Martin A (2001) *Pregnant Women, Violent Men: what midwives need to know.* Books for Midwives Press, Hale.
- Kirkwood C (1993) *Leaving Abusive Partners.* Sage, London.
- Lewis G (ed.) (2001) *The Confidential Enquiries into Maternal Deaths in the United Kingdom. Why mothers die 1997–1999.* RCOG Press, London; www.cemd.org.uk
- Lloyd A (1995) *Doubly Deviant, Doubly Damned. Society's treatment of violent women.* Penguin Books, Harmondsworth.
- McFarlane J, Parker B and Soeken K (1996) Abuse during pregnancy: associations with maternal health and infant birth weight. *Nurse Res.* **45**: 27–41.
- McWilliams M and McKiernan J (1993) *Bringing it Out Into the Open.* HMSO, Belfast.
- Martin S, English K and Andersen K (1996) Violence and substance abuse among North Carolina pregnant women. *Am J Pub Health.* **86**: 991–8.
- Mezey G and Bewley S (1997) Domestic violence and pregnancy. *Br J Obstet Gynaecol.* **104**: 528–31.
- Mirrlees-Black C (1996) *Domestic Violence: findings from a new British Crime Survey self-completion questionnaire.* Home Office Research Study 191. Home Office, London.

- Mooney J (1993) *The Hidden Figures: the North London Domestic Violence Survey.* Middlesex University Centre for Criminology, Enfield.
- Mullender A and Debbonaire T (2000) *Child Protection and Domestic Violence.* Venture Press, Birmingham.
- Radford J (1987) Policing male violence, policing women. In: J Hanmer and M Maynard (eds) *Women, Violence and Social Control.* Macmillan, Basingstoke.
- Royal College of Midwives (1997) *Domestic Abuse in Pregnancy. Position Paper 19.* Royal College of Midwives, London.
- Salzman L (1990) Battering during pregnancy: a role for physicians. *Atlanta Med.* **65**: 45–8.
- Shumway J, O'Campo P, Gielen A *et al.* (1999) Preterm labour, placental abruption, and premature rupture of membranes in relation to maternal violence or verbal abuse. *J Maternal-Fetal Med.* **8**: 76–80.
- Stark E and Flitcraft A (1996) *Women at Risk. Domestic violence and women's health.* Sage, London.
- Stenson K, Saarinen H, Heimer G and Sidenvall B (2001) Women's attitudes to being asked about exposure to violence. *Midwifery.* **17**: 2–10.
- Webster J, Chandler J and Battistutta D (1996) Pregnancy outcomes and health care use – the effects of abuse. *Am J Obstet Gynaecol.* **174**: 760–64.
- Wright S (1995) The role of the police in combating domestic violence. In: RE Dobash, RP Dobash and L Noaks (eds) *Gender and Crime.* University of Wales Press, Cardiff.

CHAPTER 8

Female genital mutilation

Comfort Momoh

Female genital mutilation (FGM) is a violation of the rights of women and children. It denies women and children security, personal liberty and the right to health. This chapter discusses the historical and social context of FGM, the different types of FGM, why it is practised and its prevalence. The effects on women's physical, sexual and psychological health are discussed, as well as issues related to childbirth and the law. The power of older women as key decision makers in perpetuating the practice of FGM is also considered. Child protection issues and the action that professionals should take when a child is at risk of FGM are addressed, as well as the role of the midwife as advocate and carer.

Introduction

All societies have norms of care and behaviour based on age, life stages, sex, gender and social class. These 'norms', often referred to as traditional practices, originate either from social or cultural objectives, or from empirical observations related to the well-being of individuals or society. Traditional practices may be beneficial, harmful or harmless. Traditional practices may have a harmful effect on health (and this is often the case in those relating to female children), relations between men and women, marriage and sexuality.

(World Health Organization, 1997: 1)

Female genital mutilation (FGM), also known as female circumcision, is considered to be a violation of women's and children's rights. A human rights perspective sets FGM in the context of women's social and economic powerlessness. FGM has no health or medical benefit, but is a deeply rooted cultural and traditional African practice that affects the health of women and children because of its short- and long-term psychological and physical effects.

The practice of female genital mutilation dates back at least 2000 years (El Dareer, 1983; Eke, 2000), and it now transcends and crosses all religious, racial and social boundaries (Webb, 1995). FGM is supported by centuries of tradition, culture and false beliefs, and is perpetuated by poverty, illiteracy, low status of women and inadequate healthcare facilities (Dorkenoo, 1995; Allam *et al.*, 1999; Eke, 2000).

It is estimated that more than 130 million girls and women worldwide have undergone female genital mutilation (World Health Organization, 1997). FGM is now becoming a growing problem in western countries due to the increasing number of immigrants. Consequently, the practice has become an issue for health and social care practitioners who may be unfamiliar with the problems and complications related to FGM. The influx of immigrants into the UK has presented challenges for midwives who must therefore develop a knowledge and understanding of FGM and its associated complications.

It is estimated that about 10 000 girls and young women in the UK are at risk of FGM. Boot (1994) has estimated that there are 3000–4000 new cases each year. In this country, FGM is seen mainly among individuals from Somalia, Eritrea, Ethiopia, Sudan, Sierra Leone and the Yemen. Despite the Prohibition of Female Circumcision Act (House of Commons, 1985), women from the UK are still taking their children back to their own countries for circumcision, and at present it is impossible to prevent this happening because it is not illegal.

Definition

The World Health Organization (WHO) defines FGM as any procedure involving partial or total removal of the external female genitalia or other injury to the female genital organs, whether for cultural or other non-therapeutic reasons.

The WHO has also classified FGM into four types (*see* Figure 8.1) as follows:

- *type 1*: excision of the prepuce, with or without excision of part or all of the clitoris
- *type 2*: excision of the clitoris, with partial or total excision of the labia minora
- *type 3*: excision of part or all of the external genitalia and stitching/narrowing of the vaginal opening (also known as infibulation)
- *type 4*: unclassified – this includes pricking, piercing or incising of the clitoris and/or labia, stretching of the clitoris and/or labia, and cauterisation by burning of the clitoris and surrounding tissue.

The procedures described above are irreversible and their effects last a lifetime (World Health Organization, 1997). Around 10% of girls and women die as a result of the short-term complications of FGM, such as haemorrhage, shock and infection. A further 25% die in the long term as a result of recurrent urinary and vaginal infections and complications during childbirth, such as severe bleeding and obstructed labour. However, these tragedies do not occur here in the UK or in other western countries.

The prevalence of FGM (*see* Table 8.1)

The actual number of women and girls who have undergone FGM is not known due to lack of systematic data collection. According to the World Health Organization (1997), the prevalence of FGM is still high in around 28–30 countries in Africa and the Middle East. However, the practice can also be traced to Latin America, India, Malaysia and Indonesia. Its incidence is estimated to range from 50% to 98% (Dorkenoo, 1995; Toubia, 1999).

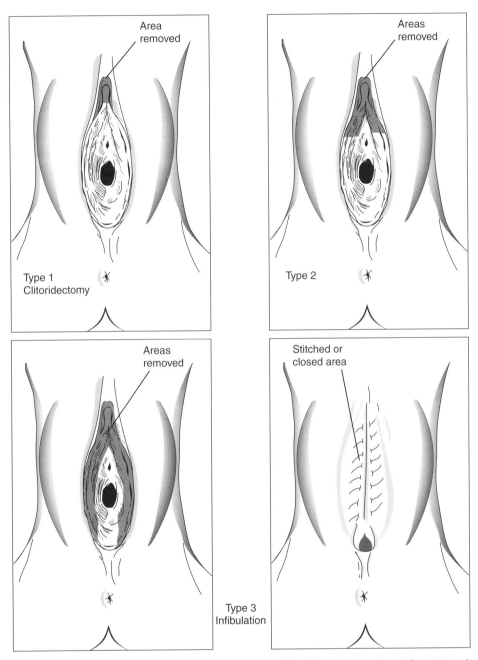

Figure 8.1   Some of the different types of female genital mutilation. (Reproduced from Momoh, 2000).

Age at which FGM is performed

The age at which FGM is performed varies according to the country, tribe and circumstances, and ranges from a few days old to adolescence, adulthood, just before marriage or after the first pregnancy. For example, Somalis tend to perform

Table 8.1   Prevalence of female genital mutilation: estimates of the extent of FGM in Africa by country (Hosken, 1993; Toubia, 1995; World Health Organization, 1998)

Country	Proportion of women affected	Number of women affected
Burkino Faso	70%	3 656 800
Central African Republic	43%	759 810
Sierra Leone	90%	2 167 200
Egypt	97%	27 905 930
Eritrea and Ethiopia	90%	26 323 250
Guinea	60%	1 999 800
Kenya	50%	6 967 500
Mali	99%	5 155 900
Niger	20%	921 200
Nigeria	40%	25 601 200
Somalia	98–100%	5 034 260
Sudan	89%	12 816 000
Tanzania	10%	1 552 000
Togo	50%	1 044 500
Djibouti	98%	248 920
Uganda	5%	513 050
Mauritania	25%	295 250
Benin	50%	1 365 000
Cameroon	20%	1 336 800
Chad	60%	1 932 000
Ivory Coast	60%	3 750 000
Ghana	30%	2 635 200
Guinea Bissau	50%	272 500
Liberia	60%	902 400
Senegal	20%	838 000
Zaire	5%	945 000

FGM on girls aged from 4 to 9 years, whereas the Ethiopian Fallashas perform the operation when the baby is a few days old (Ng, 2000). In Eastern Ethiopia, the Adere and Oromo groups perform FGM between 4 years of age and puberty, while the Amhara perform the procedure on the eighth day after birth (Missailidis and Gebre-Medhin, 2000).

How FGM is performed

The procedure is sometimes carried out using crude tools and instruments such as razors, knives and scissors. Anaesthetics and antiseptics are not generally used. However, in urban areas FGM is now more often being performed in hospitals by trained doctors and midwives. Girls may be circumcised either alone or with a group of peers from their community (Dorkenoo, 1995).

In type 3 excision or infibulation, elderly women, relatives and friends secure the girl in the lithotomy position. A deep incision is made rapidly on either side from the root of the clitoris to the fourchette, and a single cut of the razor excises the clitoris and both the labia majora and the labia minora. Bleeding is profuse, but is usually controlled by the application of various poultices, the threading of the edges of the skin with thorns, or clasping them between the edges of a split cane. A piece of twig is inserted between the edges of the skin to ensure a patent foramen for urinary and menstrual flow. The lower limbs are then bound together for 2 to 6 weeks to promote haemostasis and encourage union of the two sides (McCaffery, 1995). Healing takes place by primary intention, and as a result the introitus is obliterated by a drum of skin extending across the orifice except for a small hole (World Health Organization, 1996; Momoh, 1999; Toubia, 1999). How-ever, much will depend on the circumstances at the time. The girl may struggle ferociously, in which case the incisions may become uncontrolled and haphazard, or she may be held so tightly that some of her bones are fractured, and so the list goes on. Box 8.1 summarises the complications of female genital mutilation.

Box 8.1   Complications of female genital mutilation (Momoh, 2000)

Immediate complications	Haemorrhage from the dorsal artery, shock, pain, retention of urine, infection/tetanus that may lead to mortality
Intermediate and long-term complications	Cysts and abscesses, keloid scar formation, damage to the urethra resulting in urinary incontinence, dyspareunia, neuromata (trapped clitorial nerve), haematocolpos and sexual dysfunction

---

This procedure still continues in some villages and rural areas of some African countries, but can be performed in hospitals and cities with sterile equipment and under general or local anaesthesia to reduce the pain (Bridgehouse, 1992; Baker *et al.*, 1993). However, carrying out the procedure in hospital does not make any difference to the risk of short- and long-term complications, it violates the injunc-tion 'to do no harm' and it is unethical by any standards (Eke, 2000; World Health Organization, 2001).

Effects of FGM on women's physical, mental and sexual health

Women who have been circumcised have very specific medical, gynaecological, obstetric and psychosexual problems which doctors, midwives or other pro-fessionals are not usually trained to treat (Gordon, 1998; Morris, 1999) *(see*

Box 8.1). In most cases women do not relate the problems they are experiencing to FGM, because they will usually have been told that pain is part of growing and is therefore normal. Most of those who do relate their problems to FGM accept them as part of the natural order of things (Cameron and Rawlings-Anderson, 2001). Furthermore, it needs to be remembered that, for many women, FGM is a part of the struggle for everyday survival in areas of war and famine, where women are not well educated and there is a lack of healthcare provision (Scherf, 2000).

FGM is both unnecessary and damaging to girls' and women's physical and emotional well-being. It can also have lifelong effects, such as psychological trauma and flashbacks, on women who have undergone the procedure. Girls are usually conscious when FGM is performed with no anaesthesia, so it is not surprising that the effects of the experience remain for a lifetime. This can lead to feelings of deep anger, fear, bitterness and betrayal at having been subjected to such pain (Foundation for Women's Health Research and Development (FORWARD), 2000).

The effects of FGM on women and girls are strongly dependent on a number of factors, such as the severity and type of circumcision, the competence of the circumciser, the sanitary conditions under which the procedure was performed, and the co-operation and health of the child at the time of circumcision. All of the effects or complications that are likely to cause problems may contribute to a wide range of psychological effects, including chronic irritability, depression and anxiety, which may lead to suicide (Dorkenoo, 1995; Allam et al., 1999; Ciment, 1999; Eke, 2000; Weir, 2000).

With regard to sexual and psychological problems, anxiety due to anticipation of pain during menarche, intercourse, childbirth and medical vaginal examination has also been reported (Lightfoot-Klein, 1998). Rushwan (2000) noted that intercourse and conception may not be achieved in women with type 3 circumcision, as the tough fibrotic skin that closes the vaginal introitus could hinder penetration. He also suggests that in some women intercourse may take place through the small opening (false vagina), and that this may have detrimental effects on the woman, such as severe pain during intercourse and infertility.

The World Health Organization (1996) and Gibeau (1998) believe that many women who have undergone FGM experience various degrees of sexual dysfunction, including inability to achieve orgasm, as the clitoris is believed to be key to the normal functioning and mental and physical development of female sexuality. FGM interferes with sexual feelings and pleasure because the clitoris contains a large number of receptor nerve endings, and its removal may affect physical receptivity to sexual stimulation (Hopkins, 1999). FGM can also result in damage to the concentrated nerve complex that is responsible for clitoral erection, pelvic muscular and secretory actions and the transmission of sensory information to the central nervous system (Bridgehouse, 1992).

However, it is difficult to generalise with regard to what form of sexual dysfunction occurs. Rawlings-Anderson and Cameron (2000) published a study of 97 circumcised Sudanese women and found that 90% of these women had experienced orgasm after circumcision. However, many of these women said that their orgasms were weak, infrequent or difficult to achieve. Some women may also experience marital conflict due to some of the above sequelae (Wright, 1996).

Why is FGM performed?

The suggested reasons for performing FGM are complex, multifactorial, inter-related and interwoven with the beliefs and values that are upheld in communities. Therefore it is extremely difficult to explain exactly why this practice occurs (Rahman and Toubia, 2000). The reasons can be classified as follows: myths; social pressure; religious teaching; sex; hygiene; tradition/culture. The parents and/or relatives do not decide to circumcise their daughters with malicious intent, but regard this as an act of love and part of their culture. They do not consider it to be either unethical or immoral (Momoh, 1999; Toubia, 1999).

Historical evidence

The history of FGM is not well known, but it is thought to date back as far as the fifth century BC (Koso-Thomas, 1987). Some authors believe that it was practised in ancient Egypt as a sign of distinction (among the aristocracy), and have reported that traces of infibulation can still be found on Egyptian mummies (Izett and Toubia, 1999). Many believe that the practice evolved from early times in primitive communities that wished to establish control over the sexual behaviour of women. Such concern about women's sexual and moral behaviour does not seem to have been confined to Africa, nor is the ingenuity to curb or conceal female sexuality displayed only on that continent (World Health Organization, 1996). The early Roman technique of slipping rings through the labia majora of female slaves to prevent them becoming pregnant is an indication that FGM has been practised outside the African continent for a long time (Bridgehouse, 1992). The Scoptsi sect of Russia also performed FGM to ensure virginity (Eke, 2000).

   History also traces the practice of FGM to the UK and the USA, and evidence suggests that it was practised in the nineteenth century by gynaecologists to cure so-called 'female weaknesses' such as nymphomania, aberrant behaviour (e.g. reaching orgasm), insanity, masturbation, hysteria, epilepsy and other female disorders (Koso-Thomas, 1987; Eke, 2000).

Sociocultural reasons for FGM

FGM has formed part of the cultural identity of many groups. It is embedded in social values, beliefs and culturally defined norms, and is linked to strongly held ideas about identity, sexuality, gender and power (Rahman and Toubia, 2000). FGM may be seen as an act of love to be celebrated with ceremonial events and embraced with excitement and anticipation. It may be regarded as a rite of passage to womanhood, ensuring that daughters – as virgins – are marriage-worthy and virtuous (Momoh, 2000). Traditionally, women are said to be highly regarded within practising societies as a result of having undergone the procedure, since the belief is that unless a girl is circumcised, she will not become a mature woman, and she will lose the right to marry and bear children commensurate with others of her age group as well as her ancestors. This fear of social ostracism and being considered deviant by the community is a powerful motivating factor that ensures the continuation of the practice. Peers and family members reject girls who are not circumcised, which is disastrous for them as they have no means of security or support (Gibeau, 1998; Momoh, 1999). Furthermore, in some societies not only is circumcision positively reinforced through the social benefits described above, but it is also negatively reinforced. For example, within certain groups the greatest insult possible is to be referred to as the 'son of an uncircumcised woman' (Lightfoot-Klein, 1989).

The Foundation for Women's Health Research and Development (FORWARD) (2000) and Wright (1996) both argue that, for women who are living in a patriarchal society with no land, no education and no effective power base, marriage is their main means of survival and access to resources. In this context, one can understand why the practice of female genital mutilation continues. The World Health Organization (1996) also argues that the social reasons for FGM are centred on the dominant role of the male within the family and society, as in most African countries the head of the family is a man. Interestingly, Savane (1984) complicates the picture further by describing how university-educated women who hold administrative posts are still victims of traditional models of behaviour. She suggests that they are pulled in opposite directions by the traditional and the modern in that they aspire to the freer western philosophies but they also need the traditional structures and roles which offer them psychological security. It may be argued that they 'need the traditional structures and roles', but it would also be reasonable to assume that these women would be subjected to strong peer and family pressure to conform. It is always most difficult to become the first to deviate from the norm. However, Missailidis and Gebre-Medhin (2000) have painted a conflicting picture. In their study of three ethnic groups in Eastern Ethiopia, they found that some women felt that it made little difference to a man whether a women was circumcised or not, so long as she was a virgin. Other women felt that men still preferred circumcised women. It seems here that society acts as a mechanism to reinforce the roles of men and women in a vicious circle that perpetuates the practice of female genital mutilation.

Religion

Female genital mutilation is not associated with any one religion. Some practising communities claim its mention in the Koran or the Hadith, but it pre-dates Islam (Gibeau, 1998). However, although FGM is not cited in the Koran, Muslim principles are derived not only from the Koran but also from the anthology of Sunna (a terminology that represents words and actions attributed to the Prophet Mohammed). It is within Sunna that one finds opinions expressed with regard to FGM. Despite this, leading Islamic theologians refute the argument that the practice is based on religious doctrine (Khaled and Vause, 1996).

There is evidence that Jews, Christians, Muslims and indigenous religious groups practice FGM in Africa. However, despite the fact that FGM is not known in many Muslim countries, such as Saudi Arabia, which is the focus of Islam (Wright, 1996), it is strongly identified with Islam in several African nations. Furthermore, many members of the Muslim community believe that it is a religious obligation because it ensures 'spiritual purity' (Bridgehouse, 1992). Thus it may be that religion is being used here to legitimise FGM as a means of female social control (Lightfoot-Klein, 1989; Brooks, 1995).

Sexual reasons

There are many strange and often inaccurate reasons given for the perpetuation of the practice of FGM. Some believe that FGM reduces sexual desire and therefore preserves virginity, or that the uncut clitoris will grow large and pressure on this organ will arouse intense desire (World Health Organization, 2001). Furthermore, uncircumcised girls are believed to have an overactive and uncontrollable sex drive which will lead to the premature loss of their virginity, and this will bring disgrace to their family and damage their chances of marriage. The families in some nomadic tribes circumcise their daughters in order to prevent them from being raped in the desert while they are left alone to care for the animals.

Some socio-political theories state that FGM is perpetuated in order to oppress women and girls and control their sexuality (Lightfoot-Klein and Shaw, 1990; Boot, 1994; Khaled and Vause, 1996; World Health Organization, 1996). It is likely that FGM (as well as the use of chastity belts or the closing of the external organs with steel pins or iron tacks) is practised in order to control female sexuality and cause women to be more submissive to moral, social, legal and religious constraints, especially the constraints of monogamy. It is suggested that only by restricting the woman sexually can a man be sure that her children are his own (El Saadawi, 1980).

A narrow vaginal opening is believed by both the Somalis and the Sudanese to heighten male sexual pleasure. Unfortunately, following marriage penetration can take up to three months to achieve, and in some cases opening up is necessary before intercourse can take place. However, when Shandall (1967) surveyed 300 Sudanese husbands who had one infibulated wife and one non-infibulated wife, 266 of the husbands stated categorically that they preferred non-excised or Sunna-circumcised women sexually.

El Saadawi (1980) also suggests that men are not alone in promoting FGM to protect their economies and that of the family. There are many traditional birth attendants, nurses, paramedical staff, doctors, midwives and laywomen who make their living from circumcisions. Furthermore, they may derive much social standing and status within their community because they are upholding traditional cultural practices which are seen as vital for maintaining the social fabric of groups who may perceive themselves to be under threat from western philosophies.

Myths

Mythical reasons for FGM include the promotion of fertility, the notion that the clitoris poses a risk because it will grow and harm the baby, and the idea that FGM aids the health and survival of the child. Protagonists argue that, like male circumcision, FGM promotes cleanliness, but there is no supporting evidence for this argument (Koso-Thomas, 1987). Women in Sierra Leone were interviewed who believed that the clitoris was a source of disease and that failure to excise it would result in infertility (World Health Organization, 1996). Village communities will testify to the validity of such assumptions.

The powerful influence of older women in perpetuating FGM

In many countries, FGM is an accepted and expected custom, and for many women FGM is a fact of life – a pain that must be endured because they must conform with social expectations in order to survive. Toubia (1999) considers that traditional values and methods whereby individuals relate to each other in many African cultures are hierarchical, and therefore favour respect for authority figures and elders. Because of this social power and hierarchy, most women do not question the practice of FGM.

Women have been socially conditioned to accept FGM within social definitions of womanhood and identity, and this encourages the older women to perpetuate and continue the practice. They play a major role in the continuation of FGM because in most cases they are the key decision makers. They regard it as an important component in the process of socialisation of girls into the social, familial, sexual and reproductive roles of women, and they strongly oppose sex before marriage. They believe that circumcision increases the likelihood of achieving a favourable marriage and the family's chances of obtaining a high price for the bride (Dorkenoo, 1995). In most cultures where FGM is practised, marriage is viewed as security for life for the woman and her family.

The older women in such cultures regard FGM as a very beneficial custom and an integral part of the society's social and cultural heritage. The degree of power that is held by the older women within practising societies enables them to reinforce and pass on cultural norms from one generation to the next. They have the ability to influence members of the social network and even override the other decision makers, and because they are the custodians of family traditions they are a powerful force. The practice of FGM gives them the opportunity to exercise real power in a patriarchal culture, whereas before they were powerless and, as such, could be seen to be unwittingly colluding with their own oppression.

For an older woman to accept that FGM is a harmful practice she must accept at a psychological level that her mother did something harmful to her, and this may cause a fragmentation of her psyche. There is also the fear of allowing her daughters to remain uncircumcised, as this may lead to social ostracism from the tribe or clan on which she depends for her food, shelter and well-being. The communities, and especially the older women, therefore view FGM as an act of love and a rite of passage to womanhood, rather than as a violation of human rights or as child abuse, as it is perceived to be by the western world.

Legal issues

In some African countries, such as Ghana, Sudan and Senegal, FGM has been outlawed but the practice still continues. The arguments against FGM are based on universally recognised human rights, including the right to integrity of the person and the highest achievable level of physical and mental health (World Health Organization, 1997; Chelala, 1998; Ciment, 1999).

FGM is illegal in the UK, but despite the Prohibition of Female Circumcision Act (1985), women are still taking their children back to their own countries for circumcision and, as mentioned earlier in this chapter, it is not possible to prevent this happening because it is not illegal (Boot, 1994). Children are taken back to Africa during the summer holidays to be circumcised, and the Act alone has not brought about any change in the last 17 years. In 2001, a general practitioner was struck off the General Medical Council register for agreeing to perform female circumcision (Dyer, 2001), but this is a rare occurrence.

Although FGM is regarded as child abuse in the UK, it is important to support the family and work with them, rather than separating or arresting the parents, as they may be new to the country and unaware of the law or of the effects of FGM, due to their deeply rooted beliefs. However, if the parents are unwilling to change their practice and the child is at risk, Social Services should be informed.

The Act states that it is an offence for any person:

1 to excise, infibulate or otherwise mutilate the whole or any part of the labia majora or clitoris of another person; or
2 to aid, abet, counsel or procure the performance by another person of any of those acts on that other person's own body.
   'Anyone found guilty of performing this operation is liable to a fine or imprisonment' (House of Commons, 1985).

In 2000, the All Party Parliamentary Group on Population, Development and Reproductive Health aimed to raise awareness of female genital mutilation both in the UK and abroad, and to generate support for a prevention and eradication programme (Kmietowicz, 2000). Some of the recommendations that were made following the hearing are listed below.

• The UK Government should undertake a full assessment of local authority provision and guidance with regard to FGM, particularly with reference to child protection.
• The UK law should be amended to ensure that UK residents who take girls abroad to have them circumcised can be prosecuted under the UK law on their return, regardless of the status of FGM in the country where the circumcision took place.
• Funds should be available for non-Government organisations and for research into the prevalence of FGM in the UK.
• It should be a legal requirement for health professionals and other relevant authorities to report all incidents of FGM.
• The Act should be publicised in a media campaign.

As the raising of awareness and training are both becoming an issue with regard to FGM in the UK, many professional bodies have now created or are in the process of drawing up guidelines on FGM. The Royal College of Midwives (1998) published a position paper on FGM, and the British Medical Association (2001) has revised its guidelines.

The midwife's role

Midwives need to have a better knowledge and understanding of the cultural factors relating to FGM in order to be able to understand the reasons for it being performed and provide insightful support for women and girls who are affected by FGM. Midwives should be advocates for these women and girls, and should possess up-to-date clinical expertise in order to help these women to give birth (McCaffery, 1995; Chalmers and Kowser, 2000; Momoh, 2000). Dunkley (2000) suggests that strategies to ensure that all members of society have an equal right to health and healthcare may seem utopian, but continued efforts toward meeting this standard should be adopted and remain high on the agendas of health professionals.

Conclusion

As midwives are now caring for many refugees and immigrant pregnant women who are circumcised and from different sociocultural backgrounds, they need to be aware of issues relating to FGM in the UK. The African Well Woman's Clinic is a very good example of the way in which the needs of the community have been addressed. Advice and counselling are provided as well as the offer of de-infibulation, where the aim is to restore normal anatomy as far as is possible.

As we now live in a multicultural society, FGM is presenting a challenge for midwives that requires great sensitivity and awareness. A sensitive and caring approach by midwives is essential in order to gain the trust of these women so that they will seek help if and when it is required. This in turn should open up opportunities for midwives to empower the women with the education, advice and support that they require, both in order to help them give birth and, hopefully, to assist in the abolition of an age-old harmful practice.

- Female genital mutilation is a deeply rooted cultural practice and a violation of human rights.
- FGM continues to be a major problem in the UK, despite the law prohibiting the practice.
- FGM has no health or medical benefit for women or girls.
- Midwives need to gain knowledge and understanding of FGM in order to act as advocates and carers for these women.

Useful addresses

African Well Woman's Clinic
St Thomas Hospital
6th Floor, North Wing
London SE1 7EH
Tel: 0207 960 5595

Black Women's Health and Family Support
82 Russia Lane
Bethnal Green
London E2 9LU
Tel: 0208 980 3503

Foundation for Women's Health
Research and Development (FORWARD)
6th Floor, 50 Eastbourne Terrace
London W2 6LX
Tel: 0207 725 2606

Multi-Cultural Antenatal Clinic
Liverpool Women's Hospital
Crown Street
Liverpool L8 7SS
Tel: 0151 708 9988

African Well Woman's Clinic
Antenatal Clinic
Central Middlesex Hospital
Acton Lane
Park Royal
London NW10 7NS
Tel: 0208 965 5733

African Well Woman's Clinic
Northwick Park and St Mark's Hospitals
Watford Road
Harrow
Middlesex HA1 3UJ
Tel: 0208 869 2880

African Women's Health Clinic
Whittington Hospital
London NW10 7NS
Tel: 0207 288 3482

Eklas Ahmed
Midlands Refugee Council
5th Floor, Smithfield House
Digbeth B5 6BS
Tel: 0121 242 2200

Agency for Culture
11A Arundel Gate
Sheffield S1 2PN
Tel: 0114 275 0193

Rainbo
Queens Studios
121 Salisbury Road
London NW6 6RG
Tel: 0207 625 3400

References

- Allam MFA, de Irala-Estevez J, Navajas RF *et al.* (1999) Students' knowledge of and attitudes about female circumcision in Egypt. *NEJM.* **341**: 1552–3.
- Baker CA, Gilson GJ, Vill MD and Curet LB (1993) Female circumcision: obstetrics issues. *Am J Obstet Gynecol.* **169**: 1616–18.
- Boot J (1994) *Female Genital Mutilation.* Unpublished paper. Borough of Waltham Forest, London.
- Bridgehouse R (1992) Ritual female circumcision and its effects on female sexual function. *Can J Hum Sexuality.* **1**: 3–10.
- British Medical Association (2001) *Female Genital Mutilation: caring for patients and child protection.* British Medical Association, London.
- Brooks G (1995) The verses. *Guardian.* **11 March**: 12–19.
- Cameron J and Rawlings-Anderson K (2001) Genital mutilation: human rights and cultural imperialism. *Br J Midwifery.* **9**: 231–5.
- Chalmers B and Kowser OH (2000) 432 Somali women's birth experiences in Canada after earlier female genital mutilation. *Birth.* **27**: 227–34.
- Chelala C (1998) An alternative way to stop female genital mutilation. *Lancet.* **352**: 126.
- Ciment J (1999) Senegal outlaws female genital mutilation. *BMJ.* **318**: 348.
- Dorkenoo E (1995) *Cutting the Rose. Female genital mutilation: the practice and its prevention.* Minority Rights Publications, London.
- Dunkley J (2000) *Health Promotion in Midwifery Practice: a resource for health professionals.* Baillière Tindall, London.
- Dyer O (2001) GP struck off for agreeing to perform female circumcision. *BMJ.* **322**: 9.
- Eke N (2000) Female genital mutilation: what can be done? *Lancet.* **356 (Supplement)**: 57.
- El Dareer A (1983) Epidemiology of female circumcision in the Sudan. *Trop Doct.* **13**: 41–5.
- El Saadawi N (1980) *The Hidden Face of Eve.* Zed Press, London.
- Foundation for Women's Health Research and Development (FORWARD) (2000) *Factsheet: female genital mutilation.* FORWARD, London.
- Gibeau AM (1998) Female genital mutilation: when a cultural practice generates clinical and ethical dilemmas. *J Obstet Gynecol Neonatal Nurs.* **27**: 85–91.
- Gordon H (1998) Female genital mutilation: female circumcision. *Diplomate.* **5**: 86–90.
- Hopkins S (1999) A discussion of the legal aspects of female genital mutilation. *J Adv Nurs.* **30**: 926–33.
- Hosken FP (1993) *The Hosken Report: genital and sexual mutilation of females. Revised edition.* Women's International Network News, Lexington, MA.
- House of Commons (1985) *Prohibition of Female Circumcision Act.* HMSO, London.
- Izett S and Toubia N (1999) *A Research and Evaluation Guidebook Using Female Circumcision as a Case Study. Learning about social changes.* Rainbo, New York.
- Khaled K and Vause S (1996) Genital mutilation: a continued abuse. *Br J Obstet Gynaecol.* **103**: 86–7.
- Kmietowicz Z (2000) MP recommends tightening the law on female genital mutilation. *BMJ.* **321**: 1365.
- Koso-Thomas O (1987) *The Circumcision of Women: a strategy for eradication.* Zed Press, London.

- Lightfoot-Klein H (1989) *Prisoners of Ritual: an odyssey into female genital mutilation in Africa*. Haworth Press, New York.
- Lightfoot-Klein H (1998) The sexual experience and marital adjustment of circumcised and infibulated females in the Sudan. *J Sex Reprod*. **26**: 375–92.
- Lightfoot-Klein H and Shaw E (1990) Special needs of ritually circumcised women patients. *J Obstet Gynecol Neonatal Nurs*. **20**: 102–7.
- McCaffery (1995) Management of female genital mutilation. Northwick Park Hospital experience. *Br J Obstet Gynaecol*. **102**: 787–90.
- Missailidis K and Gebre-Medhin M (2000) Female genital mutilation declines in Ethiopia. *Lancet*. **356**: 137–8.
- Momoh C (1999) Female genital mutilation: the struggle continues. *Pract Nurs*. **10**: 31–3.
- Momoh C (2000) *Female Genital Mutilation: information for health care professionals*. King's Fund, London.
- Morris R (1999) Female genital mutilation: perspectives, risks and complications. *Urol Nurs*. **19**: 13–19.
- Ng F (2000) Female genital mutilation: its implication for reproductive health. An overview. *Br J Fam Plan*. **26**: 47–51.
- Rahman A and Toubia N (2000) *Female Genital Mutilation: a guide to laws and policies*. Worldwide Zed Books, London.
- Rawlings-Anderson K and Cameron J (2000) Female genital mutilation: a global perspective. *Br J Midwifery*. **8**: 754–60.
- Royal College of Midwives (1998) *Female Genital Mutilation (Female Circumcision)*. Position Paper 21. Royal College of Midwives, London.
- Rushwan H (2000) Female genital mutilation: management during pregnancy, childbirth and the postpartum period. *Int J Obstet*. **70**: 99–104.
- Savane MA (1984) Elegance amid the phallocracy. In: R Morgan (ed.) *Sisterhood is Global*. Penguin, Harmondsworth.
- Scherf C (2000) Ending genital mutilation: women in Africa have many other problems besides genital mutilation. *BMJ*. **321**: 570–71.
- Shandall AA (1967) Circumcision and infibulation of females. *Sudan Med J*. **5**: 178–212.
- Toubia N (1995) *Female Genital Mutilation: a call for global action*. Rainbo, New York.
- Toubia N (1999) *A Technical Manual for Health Care Providers Caring for Women With Circumcision*. Rainbo, New York.
- Webb E (1995) Female genital mutilation. Cultural knowledge is the key to understanding. *BMJ*. **70**: 441–4.
- Weir E (2000) Female genital mutilation. *Can Med Assoc J*. **162**: 1344.
- World Health Organization (1996) *Female Genital Mutilation: a report of the WHO Technical Working Group*. World Health Organization, Geneva.
- World Health Organization (1997) *FGM: a joint WHO/UNICEF/UNFPA statement*. World Health Organization, Geneva.
- World Health Organization (1998) *Female Genital Mutilation: an overview*. World Health Organization, Geneva.
- World Health Organization (2001) *A Teacher's Guide. Integrating the prevention and management of the health complication into the curricula of nursing and midwifery*. World Health Organization, Geneva.
- Wright J (1996) Female genital mutilation: an overview. *J Adv Nurs*. **24**: 251–9.

CHAPTER 9

Transition to motherhood

Nicola Winson

This chapter compares some definitions of motherhood, but focuses on the transition to the state of motherhood. Three theorists have described the process from different perspectives at different times, so that a behaviourist model, a social model and a model of feelings involved in the process will be discussed. The experience of giving birth is thought to influence a woman's transition to the state of motherhood. Postnatal events, mood and personality type can influence the woman's adaptation to this state, as it is thought can her age, although this is not yet proven in the literature. Finally, the need for social change is explored as a means of facilitating acceptance of the status of mother.

Introduction

The media portrays childbirth as a happy and joyous event (Paradice, 1995; Gibson, 2001), and society maintains and feeds the myth that mothering is both easy and natural. These sentiments do not reflect the enormous psychological adjustment that a woman undergoes to make it appear easy and natural. She has completed a complex and demanding task (Paradice, 1995). She has been financially independent, professionally competent, socially in demand and emotionally balanced with broad horizons, and she may now change into someone who is physically tired (Larkin and Butler, 2000), scarred, bruised (Ockenden, 2000), nervous, socially isolated, intellectually under-stimulated, unable to participate rationally in or digest a discussion, financially dependent, professionally non-existent, emotionally labile and hypersensitive.

The processes that occur during this transition are poorly understood, but some research has been done. This chapter will sample the antenatal literature which considers women's views about their future role change during pregnancy. The work of three major theorists will be examined as they state how these changes in role identification occur. The birthing experience is also a major influence on the transition to motherhood, and in the recent past has only been regarded as less traumatic because women now rarely die from it. Recent research demonstrates that birthing is mentally traumatic and possibly injurious both to the transition to motherhood and to the woman's mental health. Postnatally, a woman's mental health is valued less than her caring for the baby. This chapter will examine some postnatal issues, including role conflict and the effects that occur when the transition to motherhood appears to be incomplete. As the average age at which women are having children is rising, the transition to motherhood among older women will also be addressed. This social phenomenon is not the only one referred to here. Society's expectations of women, the influence of the media on women, and the control of women by society are subtle issues which will thread through this chapter.

Why study the transition process?

Why study the transition process at all when it is viewed by the media as easy and as a normal stage in family development? (Morse *et al.*, 2000). The literature answers this question by revealing that for some it is a serious challenge or even a crisis (Underdown, 1998: Morse *et al.*, 2000). Becoming a parent involves labour-intensive activity that absorbs enormous amounts of time, energy and effort almost continuously every day of the week for up to two decades (Fedele *et al.*, 1988), and it has a psychological, physiological and relational impact which will test the resources of each individual in a couple (Goldberg, 1988). It seems that the 'normative' transition has very extensive and profound dimensions. As little help with this transition seems to be available in society, clearly there is a need for healthcare professionals and midwives to understand it. Culture, as represented in part by the newspapers, tells surprising stories. The volume of personal stories that appear at least weekly in each journal is significant. 'She once confessed to being terrified of becoming a parent ... but yesterday any fear had vanished as Big Brother presenter Davina McCall described her joy at becoming a mother for the first time' (Bonnici, 2001). It seems that the transition to motherhood had taken place, but why do so many personal testimonies of it appear? If it is easy and normal, why should it be reported? If it is a trouble-free process, why should people write about it? The article quoted suggests that the public need to be told that the process of becoming a parent can be achieved by celebrities (i.e. people whom the rest of the population may regard as role models). The picture is very glamorous, which suggests the subtle message that the transition to motherhood is easy, natural and does not detract from one's public or personal appeal. This is a different idea to that offered above by Morse *et al.* (2000).

Some definitions

Transition is defined as the process of changing from one state to another (Rooney, 1999). Life is full of change – from baby to infant to child to adolescent to parent to old person. Most of these stages are marked culturally by events, celebrations and certain rituals, even if only birthday parties. They are considered to be achievements. Vehvilainen-Julkunen (1995) described transitions as forming an integral part of human development. Profound change with dramatic effects on the lives of significant others and major significance for health and welfare are other aspects of the definition of transition.

The dictionary definition (Rooney, 1999) of a mother as producing young emphasises her role as a parent, originator and protector. On chicken farms the apparatus that is used for generating warmth so that eggs can be hatched and chicks reared without a hen is called a mother! The characteristic that is required in order to mother is the ability to give physical warmth so that development occurs. Perhaps this lighthearted view has hidden depth if warmth is defined as having physical, psychological, social and emotional aspects. Schmied and Lupton (2001) consider that breastfeeding forms a major part of the definition of motherhood, and that it is central to women's experience of motherhood. Some women have portrayed breastfeeding as a crucial part of maternal identity and as being representative of good mothering. However, this perspective is not universally shared. The idea of including breastfeeding in the definition of motherhood will seem strange and inaccurate, if not oppressive, to some people. The debate about breastfeeding involving more than merely ensuring the physical survival of the infant is beyond the scope of this chapter. It could be argued that breastfeeding focuses the woman's mind more acutely on the issues and transitional processes that she is undergoing, but to suggest that it is integral to the concept of motherhood when the processes involved in the transition to motherhood are still poorly understood or researched would seem presumptuous.

Pridham and Chang (1992) quote Chick and Meleis (1986), who define the transition to motherhood as a process of personal and interpersonal change that occurs as a woman assumes maternal tasks and appraises herself as a mother. Pridham and Chang (1992) point out that previous definitions have been limited to problem solving with regard to infant care and parenting issues, and mothers have focused on assessment of their problem-solving competence, their relationship with the infant and their attention to the infant's development and individual characteristics. This definition relates to behaviour rather than to psychological attitudes, mental processes, emotional development or change. It moves current thinking beyond psychomotor skills and towards the psychological, but it still lacks information about the processes and strength of feeling that are associated with motherhood.

Maternal perceptions of the fetus before birth

Before discussing the major theorists' research on the transition process undergone by the mother during pregnancy, it is useful to consider other aspects of this transition. For example, does the ultrasound scan (USS) affect attachment? How does it affect the psychological processes of transition to the role of mother? During early pregnancy, few women are aware of more than the fact that they are feeling very sick and tired. The fetus is not a person for whom they want to care. Before the USS was available, the fetus became a person when their movements could be felt (quickening). At that point, realization of the reality of motherhood dawned. Ram and Lerman (1993) wanted to determine whether this realization (which they referred to as maternal–fetal attachment in the psychological sense rather than the physiological one) is affected by the early USS. From the sample of 139 women who completed questionnaires, it was found that early USS before or after quickening made no difference to the maternal–fetal attachment.

Verny (1988) wrote extensively about fetal life and what the fetus remembers. He stated that the interactions between the parents and the unborn child have consequences for the personality development of the child. Verny (1988) quotes research by DeCasper, who demonstrated that fetuses recognise their own mother's voice, or pieces of music that are played during uterine life.

Sorenson and Schelke (1999) wanted to know how women fantasised about their unborn child, and whether these fantasies differed according to gestational age and multiparity. A total of 184 completed questionnaires (to the open-ended question that was asked) were returned. Some women wrote full-page descriptions. No definitive pattern emerged from this study to indicate normality or abnormality. The researchers decided that the only aspect of note was that women had started the process of transition to motherhood. When these fantasies start, and what they mean with regard to women's psychological transition to the role of mother, is still unknown.

Major theories

Three theories will be discussed here. Van Gennep (1960) considered transition to be a rite of passage, and proposed a simple model. Reva Rubin (1967a) conducted qualitative research into certain behaviours and the mental processes underpinning them. Rogan *et al.* (1997) investigated the transition to motherhood with focus groups using a grounded theory approach, and they developed a model describing 'change' which has much in common with the models proposed by Rubin (1967a) and Van Gennep (1960).

Van Gennep (1960) describes how a woman exchanges one social status for another. The value of each social status will be debated later in the chapter. The woman starts as an independent person, so the first phase of the process involves separation from her former social status. She is viewed by society as different. The next phase is marginality, when the woman is between socially recognized states. This phase occurs during pregnancy. Obviously the woman starts to look different and to behave differently (perhaps with regard to her diet, alcohol consumption, energy levels and sporting activities). The third stage is that of reincorporation of the woman back into society with an altered social status. She is now a mother and has different responsibilities and priorities. Previously, society regarded her as a wife or a single employed person, but after the process of transition she is seen as neither of these. Society recognizes that her responsibilities have changed, and now changes its view of her value in terms of whether she is employable, intelligent or dependent.

Van Gennep's (1960) 'marginality' phase is considered by western society to be indicative of sexual activity, and as such has great curiosity value and is even a cause of envy for some people. In some societies pregnancy is regarded as shameful and defiling because it demonstrates that the woman has been sexually active. These two contrasting views are dependent on the social values of the culture in which they live with regard to women, pregnancy and sexuality. In one culture, men may regard women as available (or as having been so if they are pregnant) to gratify their sexual drive, whereas in another culture men may regard the sexual drive in women (as demonstrated by pregnancy) as something that needs to be guarded against because it might lead to all kinds of undesirable behaviour. It could be said that men have a poor understanding of women's sexuality, and that therefore the idea of women having a libido can be frightening. In order to control this sexual drive and avoid possibly inexplicable behaviour, men in some cultures try to suppress it or even demonise it. This attitude may be manifested by the practice of female genital mutilation to make women submissive and controllable.

Rubin (1967a) followed five primiparous and four multiparous women through their pregnancies and the first month after birth. She interviewed them on average 12 times during pregnancy and 11 times during the first month after birth, so that the process of transition could be analysed in depth. Three main topic areas emerged, namely the 'taking in' process, the self-system, and operations.

The 'taking in' process (Rubin, 1967b) is a description of how earnestly and sensitively the woman tries to understand the meaning of becoming a mother. Nothing – be it her husband's job, her sister's wedding or medical opinion – is considered relevant to her unless she can link it in some way to her maternal role. The self-system theory suggests concern for the body image, the self-image and the ideal image. The ideal image is not so much concerned with morals but with the capacity to suffer, to endure out of love for another, with gifts and giving, and so on. The self-image sees self as 'here and now' rather than in relation to the previous experiences which constituted the self-image. The body image theory focuses not on physical changes but on the body's ability to accommodate and function. Self-esteem and role achievement or failure are linked to this ability. Operations are the active processes. There are five operational levels, which from the outside inward are mimicry, role play, fantasy, introjection/projection and grief work (*see* Figure 9.1). Finally, after all of these processes have been worked through, role identity is achieved.

Mimicry is the adoption of simple behaviours, from dressing the part to following a myriad of taboos on lifting, eating, buying, and so on. Thus one sees women who have only just become pregnant wearing a maternity dress or bending backwards to see what it feels like before they have to. Role play is less symbolic and more concerned with 'acting out' situations and new role relationships. The woman searches for a young child with whom to establish a

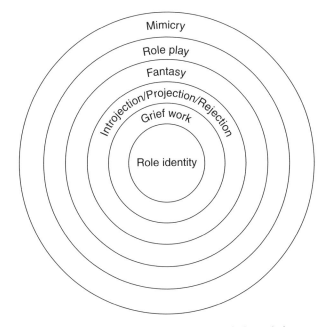

Figure 9.1   Operational level from superficial to deep psychological change.

friendship, to help them, play 'hide and seek' with them, babysit for them or even feed them. In a given situation, fantasy is concerned with the question 'how will it be for me?'. The woman asks other mothers what their labour pains were like, and what they really want to know is whether they will be able to cope or whether they will humiliate themselves by shouting or swearing. Wishes, fears and dreams indicate a deeper involvement in the forthcoming role. Information is gathered in relation to the fantasies. There may be negative fantasies as well as positive ones, and silences, loneliness and darkness may exacerbate these fantasies.

Introjection/projection/rejection refers to the manner in which the mimicry and role playing are internalised to see whether they 'fit' the woman's personality and experience. This is the most important aspect of the model. The woman has been pretending to change nappies according to the way her friends do it. At this stage she must decide for herself whether she will do things the same way. She may reject the way her friend changes nappies because she feels that disposable nappies are environmentally unfriendly. Her experience and personal philosophy have been applied to the mimicry she has been practising. If she decides to follow her role model's way of changing nappies, and that her friend's barrier cream is the most effective type available, then the mimicry and role play are reinforced. Some issues may be talked through in face-to-face conversations with a role model, but the final decision is made silently. When these decisions have been made, the woman can be said to have identified with the role that she had previously been mimicking. She no longer thinks that motherhood is something that happens to other people, but rather that it is something which is going to happen to her, and she will use the present and future tense when speaking about herself.

Grief work involves 'letting go' of a former identity. It is a review of previous attachments and associated events in the former role. Reliance on work colleagues as friends and the fun of going to the pub at lunchtime need to be stopped and grieved for because they are no longer compatible with the woman's new role. Although it is not final, some degree of resolution of the two lifestyles (i.e. that of a paid worker and that of a mother) occurs, and if it does not, there is a marked depression in role taking.

Rubin then discusses the relationship of significant others (e.g. partner and parents) to the above processes. All of the study subjects began the process by using their own mothers as models. Their peers then replaced them. Fantasies were experienced in relation to significant others at home. Husbands and partners were regarded as just that – husbands and partners – rather than as fathers. They were sometimes used not as a reference, but as a support or reinforcement.

A new theory has recently been described by Rogan *et al.* (1997) on the basis of research conducted by Barclay *et al.* (1997). They used nine antenatal focus groups with a total of 55 women to discuss the experience of becoming a mother. They concentrated on the process and after coding and categorizing, they described six stages in the process. 'Realising' occurs when the impact of the life changes that are required becomes fully apparent. Women found reality to be different from their expectation, and reported that being able to narrate their birth experiences repeatedly allowed them to move into the reality. The enormity of the impact caused women to feel unready and unprepared. Being 'drained' refers to the enormous physical, mental and emotional demands that the experience of childbirth makes upon mothers. Change is fundamentally tiring, and sleep is normally used to compensate for and adapt to it, but that is not possible for new mothers. Their lack of confidence and their awareness of the amount that they have to learn leads to the third concept, termed 'alone'. Partners are not always supportive, and new mothers are awake at unsociable hours, so the loneliness is not easily alleviated. 'Unreality' is experienced by many women, and is unaffected by attendance at antenatal classes. 'Loss' in many areas of life is also difficult to rectify. This 'loss' relates to time for partner, friends and oneself, freedom and independence, control over one's own life, and the loss of a sense of self. These losses are not reversed until the baby grows older. The final concept, namely 'working it out', seems to have been experienced by most of the women in the study after a period of time. They felt that they needed resources of personal resilience and assertiveness, and to start to trust their own judgements and feelings rather than expert opinion. This final stage of the process is not reached by all women, and some reasons for and consequences of this will be explored later in the chapter.

This social process that is experienced by so many women occurs as the mother undergoes a major reconstruction of self without being prepared, supported or recognised by society. It is increasingly challenging in contemporary western society (Rogan *et al.*, 1997). According to one feminist writer (Rich, 1976), the absence of social recognition is deliberate and aims to ensure that women remain under male control. The process of transition has been considered to be problematic, and easy transition is unusual (Oakley, 1980; Rogan *et al.*, 1997). Nuclear households which reduce women's contact with the outside world have been blamed for the difficulties in transition, which can result in 'disorientation, depression and despair' (Oakley, 1980; Rubin, 1984).

Dysphoria refers to distressed mood, and is not as serious as 'disorientation, depression and despair'. Dysphoria has been measured by Morse *et al.* (2000) at four stages during the transition process, namely 24 weeks' gestation, 36 weeks' gestation and 1 and 4 months postnatally. The number of women who experienced dysphoria (as measured using a variety of psychological tests) was 19.55% at 24 weeks, rising to 21.6% at 36 weeks before dropping to 14.9% by 4 months postnatally. This rise and fall is the only indication in the literature of the timescale of the transition process, and the only serious indication of the number of mothers for whom it may not be a 'normative stage' in family development. It may well be that if future studies replicate these data, the term 'normative' will need to be redefined and the transition issue addressed more seriously within society.

The experience of giving birth

The physical process of giving birth affects the above psychological and sociological process. The fact that a woman's emotional reaction to motherhood is affected by her delivery and care has been documented (Ball, 1987). Many women consider labour to be a challenge which they are uncertain that they can meet at the end of their first pregnancy. They have preconceived ideas which they have acquired from their mothers and friends, and from reading. Emotionally, relief that labour has started is mixed with fear of the unknown and their reaction to it, and with anticipation of seeing the child. There are insufficient words in the language to describe the psychological depth referred to earlier. In the following scenario, emotional elation and euphoria are poor descriptive words in this writer's experience. 'Within minutes a woman who has experienced natural birth is extremely engaged with her baby, talks to the baby, tries to make eye contact, and feels a happiness that she has not experienced before. What emotional elation and euphoria …' (Righard, 2001: 2). As far as western cultural values are concerned, staying in control is very important, which may explain why there are no accurate words for the 'euphoria'. They may be emotions that are out of control, but whose control? Women may be afraid of 'losing control and making a fool of themselves' (Burke, 1985: 23) by shouting, screaming and swearing. It is thought by this author and others (Burke, 1985) that the current practice of offering epidural analgesia to women who shout adds to a woman's sense of failure if she does 'lose control'. Oakley (1980) found that women who had experienced 'loss of control' were depressed after childbirth.

Another dimension of the 'control' aspect of labour has been described by Righard (2001). She believes that doctors attend normal births because they want to be in control of what is happening. They have the power to prescribe 'lying in bed', induction, Caesarean sections and electronic monitoring. By using these tools they can stay in control. If this is true, it is unlikely that many women will either be in or feel in control. Most women will avoid a power struggle in the delivery suite. Righard's (2001) observations in practice led her to point out that painkilling drugs and epidurals make women passive and that therefore, according to the doctors and some midwives, it is 'easier to have her under control'. Thus it is the emotions of anxiety, fear and intimidation that cause the woman to submit to the doctor's authority. A woman has much debriefing (i.e. telling her story) to do after birth before she can carry on the process of transition to motherhood at the same time as meeting the demands of her infant.

Receiving appropriate support in labour is known to result in a positive experience (Sosa *et al.*, 1980; Klaus *et al.*, 1986; Hofmeyr *et al.*, 1991). Both emotional well-being and the way in which women relate to their babies are affected (Gottlieb, 1978). This researcher found that positive maternal health facilitates attachment. Otamiri *et al.* (1992) looked at the effect of the type of delivery on mother–infant relationships. Women who underwent elective Caesarean sections had more doubts about their ability to care for their babies during the first few days after birth than did the mothers who had experienced vaginal deliveries. After one month the elective Caesarean section mothers were much more 'care-taking' towards their babies than the control group. It may be that the one-month measurement was made when the mothers had physical problems, and that once these were resolved they attempted to compensate for their earlier incapacity.

How traumatic birth may be has not been clearly defined because it relates to how individual women feel. Women used to die in childbirth, but today it is (according to the media) a healthy and joyous experience. Post-traumatic stress disorder (PTSD) is a condition associated with national catastrophes rather than with childbirth! Three studies have looked at childbirth and the potential stress syndrome associated with it. In one study, 6% of women were found to have the condition (Menage, 1993). In a UK study (Ayers and Pickering, 2001), it was found that 2% of women had the disorder at six weeks and 1% had it at six months. It was felt that after six months the incidence was unlikely to decrease further.

In an Australian study (Creedy *et al.*, 2000), one in three women reported a stressful birthing event with three or more traumatic symptoms such as flashbacks, re-experiencing the birth, avoidance and autonomic arousal. In that study, the level of intervention was a strong predictor of traumatic symptoms, a forceps delivery being as traumatic as an emergency Caesarean section. It is felt that after this degree of psychological morbidity, it will take the mother a long time to come to terms with her feelings, and this will need to happen before she can focus her mind on caring for herself and her baby. The transition to motherhood may thus be temporarily but hopefully not permanently suspended.

Postnatal considerations: feelings after childbirth

Anderson *et al.* (1994) measured mood antenatally and postnatally and found a correlation. They measured the desire to seek information about childcare, body image, perception of pain, tolerance and social boredom. These parameters could be used to indicate how far the mother has moved in the transition process. Anderson *et al.* (1994) suggested that if there is a negative response to these variables, then there will be a negative mood postnatally which may give rise to clinical depression or unhappiness. The mood swings were found to be more labile in pregnancy and did not improve until day 28 postnatally. Happiness in the parental relationship was associated with positive mood during pregnancy. Women who were dissatisfied with the appearance of their bodies had a lower tolerance of pain. Added to this psychological stress is cultural stress caused by the media stereotype of what is considered to be an attractive female body, namely a very slender one, which not many healthy pregnant woman can achieve. Another cultural image that women are expected to emulate is that of a fun-filled mother. Anderson *et al.* (1994) did not explore this image. It may be achievable by women who have domestic help and much free time, but not by those who return to paid employment and juggle it with childcare, as the economic climate suggests should be done.

Paradice (1995) points out that postnatal depression is not clearly understood despite being extensively studied, and that it could be a condition which arises in response to the complex life changes and demands that motherhood brings. The claim that it is a normal response is justified by hearing women's observations such as the following: 'a completely new situation', 'never fully prepared', 'not fully aware of the impact on their life', 'exhausted', 'life has changed for ever' and 'no break, even for illness'. Paradice (1995) considers that a pathological condition has been created by perceiving childbirth as a happy and joyous event. This myth that is propagated by society makes it difficult for new mothers to admit they are unhappy. Thus a pathological condition seems to have been caused by a myth. Paradice (1995) does not suggest who is responsible for generating and maintaining the myth, but the media should be named and shamed for imposing this misconception on women. Paradice does want the 'condition' to be regarded as normal so that women's experiences will not continue to be trivialised, and mothering will be acknowledged as the complex and demanding task that it really is. The clinical symptoms of depression may be slight, but the woman feels dysfunctional. As yet there is no terminology apart from a medical one (which Paradice suggests is inaccurate) to describe the condition. Medical treatment may or may not be used. Alternatively, a social management programme may be appropriate, thus taking the problem out of the clinical realm of influence and into the social realm where it truly belongs.

On a more practical level, Ockenden (2000) urges us to respect the postnatal period as an essential interval of time when the new mother needs to recover, rest and come to terms with her new life. In some Moslem, Arabic and African societies, women rest in near isolation for 40 days, during which time they receive special foods and help. In eighteenth-century England women stayed in bed for 28 days after childbirth, but in twenty-first-century England the market economy drives women to return to work. Ockenden also points out that 'Western imagery surrounding motherhood does not match reality' (Ockenden, 2000: 11). Women need realistic care for themselves, partnership with the professional, and above all for motherhood to be regarded as special. Western society is lacking in rituals which promote mothers' mental health. In cultures which do not celebrate the post-partum period, a high incidence of postnatal depression is reported.

Herbert's (1994) research reinforced the work of Rubin (1967), as it found that after birth the transition to motherhood took three months. The problems of being tired, visitors outstaying their welcome and the need to develop a new support network took at least three months to work through. Pridham and Chang (1992) used questionnaires to explore the transition to being a parent and carer. They noticed how the mothers developed and used problem solving to obtain emotional support, feedback on their performance and information. She found that better educated mothers had to be more proactive in their problem solving. They and older women reported less satisfaction with the maternal role.

One could be justified in assuming from the above that mothers' mental health may be impaired. It would be helpful to know whether or not an incomplete process of transition to motherhood has long-term effects. There is very limited literature available in the form of follow-up studies. Walker (1994) conducted a study after 8 to 10 years on 124 mothers (only 77 of whom were available) using a postal survey to assess children's social competence and behavioural problems. When compared with the maternal role indicators measured during the puerperium, there was no strong or clear prediction of the children's competence or behaviour. This finding has not been replicated in other studies.

Older women

Various researchers have used age as a variable in their research with a view to investigating whether age is relevant or affects the process of transition to motherhood. Few researchers have studied older women in their own right, yet the average age at which women start a family is rising. Randell (1993) interviewed 18 married Caucasian women at an average of 13 weeks' gestation. The average age of the women was 34 years (which might not be classed as 'older women' by some authorities). It seems that the women might have experienced problems reconciling their ideal image with their real self. They were uncertain about the way in which work colleagues would view them. Their previous identity as non-pregnant seemed to remain with them, suggesting that for them the pregnancy was not real. Another conflict was that between the need to be responsible and the urge to remain self-centred, and between having a child and being that child's mother. It may be concluded that women in western society are saying that they love their children but they find motherhood difficult. Although this research was informative, because there was no control the question arises as to whether the results would be the same or different if the average age of the women had been 24 years.

The research of Morse *et al.* (2000) into dysphoric moods (distress in antenatal women) showed that women's distressed moods in mid-pregnancy were strongly correlated with younger age and low levels of instrumental (physical) and emotional support from their partners. This suggests that younger women find the transition to motherhood more difficult. Older women's distress levels decreased more quickly during the early postnatal period, suggesting that they managed better than expected. These findings are supported by other research (Gottesman, 1992) which suggests that older women are at lower risk of postnatal depression than younger ones.

There is evidence that older women will require more medical intervention during their pregnancy (Gilbert *et al.*, 1999). Certainly they are at greater risk of having a child with Down's syndrome, but the idea that they will require more intervention gives rise to much debate. There is no doubt that pregnancy for older women is likely to be more stressful. Berryman and Windridge (1993) studied 40 nulliparous women aged 35 years or over, and asked them to complete a Maternal–Fetal Attachment Scale. Each woman was matched with a multiparous woman over 35 years of age and a multiparous woman and a nulliparous woman between 20 and 29 years of age. The unstated question related to whether their self-image was that of a woman having a baby or that of being the child's mother, and whether age made any difference. Was the transition process happening? Berryman and Windridge (1993) found that, for the multiparous mother, age had no effect. For the older nulliparous mother, there was a decreased level of attachment but it was not statistically significant. If this is true, it may be due to the failure of western capitalist society to value the woman as a mother as highly as it did the woman as a wage earner. This would make the transition to motherhood very difficult to achieve. Western society still needs to grapple with this.

Windridge and Berryman (1999) conducted a longitudinal study on 107 women to compare the birth experience and postnatal depression across age bands. The study found no age-related difference with regard to obstetric outcome. The older women were more anxious about their baby's safety, but were not more likely to develop postnatal depression.

Welles-Nystrom (1997) undertook research to examine how influential feminist thought had been with regard to women's perceptions of having children after the age of 35 years. Not all of her findings are relevant to the current topic. However, one minor finding was that American women had a more symptomatic transition to motherhood than did the Swedish women in the study. The term 'symptomatic' was not defined, but seemed to be related to 'off-line transition' behaviour, and it was found that American women over 35 years of age viewed their body changes negatively compared with Swedish women of the same age. The explanation for this was that because these women had timed their reproduction at an abnormal time in their culture, it was inevitable that the transition itself would be unusual. Welles-Nystrom (1997) postulated that the postponement of motherhood results from latent immaturity, a disturbed mother–daughter relationship or rejection of one's feminine identity. The questionnaire that was used in the research indicated that all mothers became attached to their infants with little anxiety (despite antenatal 'off-line' transition behaviour).

Conclusion

Change is part of our lives as a consequence of physical, chronological and professional development. Many girls grow up expecting to become mothers, but they do not understand how much their lives will be affected and the adaptation that they will have to experience (Gibson, 2001). 'New mothers are expected to continue with life as usual – as well as coping with the baby' (Ockenden, 2000: 10). The media dramatically misrepresent women's lives in this area. Why does western culture not recognise that motherhood can be one of the most stressful occupations? Two explanations can be offered for this. The first is that men – who are not usually the main caregivers in early infant life – control the media and cultural practices. Even the most sensitive man cannot understand the intensity of a concept for which language does not have words. For example, there is only one word for 'pain', yet pain due to contractions of labour, pain due to a dental abscess, emotional pain, pain due to terminal illness, pain due to sleep deprivation and the pain of grieving are all different, though this is not apparent in the terminology. However, this view is not well supported.

The second explanation is that the media are controlled. Women rarely exercise this control. There are few rituals and celebrations in western culture that recognise changes in women's lives. This is more of a problem in western society, because other cultures have rituals involving social recognition of women after childbirth. In Britain there used to be 'Churching of Women' after childbirth, but this is no longer practised. In other cultures, women's lives are conducted in less isolation from other women (Yearley, 1997). Understanding and support can be non-verbal, but western society communicates through newspapers, computers and mobile telephones, all means by which non-verbal communication, empathy and support are difficult to express. These means of communication are highly valued in western culture, and were developed by and are controlled by men.

The lack of recognition of the transition to motherhood means that there is no channel by which women can express themselves. In these circumstances, postnatal depression could be interpreted as a normal response (Paradice, 1994) to the buildup of fear, anxiety, responsibility, discomfort, exhilaration and guilt (Burke, 1985). It seems that the lip-service which is currently paid to motherhood must turn into reality before the role conflicts that women experience are to be resolved.

- The transition to motherhood requires psychological adjustment.
- This transition is hindered by the media's idealistic portrayal of the process of becoming a mother.
- Western capitalist society values women as earners and taxpayers rather than as mothers.
- Women are left to work through the conflict of ideas (mother versus wage earner) on their own.
- In western society, motherhood is isolating and conflict can lead to women experiencing poor mental health.

References

- Anderson VN, Fleming AS and Steiner M (1994) Mood and transition to motherhood. *J Reprod Infant Psychol.* **12**: 69–77.
- Ayers S and Pickering AD (2001) Do women get post-traumatic stress disorder as a result of childbirth? A prospective study of incidence. *Birth.* **28**: 111–18.
- Ball J (1987) *Reactions to Motherhood: the role of postnatal care.* Cambridge University Press, Cambridge.
- Barclay L, Everitt L, Rogan F *et al.* (1997) Becoming a mother – an analysis of women's experience of early parenthood. *J Adv Nurs.* **25**: 719–28.
- Berryman JC and Windridge KC (1993) Pregnancy after 35: a preliminary report on maternal–infant attachment. *Infant Psychol.* **11**: 163–74.
- Bonnici T (2001) Davina's darling. *Daily Mail.* **26 September**: 23.
- Burke B (1985) The transition to motherhood. *Nurs Mirror.* **161**: 22–4.
- Chick N and Meleis AI (1986) Transitions: a nursing concern. In: PL Chinn (ed.) *Nursing Research Methodology: issues and implementations.* Aspen, Rockville, MD.
- Creedy DK, Shochet IM and Horsfall J (2000) Childbirth and the development of acute trauma symptoms: incidence and contributing factors. *Birth.* **27**: 104–11.
- Chick N and Meleis AI (1986), Transitions: a nursing concern. In: PL Chinn (ed.) *Nursing Research Methodology: issues and implementations.* Aspen, Rockville, MD.
- Fedele NM, Godling ER, Grossman FK *et al.* (1988) Psychological issues in adjustment to first parenthood. In: GY Michaels and WA Goldberg (eds) *Transition to Parenthood: current theory and* research. Cambridge University Press, New York.
- Gibson J (2001) Motherhood: unrealistic expectations? *Pract Midwife.* **4**: 32–4.
- Gilbert WM, Nesbitt TS and Danielsen B (1999) Childbearing beyond age 40: pregnancy outcome in 20 032 cases. *Obstet Gynecol.* **93**: 9–14.
- Goldberg WA (1988) Perspectives on the transition to parenthood. In: GY Michaels and WA Goldberg (eds) *Transitions to Parenthood: current theory and research.* Cambridge University Press, New York.
- Gottesmann MM (1992) Maternal adaptation during pregnancy among adult early, middle and late childbearers: similarities and differences. *Matern Child Nurs J.* **20**: 93–105.
- Gottlieb L (1978) Maternal attachment in primiparas. *J Obstet Gynecol Nurs.* **7**: 39–43.
- Herbert P (1994) Support of first-time mothers in the three months after birth. *Nurs Times.* **90**: 36–7.
- Hofmeyr GJ, Nikodem VC and Wolman C (1991) Companionship to modify the clinical birth environment: effects on progress and perceptions of labour and breastfeeding. *Br J Obstet Gynaecol.* **98**: 756–64.
- Klaus M, Kennell J and Robertson S (1986) Effects of social support during partition on maternal and infant morbidity. *BMJ.* **293**: 5885–7.
- Larkin V and Bulter M (2000) The implications of rest and sleep following childbirth. *Br J Midwif.* **8**: 438–42.
- Menage J (1993) Post-traumatic stress disorder in women who have undergone obstetric and/or gynecological procedures: a consecutive series of 30 cases of post-traumatic stress disorder. *J Reprod Infant Psychol.* **11**: 221–8.

- Morse CA, Buist A and Durkin S (2000) First-time parenthood: influences on pre- and postnatal adjustment in fathers and mothers. *J Psychosom Obstet Gynecol.* **21**: 109–20.
- Oakley A (1980) *Women Confined. Towards a sociology of childbirth.* Martin Robertson, Oxford.
- Ockenden J (2000) After the birth is over … rest and support for new mothers. *Pract Midwife.* **3**: 10–13.
- Otamiri G, Berg G, Leijon I and Sydsjo G (1992) Mother–infant relationship: effect of mode of delivery. *J Psychosom Obstet Gynaecol.* **13**: 209–22.
- Paradice K (1995) Postnatal depression: a normal response to motherhood? *Br J Midwif.* **3**: 632–5.
- Pridham KF and Chang A (1992) Transition to being the mother of a new infant in the first 2 months: maternal problem solving and self-appraisal. *J Adv Nurs.* **17**: 204–16.
- Ram A and Lerman M (1993) Ultrasound, mother-attachment and the quickening fetus. *Int J Prenatal Psychol Med.* **5**: 127–35.
- Randell BP (1993) Growth versus stability: older primiparous women as a paradigmatic case for persistence. *J Adv Nurs.* **18**: 518–25.
- Rich A (1976) *Of Women Born.* Bantam Books, New York.
- Righard L (2001) Making childbirth a normal process (guest editorial). *Birth.* **28**: 1–4.
- Rogan F, Schmied V, Barclay L *et al.* (1997) Becoming a mother – developing a new theory of early motherhood. *J Adv Nurs.* **25**: 877–85.
- Rooney K (1999) *Encarta World English Dictionary.* Bloomsbury Publishing, London.
- Rubin R (1967a) Attainment of the maternal role. Part I. Processes. *Nurs Res.* **16**: 237–45.
- Rubin R (1967b) Attainment of the maternal role. Part II. Models and referrants. *Nurs Res.* **16**: 342–436.
- Rubin R (1984) *Maternal Identity and Maternal Experience.* Springer, New York.
- Schmied V and Lupton D (2001) Blurring the boundaries: breastfeeding and maternal subjectivity. *Sociol Health Illness.* **23**: 234–50.
- Sorenson DS and Schnelke P (1999) Fantasies of the unborn among pregnant women. *Am J Matern Child Nurs.* **24**: 92–7.
- Sosa R, Kennell J and Klaus M (1980) The effects of a supportive companion on perinatal problems, length of labour and mother–infant interaction. *NEJM.* **303**: 597–600.
- Underdown A (1998) The transition to parenthood. *Br J Midwif.* **6**: 508–11.
- Van Gennep A (1960) *The Rites of Passage.* Routledge and Kegan Paul, London.
- Vehvilainen-Julkunen (1995) Family training: supporting mothers and fathers in the transition to parenthood. *J Adv Nurs.* **22**: 731–7.
- Verny TR (1988) Some aspects of prenatal parenting. *Int J Childbirth Educ.* **3**: 19–20.
- Walker LO (1994) Maternal identity and role attainment: long-term relations to children's development. *Nurs Res.* **43**: 105–10.
- Welles-Nystrom B (1997) The meaning of postponed motherhood for women in the United States and Sweden: aspects of feminism and radial timing strategies. *Health Care Women Int.* **18**: 279–99.

- Windridge KC and Berryman JC (1999) Women's experiences of giving birth after 35. *Birth.* **26**: 16–23.
- Yearley C (1997) Motherhood as a rite of passage: an anthropological perspective. In: J Alexander, V Levy and C Roth (eds) *Midwifery Practice. Core topics 2.* Macmillan, Basingstoke.

CHAPTER 10

Maternal infant attachment

Cathy Rowan

The way you treat your child before birth and after is the way the child
will treat the world. This is the whole truth about primary prevention.
(Professor Fedor Freybergh, cited in Lee, 2000: 5)

This chapter explores some of the theories and characteristics of the nature of
the early relationship between a mother and her baby in relation to attachment behaviour. Some of the implications for midwifery practice are discussed,
including the possible effects of antenatal screening tests, the type of birth and
the effects of early separation if the baby requires special care. The implications for babies whose mothers are depressed are considered, and although no
firm conclusions can be drawn, a baby whose mother is depressed may be
affected by his or her mother's mood. Early detection and appropriate care for
these women may be important, as well as helping to facilitate the relationship
and enable the mother to understand her baby's behaviour. The woman's own
experience of mothering may affect the way in which she relates to her baby,
and in cases where difficulties are evident specialist support may be beneficial.

Introduction

The attachment relationship between mother and baby is important not only for
the physical survival of the baby in terms of the provision of food, warmth and
shelter, but also for his or her psychological well-being and development. Several
theories have been suggested that have different implications for mothers and
babies. Most would agree that the relationship which a child forms with its
primary caregiver in the first year of life is a key part of the infant's psychological
development and has implications for their future relationships, affecting their
responsiveness to others and to their own children if they become parents. Adams
and Cotgrove (1995) suggest that these patterns are established by one year of age.
Attachment between the mother and baby may begin prior to conception when the
mother is contemplating pregnancy, and it develops during pregnancy, when
the woman is coming to terms with being a mother.

Midwives and healthcare professionals are in a prime position to facilitate the
development of a positive relationship between the mother and her baby, and to
identify and support those women who may be at risk of developing difficulties in
the relationship with their baby. This chapter will examine current understanding

of maternal infant attachment and the factors which may affect this, and will discuss the implications for midwifery practice.

Mother–infant attachment: some theoretical approaches

Much has been written about the significance of early attachment between a mother and her baby, although there is not always a clear consensus. Rousseau, an eighteenth-century French writer and philosopher, was the first to use the concept of attachment in relation to the mother–infant relationship. Bowlby (1969) defined attachment as a strong affectional tie between two people, usually an infant and their mother, which develops during the first 18 months of life. Later (Bowlby, 1988) he identified the first 9 months of life as significant. Klaus and Kennell (1982) stated that the first few moments after birth are an important 'sensitive period' during which a woman is hormonally primed to accept her infant. The focus was on the mother's perspective of the attachment relationship. They found that mothers who had an extra 16 hours of contact with the baby after birth showed better mothering skills and their infant performed better on developmental skills than others who did not have this extra contact. Brazelton (1963) and Gay (1981) proposed that attachment is a mutual relationship in which both mother and child contribute, and that it takes time to develop. It is characterised by a strong orientation to each other, discriminative abilities and a desire or need to maintain proximity and contact. The pleasure and synchrony in the interaction serve as catalysts for further exploration of the relationship and its evolution towards a durable attachment (Brazelton and Cramer, 1991).

The original idea of maternal fetal attachment in humans developed from ethnological data from a variety of animal observations which suggested that there is a species-specific maternal behaviour prior to, during and immediately after birth that leads to the mother's attachment to her offspring. In animals, early removal of the offspring after parturition results in a loss of maternal behaviour. For example, a mother goat will not accept her kid if it is removed from her for more than two hours before it is one hour old. However, if five minutes of contact are allowed after birth, virtually all young are reaccepted even after three hours (Klopfer, 1971). It has been demonstrated in sheep that the longer the period of 'togetherness' before separation, the more likely it is that the mother will continue to display maternal behaviour towards her offspring after reintroduction. Poindron and Le Neindre (1979) found among sheep that when separation begins at birth and lasts for 12–24 hours, 25% of lambs are accepted by their mothers. In contrast, if a 24-hour separation begins two to four days after parturition, all ewes will reaccept their lambs. Klaus and Kennell (1982) postulated that human mothers may also perhaps show species-specific behaviours that facilitate attachment to the infant, but it is uncertain whether observations from animal behaviour can be extrapolated to humans. In an Israeli hospital, after two mothers had accidentally taken home each other's babies they were reluctant to give them up when the error was discovered at the two-week check (Klaus and Kennell, 1982).

However, the significance of the early period after birth in humans has been debated. In the 1980s, the findings of Klaus and Kennell were met with considerable criticism to the effect that the research methods were flawed, having been inspired by work with animals (Eyer, 1992). However, Korsch (1983) suggested that the critics of the bonding research were reacting as much to the exaggerated practices that had been triggered by Klaus and Kennell's work as to the research ideas. Klaus and Kennell later adapted their views, making it clear that the human experience is much less influential, and that although the early postpartum experience is significant, it is not nearly such a critical period as in animals.

Characteristics

The basis of the infant–mother attachment is thought to be biological, in that biologically determined behaviour is triggered by danger or anticipated danger to the infant, to which the infant responds by seeking greater proximity to its primary caregiver (Adams and Cotgrove, 1995). This elicits care. When the threat is resolved, the infant returns to exploration. The process is geared towards saving and maintaining life and enhancing the survival of the species. As a result of these early interactions, the child predicts and anticipates responses and develops internalised representations of these key relationships, behaving towards others in a way which has been learned. Depending on the way in which a mother responds when her infant is frightened or needs to be comforted, and how consistently she is sensitive or insensitive to her infant's needs, the infant will learn what to expect from her and other people (Gutbrod, 1999).

The maintenance of proximity between mother and baby is considered to be a requirement for the development of attachment. Early and extensive contact enables the parents to become acquainted with their infant. Feeding, embracing, rocking and maintaining prolonged visual contact foster the development of an affective tie. Seeking and maintaining proximity arouses feelings of love, security and joy (Karen, 1994). Parents who develop sensitivity in recognising the particular ways in which the infant communicates will respond appropriately by smiling, vocalising, touching and kissing until the infant signals the need to end it. By learning to decode the infant's language the parents can synchronise themselves with their baby so as to maintain certain states for longer periods of time (Brazelton and Cramer, 1991). After birth, newborns will synchronise their movements to the rhythm of a mother's voice, who in turn adapts her speech to the response that she perceives from the baby. Parents learn to rely on these responses from the infant as guides to their own behaviour. This interaction enables the infant to develop a sense of him- or herself as a separate person. Thus this sense of identity is developed from the way in which the child perceives him- or herself as a result of the mother's interactions with him or her.

A mother who has sufficient capacity for reflective self-functioning is able to consider her own mental state as well as that of her infant. This will enable her to think about the infant's internal state as separate from her own. When the infant is distressed, she will be able to respond with understanding. A mother may mirror or reflect the child's anxiety. This perception organises the child's experience and they begin to know what they are feeling. Thus the infant learns that their internal feelings are understandable and tolerable (Fonagy and Target, 1997). A mother who is unable to reflect on the infant's mind as independent from her own will be unable to provide containment when the infant is distressed, thus increasing his or her anxiety. This can lead to psychological difficulties for the child later.

Klein, a psychoanalyst, stated that infants are capable of relating to figures which are identified as separate from the self at birth, and that psychological development involves the taking into the mind from outside to create 'internal objects'. This view is supported by the work of infant researchers such as Stern (1985). Each individual lives with their own version of the world coloured by models or representations that they carry in their own mind from parental figures. Klein describes the baby's experiences as 'good' (e.g. being fed and nourished) or 'bad' (e.g. being hungry or upset). During the early months the boundaries between the baby and the mother become clearer, and by about six months the child begins to suspect that these good and bad experiences are caused by the same person. The baby needs to integrate these feelings and find a balance where the mother can be both loved and hated. The infant requires a sensitive and emotionally containing caregiver if they are to develop their own capacities to contain and assimilate experiences and feelings (Bion, 1967). If this does not occur, defence mechanisms may begin to operate, disrupting the experience of self. Subsequently, the mother and later the world may be experienced as either ideal or malign.

For mother–infant attachment to be facilitated, there needs to be emotional availability of the caregiver, emotional warmth, support-sensitive responses, appropriate stimulation, prompt responsiveness to stress, consistency over time and interactional synchrony and mutuality in the interaction (Belsky et al., 1995). Sufficient space and the ability to detach at the appropriate stage of development of the infant constitute an authentic sign of a secure attachment. A mother's most effective technique for maintaining an interaction seems to be sensitivity to her infant's capacity for attention and need for withdrawal. Infants also differ from each other. Some babies may be difficult to understand, some may take a long time to respond, and some may over-react to stimuli and react negatively with relentless crying. Parents may feel shut out or ineffective, which may have the effect of increasing their anxiety. Parents and babies need to develop an understanding of each other, and some parents may need help to understand their baby and his or her responses (Brazelton and Cramer, 1991). It may be helpful if the midwife demonstrates to the mother the ways in which the baby is demonstrating his or her ability to communicate with the mother by highlighting his or her body language.

In 1978, Ainsworth et al. developed what became known as the 'strange situation' for assessing attachment security in 12- to 18-month-old children. Parents, their infants and an experimenter were involved in separation and reunion episodes in order to cultivate attachment behaviours. Infants were classified according to how they responded to their parents during separation and especially upon reunion.

Infants who showed separation anxiety but were happy to be reunited with their parents were termed secure. Insecure infants were those who showed distress during separation and ignored their parent upon reunion, and those who were extremely distressed during separation and unable to be comforted (Gutbrod, 1999). It is as if children evolve attachment patterns that are optimal for ensuring their survival in that environment (Thompson and Calkins, 1996). However, such strategies of emotional regulation may make the adult or child very vulnerable and lead to psychological difficulties later. Moreover, focusing on the strange situation as a measure of attachment behaviour ignores the possible influence of temperament and the child's familiarity with separations.

Within the scientific literature pertaining to attachment, very few factors have been singled out as being significantly associated with the development of a strong link between parents and their baby. Much that has been written adopts a largely white, middle-class view of motherhood. However, regardless of different parenting styles, which may vary according to historical period and culture, children have grown and developed normally. Tizard (1991) states that a child's relationship with his or her mother is only one of a number of significant relationships that are established in childhood. He also argues that children are resilient and have the ability to overcome the ill effects of negative periods in their development.

It may be that the infant has the capacity to interact and form bonds with more than one person (Bowlby, 1969; Brazelton and Cramer, 1991). Families, too, share working models of how to behave, and Byng Hall (1991) terms these 'family scripts'. Children may therefore be able to view their whole family (rather than just their mother or father) as a secure base from which to explore their environment, secure in the knowledge that they can seek proximity and reassurance at times of stress.

Attachment in pregnancy

The relationship between the mother and her baby begins in pregnancy or even before the child is conceived, when the woman has ideas of what her child may be like. During the first stage of pregnancy, the woman is coming to terms with becoming a mother, and parents usually look forward to becoming attached to their infant before his or her birth. Some of the mother's feelings about the baby will depend on her individual situation and whether she has the support of her partner. Cranley et al. (1983) found an association between maternal attachment scores and level of social support. There is a growing awareness of the baby in the uterus as a separate individual, which usually starts with quickening. From the baby's point of view, he or she may become aware of the sounds, activities and rhythms of the mother's world prior to birth.

The experience of screening and diagnostic tests for fetal abnormalities may have a complex effect on the woman's feelings about her baby. A positive association between attachment during pregnancy and the presence of fetal activity and ultrasound movements has been demonstrated by Heidrich and Cranley (1989). Lumley (1990) suggests that scans performed early in pregnancy may slightly improve maternal fetal bonding, but those performed after quickening are not associated with attachment. Ram et al. (1993) suggested that ultrasound examination during pregnancy was associated with a significant increase in maternal fetal attachment, but that this change was mainly due to the effect of ultrasound scanning on women who had experienced quickening before the scan. There was no difference in attachment scores in the subgroup of women who had not experienced quickening prior to the scan. Short-term positive effects on maternal health behaviour, such as a reduction in smoking, have been detected when detailed information was given during the scan (Reading et al., 1982). Hyde (1986) confirmed the anxiety-allaying effect of ultrasound scans, but reported that not all women found them reassuring. Lumley (1990) suggested that maternal anxiety may be increased by scanning and then allayed by positive feedback. A trial by Kemp and Page (1987) found a significant association between ultrasound scans and attachment, although this was much smaller than the association of attachment with the presence of fetal movement. The study did not specify the timing of the ultrasound scans. Some parents may be disappointed when they discover the sex of the baby. The work of attachment takes time, and early attempts to consolidate it may be rejected (Brazelton and Cramer, 1991). Kemp and Page (1987) concluded that ultrasound scans may hasten but do not substantially alter the development of attachment in the long term, although the skill and communication of the operator may affect the mother's perceptions.

The midwifery literature reflects an increasing awareness of the psychological costs of screening (Grayson, 1996; Massey-Davis, 1998). Although screening tests for fetal abnormalities may be reassuring for some women, the resultant anxieties may postpone the maternal fetal attachment process during the antenatal period. Care that focuses on potential abnormalities may undermine a woman's knowledge and her confidence in her ability to produce a fit and healthy baby. Statham and Green (1993) described the psychological effects, such as increased anxiety, experienced by women who receive a result that indicates increased risk. In the study by Fairgreave (1997) of women at greater risk of having a baby with an abnormality, 89.4% of women expressed worry or apprehension prior to the results of amniocentesis. For the remainder of the pregnancy, 14% of the women constantly worried and 44.7% occasionally worried. Farrant (1980) commented that while they were waiting for the results, women smoked more and took tranquillisers. Green et al. (1996) found that women who received a false-positive result continued to show raised anxiety levels during pregnancy, even when subsequent diagnostic tests showed that there was no problem. A lack of privacy, confidentiality or sensitivity in relaying test results can also cause distress.

Concern has now been expressed about the possible psychological, emotional and physical effects of prenatal experiences on postnatal life (Lee, 2000). Some degree of anxiety may be a normal part of pregnancy, but increased anxiety levels may be harmful. Teixeira et al. (1999) showed an association between maternal anxiety in pregnancy and increased uterine artery resistance index, suggesting a mechanism whereby the psychological state of the mother may affect fetal growth and development. Hall et al. (2000) found that mothers who were given a false-negative result had higher parenting stress levels and more negative attitudes towards their children, and had a greater tendency to blame others, than those who declined the test. They suggested that a false-negative result seems to have a small adverse effect on parental adjustment which is evident from two to six years. The false-positive test can make a woman detach from her baby as a means of coping should she need to terminate the pregnancy (Lawrence, 1999). For example, if further tests prove that the baby does not have Down's syndrome, such mothers may have great difficulty in reforming an emotional attachment to their unborn baby. Robinson (2001) has postulated that the unborn child could be sensitive to the temporary rejection by its mother which is brought about by prenatal screening, and that this could have an ongoing effect. If the uterus is becoming an insecure place for the baby to be, one of the consequences could be suppressed anger in the unborn child (Lee, 2000).

The offer of screening tests and their acceptance by the mother can lead to some distressing findings, and mothers need to be informed that the tests have limitations as well as benefits. Professionals need up-to-date information and also skills in developing a more facilitative style of counselling to improve the mother's understanding. They need to be able to recognise and refer those women who may be unsure or anxious about the test, and who need help to explore the implications for themselves in more depth.

Parent education may provide opportunities for pregnant women to share their experiences, which may help to reduce some of their anxiety. Rosser (1999) suggests that pregnant women should be offered opportunities to enjoy themselves in pregnancy, such as yoga or aquanatal classes. Michel Odent advocated weekly singing groups!

The effect of labour

The mother's active participation and involvement during labour set the stage for the reception of the baby at birth. Emotional support during labour, analgesia, interventions, episiotomies and instrumental delivery may all affect the mother's state postnatally and do not allow her the maximum opportunity to feed, feel and hold her baby (Hillan, 1992b). If opiate analgesia is given to the mother during labour, this may affect both the responsiveness of the baby after birth and the ability of the mother to adjust to the baby (Belsey *et al.*, 1981). Redshaw (1982) suggests that it may be the mother's lack of participation in the care of her baby immediately after birth which contributes to the psychological separation of mother and baby that has been ascribed to analgesia given during labour.

Home birth may offer the optimal setting for early bonding to occur. The familiar, safe and relaxed environment, with little or no intervention, allows natural attachment processes to take place immediately after birth. Stevenson (1997) states that it is often at the time of the birth that the mother has a spontaneous, automatic, overwhelming feeling of love and protectiveness towards her new baby, particularly in the first hour after birth, and it is important for her to see and touch the baby. Bonding between parents and their infants can be enhanced by giving them the opportunity to feed, feel and hold their baby after birth, when the baby is often wide awake, settled, calm and interested in his or her surroundings. Within minutes the baby can show his or her preference for contact with people rather than with objects. The baby will turn their head to the sound of someone's voice, and will also be attracted to faces (Murray and Andrews, 2000). It has been suggested that early contact influences the way in which the mother interacts with her infant throughout the first year of life.

The performance of Caesarean section will inevitably influence the amount of contact that the mother has with her baby immediately after delivery, and reactions are likely to be affected by the stress associated with the operation. A large study (Hillan, 1992a) found that morbidity among women following a Caesarean birth included tiredness, backache, headaches, sleeping difficulties and depression. It is difficult to determine the effect of Caesarean birth on the mother–baby relationship. Hillan (1992b) compared 50 primigravid women who gave birth by Caesarean section with 50 women who delivered vaginally by collecting data from interviews on day 3 or 4 postnatally and again 6 months after the birth. She found that women who delivered by Caesarean section took significantly longer than those who gave birth vaginally to feel close to their infants, and these differences persisted for several months after the birth. Only 43% of mothers stated that they felt close to the baby immediately, compared with 64% in the control group. Cranley *et al.* (1983) found that by two months there was still a difference. Those women who had had a Caesarean birth did not feel as close to the baby. Among those who had

had an emergency Caesarean section as opposed to an elective one the problem seemed to be worse. It may be that a period of physical and emotional 'self-repair' following any traumatic birth makes the mother less available to her infant. After a long and difficult labour she may have feelings of rejection and resentment which she may find difficult to acknowledge.

However, it is difficult to draw firm conclusions from these studies, and for some mothers maternal affection may be lacking after any form of birth. Some of the effects of a Caesarean section may be mitigated by preparation. A woman who has read about it, discussed and prepared herself may feel very differently to a woman who was faced with a rapid decision after a long labour. Cranley *et al.* (1983) suggested that women who have regional analgesia and remain conscious throughout the procedure feel more in control of their situation and benefit from early parent–infant contact. The midwife is in a key position to promote early contact between mother and baby, whatever the type of birth. It may help some women if they are given the opportunity to clarify any confusion, reconstruct their experiences and express their feelings, which may facilitate adjustment during the postnatal period.

The infant who requires special care

Early and prolonged separation of the mother from her baby may hamper the attachment process and play a part in later parenting difficulties. Many studies have highlighted the fact that a lengthy stay in the neonatal intensive-care unit denies the mother a close relationship with her infant, which may jeopardise the development of attachment (Dormire *et al.*, 1989; Coffman, 1992). The mother's confidence and self-esteem may be shattered by feelings of inadequacy because she could not achieve a full-term pregnancy, and a premature infant has limited abilities to show a response to parental love. Fear of the baby dying as well as the presence of incubators and other technology can have a negative effect on the bonding process. Dawson (1994) found that parents may become overwhelmed by the noise, monitors and flashing lights and be unable to focus on their infant. Hunter *et al.* (1978) found an eightfold increase in the incidence of maltreatment for premature and ill newborns.

If the baby has a defect or a malformation, the formation of an attachment can be difficult because the parents are going through a grieving process for their 'perfect' child, and they may also feel guilty. On the other hand, increased contact with the infant has been associated with increased attachment behaviours (Norr *et al.*, 1989). Good social support may aid positive maternal role function (Bass, 1991). Providing information and helping the parents to develop caregiving skills are also important. Attempts to support parents whose baby is born prematurely and to facilitate the development of the early attachment have been shown to produce positive results (Meyer *et al.*, 1994; Als, 1997).

As mentioned previously, the evidence for an extremely short 'critical' period in human parents is inconclusive, and the guilt and anxiety generated by this belief may be an unnecessary burden on parents. Infants and their parents are considerably more resilient and flexible than they are often given credit for, as is evidenced by their ability to cope with very different experiences of birth. Although a

Caesarean birth or preterm delivery may cause some problems, this does not necessarily mean that the relationship between the mother and her infant is permanently affected or that the child will experience emotional difficulties later (Redshaw, 1982).

Infants of depressed mothers

Infants are prepared for an environment of human care and are highly sensitive to the quality of their interpersonal contacts, demonstrating sensitivity to the emotional states of others (Murray, 1992). They come into the world ready to respond to people. An association has been found between depression in the mother and insecure attachments (Martins and Gaffan, 2000). Murray and Trevarthen (1985) demonstrated that when the mother was interacting with her infant normally, the baby responded with positive emotions, by smiling and adopting a relaxed posture. If the mother had an expressionless face, as she might do if she was feeling unhappy or depressed, the relaxed expression of the baby faded. Tronick *et al.* (1986) asked the mothers in their sample to act as if they were depressed. The mothers still talked to their infants, but their interaction was less lively. The researchers reported that the infants also began to look depressed. Murray and Stein (1989) found that if mothers maintained a blank facial expression, the babies initially protested, then became distressed and eventually withdrew. When the babies became disappointed and withdrawn, the mothers became agitated and depressed as well (Brazelton and Cramer, 1991). Thus it would seem that the emotional state of either the mother or the baby will affect the other in turn.

Mothers who are depressed may create insecure attachments to their infant (Byng Hall, 1991) because they often cause a violation of their baby's expectancy. When they are able to interact normally, they set up expectancy in the babies. Their later withdrawal leaves the baby in a state of depression and hopelessness, confused by the contradiction. Field (1984) found that the behaviour of the infant appeared to mirror that of the mother. Cohn *et al.* (1990) studied a cohort of depressed and non-depressed mother–infant dyads and found that depression had a negative influence on the behaviour of both. Studies on the impact of postnatal depression on the mother–child relationship have shown that depressed women have difficulties in sensitively attuning their responses to the infant and in keeping their infant's experience in mind, rather than being preoccupied with their own concerns. Murray (1992) studied women with a previous history of depression and a control group followed up to 18 months, and found that infants of postnatally depressed mothers performed less well on object concept tasks, and showed mild behavioural difficulties and more insecure attachments.

A number of studies have assessed the longer-term impact of maternal depression by interviewing the mother later about the child's current behaviour (Williams and Carmichael, 1985; Caplan *et al.*, 1989). However, these studies have methodological limitations and yielded inconsistent findings. The balance of evidence suggests that although mild levels of difficulty may be evident, serious behavioural disturbances are not a significant consequence of postnatal depression (Murray and Stein, 1989). However, in a four-year follow-up of a postpartum sample, Cogill *et al.* (1986) found that children of postpartum depressed mothers were significantly delayed in terms of cognitive development compared with controls. Stein *et al.* (1991) found that at 19 months, mother–infant interactions were less effectively positive and less mutually responsive in cases where the mother had suffered from depression during the postnatal period than in cases where the mother had not been depressed. Murray *et al.* (1999) found that there were more behavioural disturbances at home and less creative play when the child was five years of age if the mother had been depressed, and there was an increase in difficulties for the child at school (Sinclair and Murray, 1998). Carter *et al.* (2001) found that boys were at greater risk of being affected by maternal depressive symptoms than girls, but they suggest that caution is needed in interpreting these findings. The results with regard to the remission from depression on interaction are inconclusive. Stein *et al.* (1991) found that poor interaction was present at 19 months regardless of whether the depression had remitted by then. However, Campbell *et al.* (1995) found that the characteristics in remitted mothers were better than those in still depressed mothers at 6 months.

Holden *et al.* (1989) observed a considerable improvement in maternal mood in women who were treated over eight weekly sessions by health visitors trained in non-directive counselling. Seeley *et al.* (1996) demonstrated the benefits of increased health visitor intervention following specific training in cognitive behavioural counselling skills. The difficulties experienced and relationship problems were significantly less in the group which had received additional input from the health visitor. Antidepressant medication may also be effective, but the majority of women are likely to prefer 'talking' therapy (Chilvers, 2001). Murray (1992) concluded that even if postnatally depressed mothers recover from their depression within the first three months, this does not bring about an improvement in the mother–infant relationship, and that the focus on therapeutic intervention should extend beyond maternal depressive symptoms to the infant–mother relationship. However, there may be other causal factors with regard to mood disorder, such as difficult social circumstances in terms of poverty or loneliness. Maternal and infant characteristics may also interact. Maternal depressive symptoms, if combined with vulnerabilities in the baby (e.g. premature birth), may increase a child's risk of developing unfavourable patterns of attachment (Poehlmann and Fiese, 2001).

Little information is available on the impact of more comprehensive treatment approaches on the longer-term outcome of mothers and babies. Psychotherapy has been shown to change a mother's depressive behaviour, with beneficial effects on the child (Teti and Gefland, 1997). Cramer *et al.* (1990) used a psychodynamic treatment to focus on the mother's internal representation of the baby in her mind, and to explore the links with the mother's unresolved conflicts in relation to her own childhood. This approach has shown promising results.

The leading cause of maternal death today is suicide (Lewis, 2001). Women with a past history of mental illness (puerperal or non-puerperal) face a risk of recurrence of between one in two and one in three following birth. Staff, including midwives, often underestimate symptoms of depression or psychosis. It was found that half of all women who died from psychiatric illness in the postnatal period had a previous history of mental illness (Lewis, 2001). The report recommends that 'a relatively simple procedure should be instituted in every antenatal clinic to identify women at risk of postnatal psychiatric illness and/or self-harm'.

The relevance of the mother's own experience of attachment

It is believed that parents' own attachment experiences in childhood influence their internal model of attachment as adults, which in turn influences whether their infant develops a secure or insecure attachment relationship with them (Bowlby, 1988). A study by Fonagy *et al.* (1991) of 100 women showed that the mother's account of her childhood may be an indicator of subsequent attachment behaviour with her own children. Steele *et al.* (1996) interviewed mothers during pregnancy about their childhood attachment and were able to predict quite accurately which mothers would have an insecurely attached child 15 months later. Brazelton and Cramer (1991) suggest that mothers can tolerate the tremendous selfishness of babies because, in caring for them, they are vicariously satisfying their own selfish needs and wishes, and that these energise a woman's capacity to mother and nurture and set the stage for attachment to the baby.

However, if the mother's dependency needs are too great (e.g. if she is very young), she may regard her baby as a rival, she may treat him or her as an envied sibling, and mothering may seem very difficult. Parents may re-establish old patterns of the past (positive or negative) through their children. Some children may be viewed as a replacement parent. Unresolved loss or mourning can be projected on to the newborn and expressed as an obsessive fear that the child will die. Family therapy may help to identify and resolve some of these issues. However, if the mother can regain or retain access to unhappy memories and reprocess them in such a way that she can come to terms with them, she will be just as able to respond to her child as a woman whose childhood was happy (Bowlby, 1988). Fonagy *et al.* (1997) concluded that individuals who have overcome adversity from their childhood have broken the inter-generational transmission of insecurity.

Life events

Life events and stresses will also influence the mother, and even the most securely attached mother may become highly stressed in difficult circumstances (e.g. poverty, bereavement, difficult relationships). The mother's stress levels may have a negative effect on the child's well-being and sense of security (Belsky *et al.*, 1995). There may also be a number of contextual variables which may affect the infant's emotional well-being, such as the mother's personality, the infant's temperament, the quality of the relationship with her partner and social support, as well as the relationship between work and family. However, significant characteristics of the infant's emotionality (e.g. irritability) can be substantially modified by the mother's behaviour and personality, as well as by the quality of the relationship between the mother and her partner (Nachmias *et al.*, 1996). Women who receive strong support from a partner may be more responsive to their infants.

Women from families where one or both parents had died have been shown to interact significantly less with their 20-week-old babies (Hall *et al.*, 1980). Mothers who feel unsupported and those from a difficult family background or whose pregnancy was unwanted may be particularly vulnerable. A parent who has ambivalent feelings about their child may give inconsistent messages to the infant, which may lead the child to feel that its world is unpredictable and insecure.

Vulnerable parents may also include substance abusers, teenage mothers and those with a learning disability. Insecure attachments are considered to increase internalised feelings of helplessness and low self-esteem, which are linked to depression in adults.

Attachment and the effects of fertility treatment

Individuals who are undergoing treatment for infertility are known to experience physical pain and psychological distress, and adoption procedures can be prolonged and emotionally stressful. Holditch-Davis *et al.* (1998) examined the early parent–infant interactions in infertile couples who became parents through pregnancy or adoption. Two groups of infertile couples (30 couples who achieved pregnancy and 21 couples who adopted, and a group of 19 couples without fertility problems) were observed interacting with their babies 7 days and 21 days after the birth (or adoption) and a week later. The behaviours of the mother, father and infant were recorded. The findings suggest that neither infertility nor adoption *per se* impairs early parenting, but additional research is needed to determine whether the experience of infertility and adoption might have a greater impact as the child matures. It may also be useful to explore the effect of particular fertility treatments and the length of time spent trying for a child, and the effect of different types of adoptions. McMahon *et al.* (1999) found that IVF mothers were more anxious and talked less to their unborn child, but also reported positive idealised attitudes to pregnancy. Previous studies did not find any difference compared with control mothers on self-reports of attachment to their unborn babies (McMahon *et al.*, 1997a), or any differences in maternal sensitivity at 4 months postpartum (McMahon *et al.*, 1997b). In their pilot study, Dunnington and Glazer (1991) found that previously infertile mothers had lower postpartum maternal identity scores and less self-confidence in performing mothering tasks. However, Gibson *et al.* (2000) found no evidence that the early anxieties and concerns of IVF mothers translated into negative socio-emotional sequelae for their relationship with their infants at 12 months of age.

The issues with regard to surrogacy are more complex. Although the Surrogacy Arrangements Act (1995) makes commercial surrogacy illegal, non-commercial and privately arranged surrocacy is legal. It is speculated that surrogate mothers do have attachment feelings for their fetus, and that giving up the baby could be difficult and emotionally damaging, and for some mothers impossible (Winston, 1994). However, it may be that the surrogate mother is able to dismiss her feelings of attachment (Smith, 1998). Furthermore, it may be easier to hand over the child after birth because of the lack of a genetic connection (Singer and Wells, 1984). A study by Snowdon (1994) found that it was more difficult for the surrogate to give up the baby if it was her own ovum, and that gestational surrogacy was less of a bond. However, other researchers suggest that many surrogate mothers deny their true feelings (Fischer and Gillman, 1991). Chestler (1988) warns that surrogates tend to exhibit a high degree of dissociation from their feelings, their bodies and reality. It is clearly important that there is adequate support, counselling and monitoring of surrogacy arrangements. Midwives need to be aware both of their own feelings and of the fact that the feelings of the surrogate may be unpredictable.

With regard to the parents of children conceived as a result of surrogacy arrangements, Snowdon (1994) found that genetic and gestational connections mean different things to different women, and that it is the emotional investment a woman has in pregnancy that is of consequence. For some, the genetic link was not crucial in defining the relationship to a child. Another finding was that adoption was more balanced because the child would not be genetically linked to either partner.

Promoting the mother–baby relationship

If a mother is finding it difficult to relate to her baby, it cannot be concluded from the available research that there will be lasting negative consequences for the child. However, it is clear that babies come into the world ready and willing to be sociable, and they seem to enjoy interacting with people. There is some evidence that the quality of early relationships may have later consequences for cognitive, emotional and social development. Helping parents to recognise the potential of their baby may help them to realise that there is a point in interacting with their baby (Paradice, 1993). Promoting early contact between the mother and baby at birth by giving them time together and keeping the baby with the mother during the postnatal period is helpful. It may also be useful to emphasise the importance of parental response to infant cues, and to highlight the infant's abilities and his or her attempts to communicate (e.g. through smiling and eye contact).

What might seem at first glance to be random and confused infant behaviour is in fact highly organised. The most dramatic of the baby's abilities, even in the first weeks of life, are his or her social responses. By watching the subtle changing pattern of a baby's expression and movement, and by appreciating the significance of these cues, parents can become aware of the richness of the baby's experience and can be guided to help their infant (Murray and Andrews, 2000). Tiny babies as young as half an hour old can copy facial gestures such as tongue protrusion (Meltzoff and Moore, 1977). Infants seem to quickly recognise and prefer aspects of their mother or primary caretaker, such as her voice and her face (Field and Fox, 1985). Face-to-face play with babies in the second and third months can seem like a musical duet where the baby's initiative is taken up by the parent who, quite unconsciously, mirrors and develops the baby's original communication.

Babies are also attracted to particular types of visual stimulation, as well as to people's faces. They will look intently at patterns that have strong clear contrasts. The optimum distance for them to focus is 22 cm. Mothers can be made aware of the various ways in which the baby is communicating with them. Giving care that is sensitive to the baby's unique signals, reliable and predictably structured will help the baby to build up a sense of a familiar world where events can be anticipated, and in which minor delays and difficulties can be more easily tolerated.

Conclusion

It may be concluded that early contact does seem to facilitate mother–infant attachment under certain conditions with certain groups of individuals. Because of the subtleties of the behaviours involved, socio-economic status, age, feeding methods, behaviour of the baby and so on, it is not possible to make generalisations. The ability of the mother to develop a healthy relationship with her baby will be influenced by many factors, extending back to the relationship which the mother had with her own parents. Our ideas about the nature of the relationship between mother and baby are also shaped by our culture, and there are many dimensions to the nurturing of children. Focusing on the early bonding experience may over-simplifiy complex issues and put unnecessary blame on the mother.

However, it may be that in stressful or traumatic circumstances the child who feels insecure may be more vulnerable to emotional difficulties, have low self-esteem and find it difficult to trust others. Early interventions by healthcare professionals may help to prevent the formation of insecure attachment patterns in some women and increase the likelihood of transmission of secure attachments across the generations (Adams and Cotgrove, 1995). Working in partnership with mothers, considering the way in which screening tests are presented, providing flexible and humane care during labour and promoting early contact with the baby may be beneficial to the developing relationship between mother and baby. It may also be appropriate not to insist that there is only one way to care for the baby, in order to avoid lowering the mother's self-esteem and confidence.

It is important to acknowledge that some women never themselves experienced quality mothering or secure attachment as children. For them, the task of mothering may seem overwhelming and highly frustrating and they may need extra support. It may be possible to identify those at risk of postnatal depression before delivery (e.g. those with a poor partnership/marital relationship, social and economic stress or a previous psychiatric history). O'Hara (1997) found that mothers who are experiencing negative life events are more likely to become depressed. Paying close attention to vulnerable mothers during the postnatal period may be important. Facilitating early contact after birth and helping the mother to understand the ways in which the baby is attempting to communicate with her may promote the development of a healthy relationship. Extra support may range from increased education, extra visits, recognising and reducing stressful demands and increasing emotional support, through to individual or group counselling or psychotherapy (Raphael-Leff, 1990). The midwife is in a key position to recognise the individual needs of each mother.

- Midwives should work in partnership with mothers, enabling them to make choices with regard to their care, and to increase their self-esteem and confidence.
- Midwives should identify those mothers who may require extra support during pregnancy and the postnatal period, and continuity of care for such women should be promoted.
- For women with a past history of severe mental illness, clear multi-disciplinary planning should take place because of the risk of recurrence.
- Where possible, early contact between the mother and her baby after birth should be encouraged.
- Teaching the mother about the abilities of her baby and encouraging recognition of the baby's communication skills may promote healthy development of the relationship between mother and child.

- Women with a history of depression or psychiatric illness should be identified and given appropriate support.
- Women who may become or who are depressed during pregnancy or after the birth should be identified and offered appropriate support. This may include psychological treatment.
- Attention should be given to the mother's emotional well-being at the six-week check.

References

- Adams L and Cotgrove A (1995) Promoting secure attachment patterns in infancy and beyond. *Prof Care Mother Child.* **5**: 158–60.
- Ainsworth MA, Blehar M, Waters E and Wall S (1978) *Patterns of Attachment: a psychological study of the strange situation.* Lawrence Erlbaum Associates, Hillsdale, NJ.
- Als H (1997) *Earliest Intervention for Preterm Infants in the Newborn Intensive Care Unit.* Paul H Brookes Publishing Company, London.
- Bass LS (1991) What do parents need when their infant is a patient in the NICU? *Neonat Network.* **10**: 25–34.
- Belsey EM, Rosenblatt DB, Leberman BA *et al.* (1981) The influence of maternal analgesia on neonatal behaviour. 1. Pethidine. *Br Obstet Gynaecol.* **88**: 398–406.
- Belsky J, Rosenberger K and Crnic K (1995) The origins of attachment security: classical and contexual determinants. In: S Goldberg, R Muir and J Kerr (eds) *Attachment Theory: social, developmental and clinical perspectives.* Analytic Press, London.
- Bion W (1967) A theory of thinking. In: W Bion and W Ruprecht (eds) *Second Thoughts (selected papers on psychoanalysis).* Heinemann, London.
- Bowlby J (1969) *Attachment and Loss. Volume 1. Attachment.* Basic Books, New York.
- Bowlby JA (1988) *A Secure Base: clinical application of attachment theory.* Routledge, London.
- Brazelton TB (1963) The early mother–infant adjustment. *Pediatrics.* **34**: 931–7.
- Brazelton TB and Cramer MD (1991) *The Earliest Relationship.* Karnac Books, Addison-Wesley, New York.
- Byng Hall J (1991) The application of attachment theory to understanding and treatment of family therapy. In: CM Parkes, J Stevenson-Hind and P Marris (eds) *Attachment Across the Life Cycle.* Routledge, London.
- Campbell SB, Cohn JF and Meyers T (1995) Depression in first-time mothers: mother–infant interaction and depression chronicity. *Dev Psychol.* **31**: 349–57.
- Caplan HL, Cogill SR, Alexandra H, Robson KM, Katz R and Kumar R (1989) Maternal depression and the emotional development of the child. *Br J Psychiatry.* **154**: 818–23.
- Carter A, Garrity-Roukous E, Chazan-Cohen R, Little C and Briggs-Gowan M (2001) Maternal depression and comorbidity: predicting early parenting attachment, security, and toddler socio-emotional problems and competencies. *J Am Acad Child Adolesc Psychiatry.* **40**: 18–26.
- Chestler P (1988) *Sacred Bond: motherhood under seige.* Virago, London.

- Chilvers C (2001) Antidepressant drugs and generic counselling for treatment of major depression in primary care: randomised trial with patient preference arms. *BMJ.* **322**: 772–5.
- Coffman S (1992) Parent and infant attachment: review of nursing research 1981–1990. *Pediatr Nurs.* **18**: 421–5.
- Cogill S, Caplan H, Alexandra H, Robson K and Kumar R (1986) Impact of postnatal depression on cognitive development in young children. *BMJ.* **292**: 1165–7.
- Cohn J, Campbell S, Matias R and Hopkins J (1990) Face-to-face interactions of postpartum depressed and non-depressed mother–infant pairs at 2 months. *Dev Psychol.* **26**: 15–23.
- Cramer B, Robert-Tissot C, Stern DN *et al.* (1990) Outcome evaluation in brief mother–infant psychotherapy: a preliminary report. *Infant Ment Health J.* **11**: 278–300.
- Cranley MS, Hedahl KJ and Pegg SH (1983) Women's perceptions of vaginal and Caesarean deliveries. *Nurs Res.* **32**: 10–15.
- Dawson B (1994) Put the parents and baby first: nurse/parent relationships in neonatal intensive care. *Prof Nurse.* **10**: 30–35.
- Dormire SL, Strauss SS and Clarke BA (1989) Social support and adaptation to the parent role in first-time adolescent mothers. *J Obstet Gynecol Neonatal Nurs.* **18**: 327–37.
- Dunnington R and Glazer G (1991) Maternal identity and early mothering behaviour in previously infertile and never infertile women. *J Obstet Gynecol Neonatal Nurs.* **20**: 309–17.
- Eyer D (1992) *Mother–Infant Bonding.* Yale University Press, New Haven, CT.
- Fairgreave S (1997) Screening for Down's syndrome: what women think. *Br J Midwif.* **5**: 148–51.
- Farrant W (1980) Stress after amniocentesis for high serum alpha-feto protein concentration. *BMJ.* **281**: 452.
- Field T (1984) Early interactions between infants and their postpartum depressed mothers. *Infant Behav Dev.* **7**: 517–22.
- Field TM and Fox N (1985) *Infant Social Perception.* Ablex Publishing Company, Norwood, NJ.
- Fischer S and Gillman I (1991) Surrogate motherhood: attachment, attitudes and social support. *Psychiatry.* **54**: 13–20.
- Fonagy P and Target M (1997) Attachment and reflective function: their role in self-organisation. *Dev Psychopathol.* **9**: 679–700.
- Fonagy P, Steele H and Steele M (1991) Maternal representations of attachment during pregnancy predict the organisation of infant–mother attachment at one year of age. *Child Dev.* **62**: 891–905.
- Fonagy P, Steele M, Steele H and Target M (1997) *Reflective Functioning Manual Version 4.1 for Application to Adult Attachment Interviews.* University College London Psychoanalysis Unit, London.
- Gay J (1981) A conceptual framework of bonding. *J Obstet Gynecol Neonatal Nurs.* **10**: 440–44.
- Gibson F, Ungerer J, McMahon C, Garth L and Saunders D (2000) The mother–child relationship following *in vitro* fertilisation (IVF): infant attachment, responsivity, and maternal sensitivity. *J Child Psychol Psychiatry.* **41**: 1015–23.
- Grayson A (1996) The triple test decision. *Modern Midwife.* **6**: 16–19.

- Green JM, Statham H and Snowdon C (1996) *Pregnancy is a Testing Time. Report of the Cambridge Prenatal Screening Study.* Centre for Family Research, University of Cambridge.
- Gutbrod T (1999) Mother and infant relationships. *Int J Altern Compl Med.* **17**: 18–19.
- Hall F, Pawlby SJ and Wolkind S (1980) Early life experiences and later mothering behaviour: a study of mothers and their 20-week-old babies. In: D Shaffer and J Dunn (eds) *The First Year of Life.* John Wiley and Sons, New York.
- Hall S, Bobrow M and Marteau TM (2000) Psychological consequences for parents of false-negative results on prenatal screening for Down's syndrome: retrospective interview study. *BMJ.* **320**: 407–12.
- Heidrich SM and Cranley MS (1989) Effect of fetal movement ultrasound scans and amniocentesis on maternal fetal attachment. *Nurs Res.* **38**: 81–4.
- Hillan EM (1992a) Short-term morbidity associated with Caesarean section. *Birth.* **19**: 190–4.
- Hillan EM (1992b) Maternal infant attachment following Caesarean delivery. *J Clin Nurs.* **1**: 33–7.
- Holden J, Sgovsky R and Cox J (1989) Counselling in a general practice setting: controlled study of health visitor intervention in treatment of postnatal depression. *BMJ.* **298**: 223–6.
- Holditch-Davis, Sandelowski M and Harris B (1998) Infertility and early parent–infant interactions. *J Adv Nurs.* **27**: 992–1001.
- Hunter RS, Klostron N, Kraybill EN and Loda F (1978) Antecedents of child abuse and neglect in premature infants. A prospective study in a newborn intensive care unit. *Paediatrics.* **61**: 629–35.
- Hyde B (1986) An interview study of pregnant women's attitudes to ultrasound scanning. *Soc Sci Med.* **22**: 587–92.
- Karen R (1994) *Becoming Attached: unfolding the mystery of the infant–mother bond and its impact on later life.* Warner Books, New York.
- Kemp VH and Page CK (1987) Maternal prenatal attachment in normal and high-risk pregnancies. *J Obstet Gynecol Neonatal Nurs.* **16**: 179–84.
- Klaus MH and Kennell JH (1982) The family during pregnancy. In: MH Klaus and JH Kennell (eds) *Parent Infant Bonding.* CV Mosby Company, St Louis, MO.
- Klopfer PH (1971) Mother love: what turns it on? *Am Sci.* **49**: 404–7.
- Korsch B (1983) More on parent infant bonding (editorial) *J Pediatrics.* **102**: 249–50.
- Lawrence S (1999) Counselling for Down's syndrome screening. *Br J Midwif.* **7**: 368–70.
- Lee B (2000) Attached or detached? Aspects of baby–parent attachment. *R Coll Midwives J.* **3**: 158–9.
- Lewis G (ed.) (2001) *Why Mothers Die. The Fifth Report of the Confidential Enquiries into Maternal Deaths in the United Kingdom (1997–1999).* Royal College of Obstetricians and Gynaecologists, London.
- Lumley J (1990) Through a glass darkly: ultrasound and prenatal bonding. *Birth.* **17**: 214–17.
- McMahon CA, Ungerer JA, Beaurepaire J, Tennant C and Saunders D (1997a) Anxiety during pregnancy and fetal attachment after IVF conception. *Hum Reprod.* **12**: 176–82.

- McMahon CA, Ungerer J, Tennant C and Saunders D (1997b) Psychological adjustment and the quality of the mother–child relationship at four months postpartum after conception by *in vitro* fertilisation. *Fertil Steril.* **68**: 492–500.
- McMahon CA, Tennant C, Ungerer J and Saunders D (1999) 'Don't count your chickens': a comparative study of the experience of pregnancy after IVF conception. *J Reprod Infant Psychol.* **17**: 345–56.
- Martins C and Gaffan EA (2000) Effects of early postnatal depression on patterns of infant–mother attachment: a meta-analytic investigation. *J Child Psychol Psychiatry.* **45**: 737–46.
- Massey-Davis L (1998) A woman's right not to choose. *Pract Midwife.* **1**: 23–5.
- Meltzoff AM and Moore MK (1977) Imitation of facial and manual gestures by human neonates. *Science.* **198**: 75–8.
- Meyer EC, Coll CT, Lester BM, Boukydis CF, McDonough SM and Oh W (1994) Family-based intervention improves maternal psychological well-being and feeding interaction of preterm infants. *Pediatrics.* **93**: 241–6.
- Murray L (1992) The impact of postnatal depression on infant development. *J Child Psychol Psychiatry.* **33**: 543–61.
- Murray L and Trevarthen C (1985) Emotional regulation of interaction between two-month-olds and their mothers. In: T Field and W Fox (eds) *Social Perception in Infancy.* Ablex Publishing Company, Norwood, NJ.
- Murray L and Stein A (1989) The effect of postnatal depression on the infant. *Balliere Clin Obstet Gynecol.* **3**: 921–31.
- Murray L and Andrews L (2000) *The Social Baby.* CP Publishing, Richmond.
- Murray L, Sinclair D, Cooper P, Ducournay P and Turner P (1999) The socio-emotional development of 5-year-old children of postnatally depressed mothers. *J Child Psychol Psychiatry.* **40**: 1259–71.
- Nachmias M, Gunnar M, Mangelsdorf S *et al.* (1996) Behavioural inhibition and stress reactivity: the moderating role of attachment security. *Child Dev.* **67**: 508–22.
- Norr KF, Roberts JE and Freese U (1989) Early postpartum rooming in and maternal attachment behaviours in a group of medically indigent primipara. *J Nurs Midwifery.* **34**: 85–91.
- O'Hara M (1997) The nature of postpartum depressive disorders. In: L Murray and P Cooper (eds) *Postpartum Depression and Child Development.* Guildford Press, London.
- Paradice R (1993) How important are early mother–infant relationships? *Health Visitor.* **66**: 211–13.
- Poehlmann J and Fiese BH (2001) The interaction of maternal and infant vulnerabilities on developing attachment relationships. *Dev Psychopathol.* **13**: 1–11.
- Poindron P and Le Neindre P (1979) Hormonal and behavioural basis for establishing maternal behaviour in sheep. In: Zichella and R Panchari (eds) *Psychoneuroendocrinology in Reproduction.* Elsevier/North Holland Biomedical Press, Amsterdam.
- Ram A, Lerman M, Retzoni N and Tyano S (1993) Ultrasound, mother–infant attachment and the quickening fetus. *Int J Prenatal Perinatal Psychol Med.* **5**: 127–34.
- Raphael-Leff J (1990) Psychotherapy and pregnancy. *J Reprod Infant Psychol.* **8**: 119–35.
- Reading AE, Campbell S, Cox DN and Sledmore CM (1982) Health beliefs and health care behaviour in pregnancy. *Psychol Med.* **12**: 379–82.

- Redshaw M (1982) The influence of analgesia in labour on the baby. *Midwife Health Visitor Commun Nurse.* **18**: 126–32.
- Robinson J (2001) Does prenatal screening provoke anticipatory grief? *Br J Midwifery.* **9**: 307–11.
- Rosser J (1999) Anxiety and pregnancy: bad for women, bad for babies. *Pract Midwife.* **2**: 4–5.
- Seeley S, Murray L and Cooper P (1996) The outcome for mothers and babies of health visitor interventions. *Health Visitor.* **69**: 134–8.
- Sinclair D and Murray L (1998) Effects of postnatal depression on children's adjustment to school. *Br J Psychiatry.* **172**: 58–63.
- Singer P and Wells P (1984) *The Reproductive Revolution: new ways of making babies.* Oxford University Press, Oxford.
- Smith M (1998) Maternal–fetal attachment in surrogate mothers. *Br J Midwifery.* **6**: 188–92.
- Snowdon C (1994) What makes a mother? Interviews with women involved in egg donation and surrogacy. *Birth.* **21**: 77–83.
- Statham H and Green G (1993) Serum screening for Down's syndrome: some women's experiences. *BMJ.* **307**: 174–6.
- Steele H, Steele M and Fonagy P (1996) Associations among attachment classifications of mothers, fathers and their infants. *Child Dev.* **67**: 541–55.
- Stein A, Gath DH, Buxcher J, Bond A, Day A and Cooper PJ (1991) The relationship between postnatal depression and mother–child interaction. *Br J Psychiatry.* **158**: 46–52.
- Stern D (1985) *The Interpersonal World of the Infant.* Basic Books, New York.
- Stevenson J (1997) Pondering about bonding. *Midwif Matters.* **74**: 20–22.
- Teixeira J, Fisk N and Glover V (1999) Association between maternal anxiety in pregnancy and increased uterine artery resistance index: cohort-based study. *BMJ.* **318**: 153–7.
- Teti DM and Gefland DM (1997) Maternal cognitions as mediators of child outcomes in the context of postpartum depression. In: L Murray and PJ Cooper (eds) *Postpartum Depression and Child Development.* Guildford Press, London.
- Thompson RA and Calkins SD (1996) The double-edged sword: emotional regulation for children at risk. *Dev Psychopathol.* **8**: 163–82.
- Tizard B (1991) Working mothers and the care of young children. In: E Lloyd, A Phoenix and A Wollett (eds) *The Social Construction of Motherhood.* Sage, London.
- Tronick EZ, Conn J and Shea J (1986) The transfer of affect between mother and infants. In: TB Brazelton and MW Yogman (eds) *Affective Development in Infancy.* Ablex Publishing Company, Norwood, NJ.
- Williams H and Carmichael A (1985) Depression in mothers in a multi-ethnic urban industrial municipality in Melbourne: aetiological factors and effects on infants and preschool children. *J Child Psychol Psychiatry.* **26**: 277–88.
- Winston R (1994) *Infertility: a sympathetic approach.* Optima, London.

CHAPTER 11

The medicalisation of childbirth

Alyson Henley-Einion

Childbirth in the UK takes place within a medical context, and is defined by medical norms. As such it is no longer a purely social or personal event, nor is it the specific province of women. This chapter explores the roots of the medicalisation of childbearing, related to advances in science and medicine which are reflected in the status of these disciplines within society. Midwives, whose role is primarily to care for women with healthy pregnancies and births, straddle the divide between the natural and medical, and must be competent in both areas. The status of midwives as employees and representatives of the institution of the hospital or National Health Service (NHS) Trust is explored, together with the effects of their drive towards professionalisation, in particular the dilution of their role and a deskilling in relation to natural birthing in favour of the acquisition of technical skills. The medical definition of birth as the dominant paradigm (both within healthcare services and within the media) is discussed alongside an examination of the social and cultural forces which have led to birthing women demanding medical birth. Sociological, midwifery and feminist theory is used to explore these issues.

Introduction

Most women's experiences of childbearing in the UK today are medicalised, as birth takes place predominantly in a hospital, on a maternity ward and in the presence of doctors. Doctors may not be physically present in the room during the actual labour, but the maternity unit and the labour ward are their domain. The act of birth is surrounded by all of the symbols of the medical profession and all that it stands for – science, power and knowledge.

The medicalisation of childbirth can essentially be broken down into a process which has led to childbirth becoming a medical event rather than a social one, in which human experiences are redefined as medical problems (Becker and Nachtignall, 1992). In this instance it concerns the experiences of women and their partners on becoming pregnant and giving birth. Today any pregnant woman who is asked what she anticipates in relation to labour and birth will include the word 'hospital' in her reply. Part of her childbirth classes will prepare her for her experience of the hospital, introducing her to the delivery room and the machinery and technology which will supposedly offer her a better and safer birth. It has also been described as the expansion of medical jurisdiction into the realms of previously non-medically defined problems (Gable and Calnan, 1989). Nowhere is this more apparent than in relation to birth.

The critiques of medicalisation are many and varied. They stem from midwifery, feminist and social theory. The cultural and social meanings of birth and its surrounding rituals have developed in parallel with the relentless march of progress into our technologically dominated present. In the western world, medical frames of reference and knowledge have been accepted and legitimated within a system of maternity care which has brought about not only a surge in engineering obstetrics but a steady erosion of maternal choice, control and satisfaction in relation to many aspects of pregnancy and labour, usually justified in the name of safety (Cahill, 2001). Illich (1976) associates medicalisation with industrialisation, and this culture is based on the industrialisation of all areas of human experience. An example of this can be seen in the following quotation:

> The first stage of labour can be likened to a vehicle going up a hill: the steepness of the hill is the amount of pelvic resistance, the engine is the uterine contractions, and the vehicle is the fetus.
>
> (Fay, 2001: 8)

The text goes on to describe what happens if the progress is unsatisfactory, in which case oxytocin augmentation may be used, which is likened to 'putting the foot down on the accelerator' (Fay, 2001: 8). Women and their lived experiences do not seem to fit in here.

Feminist writing refers to the way in which women's social experience (including their health and healthcare) are mediated by the institutions of patriarchy, usually in oppressive ways (Annandale and Clark, 1996). These institutions must then be the focus of much of the discussion of the medicalisation of childbearing. Sociological theories such as functionalism relate women's experiences of childbearing to specific behavioural directives which are related to roles and norms that are gender specific (Haralambos and Holborn, 1995). These theories have much to contribute to the debate over the medicalisation of childbearing. This chapter aims to use some of these theories as a basis for discussion of the historic and current medicalisation of childbearing.

Childbirth is in itself a natural physiological process. Prior to the advent of scientific medicine, birth was a social event, and the only 'intervention' was the presence of a midwife, who provided social support and had the experience of having attended other births, so possessed knowledge of childbirth and its processes. The social setting in which birth now occurs is one where the dominant culture is that of science. Midwives are part of this scientific movement. Women continue to give birth within an obstetric regimen which has to a considerable degree been able to resist or dilute alternative approaches to care (Campbell and Porter, 1997). Obstetrics, the dominant form of knowledge, is regarded as mainstream, *malestream* knowledge, whereas natural childbirth is labelled as 'alternative'.

The care that is given to labouring women is prescribed by doctors, and the interventions that are used to achieve 'normal' birth are based on western notions of time and scientific calculations. Pregnancy and birth, the latter being possibly the most potent and powerful natural event of a woman's life, are regularised and constantly scrutinised by medical professionals, acting on a definition of childbirth as hazardous (Fox, 1999). The dominant philosophy is one of risk prediction (Rothwell, 1995) and, because there is the potential for all pregnant women to experience obstetric complications, they are all considered to require surveillance by doctors. This has alienated women from a potentially empowering experience.

This chapter aims to explore these issues through an examination of the history of obstetrics and midwifery — that is, the recorded history of birth. This approach is perilous because those who hold knowledge and power also control who records history and the events of people's lives. However, Oakley (1990) highlights a feminist concern with the social structure of science as representing an inherently sexist, racist, classist and culturally coercive practice and form of knowledge. Thus the motivation for a deconstruction and analysis of medicalised childbearing is fundamentally to determine how it has affected birthing women. Studies of the way in which women experience the maternity services have long revealed an iceberg of dissatisfaction (Kirkham, 1986; Oakley, 1990; Kitzinger, 1992). If this iceberg is to be melted, an evaluation of its extent is necessary, and this understanding must be used to set up measures to redress the balance.

Childbearing: a history of the rise of science, technology and obstetrics

Medicalisation and control of childbirth are inextricably linked with patriarchy. Patriarchy in the western world can be dated to the rise of Christianity, whose moral and ethical codes underpinned social structures and teachings in Europe and the New World. The Bible provides the first evidence of a formal definition of the role of man as provider and controller, and of woman as childbearer and supporter, as follows:

> I will greatly multiply thy sorrow and thy conception; in sorrow thou shalt bring forth children: and thy desire shall be subject to thy husband, and he shall rule over thee.
>
> Genesis 3: 16

Women's roles were clearly delineated within this one verse. As such, the Bible has formed the basis of the nuclear family unit, and its teachings have been disseminated over the last two millennia both by the Church and by secular governments.

The rise of medicine as a political and social force within the female sphere of motherhood can be traced back as far as the fourteenth ecntury. Physicians, who had been trained at universities, managed to gain approval from the Church and set out to shake the faith of the people in traditional remedies (Towler and Bramall, 1986). This was the beginning of medicine's assumption of authority over the mysteries of the body, health, birth and death.

Historical analyses show that, until the seventeenth century, childbirth in Britain was firmly located within the domestic arena (Cahill, 2001), with women being attended by lay midwives, family and close friends. The seventeenth and eighteenth centuries saw a rise in the power and status of the medical profession, which was achieved largely by the denigration and usurping of traditional or non-licensed practitioners such as midwives. Since this time, medicine and religion together have systematically devalued female roles and traits and excluded women from power in society through the dissemination of patriarchal ideology (Cahill, 2001).

The explosion of scientific knowledge, especially in the fields of physiology and anatomy, attracted men to the practice of midwifery. With the application of their knowledge as physicians and their skills as surgeons (using their newly acquired forceps), these 'men-midwives' changed irrevocably the nature and pattern of midwifery practice (Towler and Bramall, 1986). The separation of caring and curing in the healing arts arose from the Cartesian notion of the separation of the mind and the body, and the concept of the body as a machine (Achterberg, 1990). This was followed by a change in the role and function of women within the sphere of pregnancy and birth, and it consolidated the value of professional versus lay birth attendants.

The popularity of 'men-midwives' and male medical practitioners among the upper classes, who set the standards for the rest of society, led to a social 'shift' in the frames of reference and behaviours surrounding birth. The use of the term 'brought to bed' in accounts of childbirth among the gentry implies that this class abandoned the traditional birth chair for the bed, and at the same time they abandoned the traditional midwife for the male accoucheur (Towler and Bramall, 1986). Therefore the role of women as childbearers changed from active to passive.

The first 'lying-in' hospitals were established in the middle of the eighteenth century, reflecting the shift in emphasis from birth as a home-based family event to birth as a hospital-based medical event. It was only in the late nineteenth and early twentieth centuries that pregnancy on the whole became viewed as a condition that warranted some kind of supervision, stemming from the need to reduce an unacceptable level of maternal mortality (Field, 1990). This was complemented by the introduction of X-rays between 1900 and 1910. These enabled doctors both to measure the size of the pelvis and to obtain for the first time graphical information about the fetus (Oakley, 1984). Such technical developments in turn began to define the form that antenatal care would subsequently assume (Field, 1990), in that surveillance of the fetus became an important factor.

Political moves to regularise the practice of midwifery, instigated and controlled by the medical profession, brought about legislation that established the role of the midwife as a provider of care, but within strict boundaries. In ultimately limiting the midwives' role to attendance only at *normal births* (eventually enshrined in the 1902 Midwives Act), medicine operated a demarcating strategy to define this 'subordinate' group's sphere of practice and competence (Cahill, 2001). In the UK, the profession began its life as an acceptable occupation under medical control. The Central Midwives Board established in 1902 was, by law, made up of doctors, who were also responsible for the education of midwives and presided over their final examination (Boyle, 2000). The earliest midwifery textbooks were written by doctors, so it is hardly surprising that the values of the medical profession have been ingrained in midwifery (Boyle, 2000).

The twentieth century saw the greatest and most rapid advances in obstetric medicine and reproductive technology, mirroring advances in science and industry in general. The formation of the National Health Service (NHS) consolidated the medical status of pregnancy and birth, by assuming responsibility for the health of everyone, for the treatment of their illnesses, and for ushering them to and from this world. Thus the shift from home to hospital occurred at both ends of life, and for any time in between when health was less than optimal.

Advances within the pharmaceutical industry added a new twist with the increase in availability of contraceptive drugs, which was a positive and welcome option for large numbers of women, but had an interesting 'side-effect'. The practice of birth control led to a steady decline in the birth rate, and this resulted in a reduction in women's personal experience of, knowledge of and self-confidence in giving birth. Women were no longer witnessing births within extended families. The growing complexity of childbirth management meant that women's knowledge, gained through personal experience and passed on to others, was less applicable to the newer, more medicalised approach. The net effect was a greater reliance on 'experts' in the mechanics of childbirth to educate women about reproduction, and to replace 'old wives' tales' with the latest scientific knowledge (Simkin, 1996). Thus the concept of authoritative knowledge developed (Davis-Floyd and Sargent, 1997; Jordan, 1997), reflected in the status of those who hold that knowledge in our society.

Following the introduction of the NHS, maternity care became more and more fragmented. As Field (1990) has shown, the main developments in antenatal care in the UK since the 1960s have been an extension of hospital antenatal clinics, a decline in community clinics and a decline in general practitioner care, perpetuating and consolidating the shift from social birth to hospital (and therefore medicalised) birth. Thus birth has moved from the home to the hospital, and from a natural phenomenon to a medical event. It is also an extension of our cultural dependence on professional healthcare (Oakley, 1979; Davis-Floyd, 1990).

Not all aspects of the medical management of pregnancy and birth are negative. Biomedicine has contributed to higher maternal and fetal survival rates due to a number of factors. The availability of safe blood transfusions has redressed a major risk factor in giving birth, namely the risk of haemorrhage. Medical and surgical advances, especially the use of general anaesthesia for Caesarean section, mean that women and babies with complications can be treated effectively. Antibiotics have proved invaluable for the treatment of puerperal fever. The issue is not that medicine has no place within maternity care, but that *all* pregnancies are medically managed, *all* of them are viewed as inherently pathological or risky, and normality is only ever defined in retrospect.

Another possible benefit of the medicalisation of reproduction is that women can be freed from biological determinism – they can control their own fertility. Women have achieved some control over their reproductive activities through the availability of effective contraception. It could be argued that this is no less a product of the medicalisation of childbearing than is assisted conception. For the first time in our history, women can make fundamental changes to their biological destiny (Challoner, 1999). The concern is not what is available, but who controls it and for whose ultimate benefit.

Biomedicine as a male-gendered profession

A clear line of demarcation tends to be drawn in the literature between obstetrics and midwifery, each being portrayed as a unitary and internally coherent body of thought and practice which is at odds with the other (Annandale and Clark, 1996).

In this instance, it seems to be a gendered debate. The medical profession and its scientific philosophies are gendered male by their history and development, and this situation is not altered by the presence of female doctors. The profession of medicine is masculinist, in that it purports to be objective and objectivist, rational and measurable, and female doctors are socialised through their training into this mode (Davis-Floyd, 1990). Male thought is predominantly equated with scientific thought, despite the fact that, in the case of obstetrics, much practice is not based on research evidence (LoCicero, 1993). From a political standpoint, this situation appears to have been exacerbated by the governmental tendency in the last 50 years to allocate power to doctors in the management of health and repro-duction, thus creating a cultural norm of high-tech medical management of preg-nancy and birth (Mason, 2000).

Informed choice: an illusion?

The *Changing Childbirth* Report (Department of Health, 1993) emerged in response to political and public pressure to promote choice, control and informed consent for expectant mothers. This has put the concepts of choice and control in the main frame, but midwives and obstetricians offer only an illusion of choice. Ultimately, a woman cannot exercise informed choice because the information that is given is controlled and restricted by the institution, the medical profession and some midwives. Furthermore, the information and descriptions that are provided for women do not allow them to exercise an informed choice, because the language can only be understood by the initiated (Foucault, 1976). Women are choosing medical interventions such as epidural analgesia, and booking Caesarean sections for first pregnancies, not fully understanding the interventions and procedures or their implications. True choice is not offered, and the only real options are those related to a technological labour and birth. Normal labour now consists of electronic monitoring of fetal heart rate, the use of epidurals and the routine use of surgical and medical interventions to speed up the process. Normal labour involves removing the woman from her familiar surroundings and her usual support network, to labour in a clinical setting where every appliance, uniform and explanation speaks of science, medicine and doctors. Choice, in this context, would not appear to be between natural and interventionist birth, but between normal medical labour and complicated medical labour.

The critical issue at the beginning of the twenty-first century is this – some women are *choosing* medical birth themselves, sometimes even elective Caesarean births. It is imperative that the fact that it is women who give birth is not overlooked. If women are to be educated about the normal processes of birth and offered a true choice, it is necessary to challenge why they choose medicalised birth. Furthermore, it is necessary to challenge the underlying fears that motivate them to make such choices, while at the same time respecting their right to choose (Pike-Urlacher, 1998).

Such fears may be linked to the patriarchal nature of science, which has con-trolled women both overtly and subtly. This control continues in the most insidious ways, through popular acceptance produced by socialising agents such as hospitals (Davis-Floyd, 1990). Counter-cultures and opposing political and social movements remain on the fringes. The lived experience of midwifery is becoming merely the largely unresearched antithesis of obstetrics (Annandale and Clarke, 1996).

Midwifery or obstetrics?

Midwifery and obstetrics appear to stand on either side of a clearly demarcated divide. Traditionally, and legally, the midwife deals with the 'normal' while the obstetrician deals with the abnormal, in the form of medical conditions that are affecting pregnancy, or complications of pregnancy. However, in order to practise within the dominant paradigm, the midwife must straddle this divide, working within an obstetric framework and using obstetric terminology and technology, which defines all pregnancies as inherently problematic and potentially dangerous. The obstetrician/midwife divide appears to mimic the two competing models of childbirth, namely the biomedical/technocratic model and the natural/holistic model (Viisainen, 2001).

However, the medical model dominates all aspects of pregnancy and birth. Births in the UK take place in hospitals. Midwives are trained within hospitals, must become as conversant with the pathology of pregnancy and birth as with its natural processes, and must be skilled in the use of medical technology and assistance with medical and surgical procedures. This is in part due to the constant struggle for professional survival that midwifery must engage in. The 'experts' in normal birth can no longer solely concern themselves with the predominantly supportive role of the 'classic' midwife. In their drive to gain recognition as both a profession and an academic discipline, midwives have adopted the common understanding that scientific knowledge developed through research is superior to other forms of knowledge, being objective, impersonal, value-free, theoretical, generalisable and universal (Bjornsdottir, 2001). In the gaining of these new skills and status, there has been a concurrent de-skilling of midwives in the traditional arts of midwifery (Sandall, 1991).

One by-product of this process of medicalisation and regulation of the women who provide care during childbirth has been not just the restriction of their roles as midwives, but the demand that in order to fulfil their role they must commit to midwifery at the expense of their domestic lives (Ball et al., 2002). A new stressor now exists for the 'professional midwife', as it seems that she must approach her work in the same way as men are expected to – as her primary occupation. Within UK maternity care there are some midwives who do this and other midwives who do not. The midwives who conform to a capitalist patriarchal model, ordering their lives into 'work first, family later' mode, are those who advance up through the ranks (and pay-scales). They achieve positions where they potentially possess the power and influence to change birth for the greater benefit of all women (but they do not necessarily do this). Those who 'opt out', putting family life before work, are left out in the cold, and experience what Kirkham and Stapleton (2000) have described as 'horizontal violence' from colleagues who regard them as not complying with expected behaviours. Sandall (1995) describes the situation as consisting of a divided workforce composed of an elite core and a casualised periphery based on the ability to give a full-time flexible commitment to work. The medical model has imposed upon women a structure which makes the combination of motherhood and midwifery untenable unless one has a surfeit of family support and childcare. This reinforces the status of caring, co-operation and community within the birth arena as the lowest status of all. In this case, midwives have been disempowered by the institution and the system in much the same way as have childbearing women.

The technology question

Technology is a central question in any examination of the medicalisation of childbearing, because medicine and technology are inextricably linked. The advent of technology within society has resulted in a change in women's perceptions of pregnancy, birth and motherhood. Much of this is due to advances in communications technology, such that most women have access to or are exposed to topical information about new or impending motherhood and its medical treatment, usually through all imaginable media. The dissemination of such information is in itself a means of constructing social identities and expectations about birth and the transition to motherhood. It seems that obstetric technology is now a part of normal birth.

Given the available evidence that medicalised childbirth may not be the optimum approach for all women, the continued aggressive promotion and use of technologies for normal birth might seem remarkable. However, this can again be shown to derive from social and societal forces and cultural trends, both within medicine and in the wider world.

Electronic fetal monitoring (EFM) is a prime example. EFM uses a beam of ultrasound to record the fetal heart rate, and a pressure sensor to monitor uterine contractions. The woman is usually immobilised on a bed while monitoring takes place. EFM was originally designed for high-risk labours (Basset *et al.*, 2000), but is now used throughout pregnancy and birth from as early as 23–24 weeks' gestation. It is the primary tool for diagnosis of fetal well-being. From the mid-1970s, clinical trials using sophisticated study designs and increasingly 'high-risk' patients indicated that EFM provided no benefit with regard to fetal or maternal outcome compared with midwife intermittent auscultation. Several large, well-conducted, randomized clinical trials that were undertaken in the 1980s support this view (Basset *et al.*, 2000).

Thus according to their own criteria of scientific knowledge, obstetricians know that the value of EFM from a clinical viewpoint is questionable, yet they continue to use it as the most appropriate clinical tool for assessing fetal well-being in normal labours, as do midwives. A number of factors contribute to its use. It is used as a means of reassuring the mother. Emotional stress, anxiety and fear are addressed by the employment of medical interventions instead of giving emotional support, thereby increasing the woman's reliance on medicine and obstetrics. Furthermore, EFM is linked to capitalism, another product of a patriarchal society, whereby the makers of these costly machines perpetuate their use by investing in the hospitals which use them, in a blatant form of product placement. EFM is also linked to the rise in defensive medicine, a social phenomenon which has increased enormously in recent years. DeVries (1993) suggests that midwives gain power, status, prestige and respect from the public by offering the 'best' means of risk reduction, which means understanding and using obstetric technology. Midwives themselves become as eager as doctors to promote the use of these technologies.

Legally, the fetus has no rights, but this fact is not reflected in practice. There have been cases of women being forced to undergo Caesarean section against their will, which have clearly highlighted the fact that women's rights of control over their own bodies can be superseded in favour of fetal rights. Iphofen and Poland (1998) suggest that the use of technologies such as EFM creates a more direct relationship between wider society, medicine and the fetus, which further marginalises the role of women.

It is hardly surprising that with these types of social and legal interactions, compounded by the pressures exerted by the medical profession, women perceive that they are placing their child's health status first in their list of priorities, and they buy into the medico-legal model. The underlying capitalist nature of bio-medicine and reproductive technology is reflected in a woman's desire to 'have' (a capitalist term) a child of her own (Oakley, 1993).

The media: defining cultural norms

Technological advances outside the realm of medicine seem to have brought about popular acceptance of and even enthusiasm for medical birth. One of the strongest influences on the acceptability of medical birth seems to be the media (a product of our technological society, which is highly successful at perpetuating itself by making us think that we cannot live without it). Newspapers, magazines, and current affairs programmes and talk shows on television all sensationalise and standardise birth and present a view of this experience that is biased in favour of the dominant culture.

The influence of the popular press on common understanding and awareness of birth and current issues within the health services is well documented. However, the way in which such stories are presented is generally influenced by the style popularised by this type of journalism. In June 2001, the *Daily Mail* carried the front-page headline 'The Demise of Natural Childbirth' (Marsh, 2001), making many of the criticisms raised in this chapter, but in much more emotive language – for example, 'Doctors are accused of meddling with motherhood', 'alarming rises in induced and Caesarean births' (Marsh, 2001: 1). Inside this same edition, the headline is 'The "social" Caesareans', and the article mentions the rise in the rate of Caesareans in the UK and the fact that it is one of the highest in Europe (Marsh, 2001). Within the confines of the genre and style, it does what such an article should do – it challenges the dominant paradigm. However, the very nature of this genre results in the reader 'oohing' and 'aahing' over such an article and taking it with a pinch of salt, or at the very least regarding it as a news story, rather than a social and personal crisis. A more positive article was that by Kitzinger (2001), entitled 'The Great Childbirth Blackmail'. It succinctly and clearly illustrated the ways in which women are pressured to undergo intervention without a true knowledge or understanding of the risks involved. However, it was placed within the *Femail* section of the *Daily Mail*, which then proscribed who would read it, making it little more than 'girl talk'.

In recent years, rapid advances in communications and entertainment technologies have brought vast amounts of information from all over the developed world into the home of the average person. Satellite and digital television is one culprit that is particularly guilty of advertising birth in all its medical glory. During prime viewing time, programmes (the majority of which are American) are aired showing medical birth stories (e.g. *A Baby Story*, *Birth Day*). Even in cases where the mother has planned for normal birth by taking Lamaze, yoga, exercise or birthing classes, the end result has been hospitalised, physician-controlled birth. The women labour in bed, attached to EFMs, have epidurals and oxytocin drips, and deliver in the lithotomy position. The fetus and its well-being are emphasised constantly, as is the use of technology and medication. The UK-made programmes feature hospitals and hospital births, and highlight women who had aimed to have a natural birth and were thwarted by nature, then availing themselves of every obstetric service available. Some of the programme content is useful and can help to demystify the processes of hospitalisation in relation to birth. However, it glamorises and glorifies the role of medicine in pregnancy, and it often features women and families who have overcome adversity through medical intervention, rather than focusing on the normal aspects of birth. The reason for this is straightforward – dramatic rescues and the mobilisation of medical science and technology make for higher viewing rates, and normal labours have none of the on-screen drama that medical interventions present.

What are the effects of this constant exposure to high-risk pregnancies and medically managed births? First, women may begin to view their pregnancies as inherently risky, potentially problematic and having an uncertain outcome both for themselves and for their babies. This leads to a greater dependence on science and medicine to reassure and support them, and perhaps a desire to access all of the available medical interventions (hence the need in some cases to give birth by elective Caesarean section). Secondly, women only view birth from a medical perspective, so medical birth becomes the norm, and home birth is reinforced as the rare, unsafe alternative.

Conclusion

The modern environment of birth is the institution – the hospital – with its own set of rules, standards of behaviour, language and technology. In order to function within this system, the woman and her partner must comply with and conform to these rules and standards and attempt to communicate using the same codes and language. Importantly, they must also respect and value the technology surrounding them. Birth is viewed in terms of pain and effort, and anything that might ease the process for the mother is desirable, so long as the infant can be brought safely through the birth (Simkin, 1996). An alternative social paradigm of birth would celebrate the activities of birth as much as the outcome, and would focus on the mother's change of role and identity in the long term, instead of focusing on the birth as the finite event.

Combating the entrenched norms of pregnancy and birth is a much greater task than simplistic opposition to medical control and technological supremacy, because becoming pregnant and giving birth are complex social processes (Kent, 2000). If clinical care is to be truly effective, then it must be inclusive rather than exclusive, and it should be the result of the contributory work of women who give birth, as well as those who seek to control it.

There can be no excision of biomedicine, science or technology from the human experience of birth. Indeed, despite their drawbacks, these disciplines have much to offer society and the families whose interests are jointly vested in the reproductive process. Therefore childbirth will continue to be influenced, affected and enhanced by science. A continued assertion of the importance of the natural, the status of the mother and her independence is necessary, and to achieve this it may be necessary to embrace certain aspects of medicalisation. Rothwell (1995) suggests that women should oppose medical intervention in childbearing, using the language of science, medicine and obstetrics. The assertion of midwifery as a profession that is on a par with obstetrics is one such move, but so far it appears that this has been detrimental both to midwives and to mothers by removing them from natural birth, and adding to the perception of birth as a medical event. However, fundamental changes are needed in the power associated with and the popular attraction of science and scientific knowledge (Basset *et al.*, 2000). Perhaps the assertion of knowledge from more human sources, involving a holistic model of data generation and validation, should take place alongside pure science, at least with regard to health, which is after all about people.

Is there any way in which birth within the NHS can be anything other than medicalised? Is there room within the institution as a system, organisation and structure for woman-centred, woman-controlled birth? Moves have been made in this direction, and not only by the fringe groups of feminists who contribute to the political and medical debates. The *Changing Childbirth* Report (Department of Health, 1993) enshrined all of the principles of woman-centred maternity care within the NHS, and as a document it was ground-breaking. The extent to which its principles have been put into practice and its goals have been achieved is debatable. However, changes have been made to the physical environment of hospital birth, in the form of natural birthing rooms in which the most obvious technology is removed or concealed, and with comfortable, 'home-like' furniture and the availability of birth stools, birth pools, bouncy balls and bean bags. This may be regarded as an improvement, However, it could equally be argued that it is an illusion of power, in much the same way as birth plans promise women choice which does not exist in reality (Foucalt, 1976). Thus an illusion of the natural is provided while remaining under the supervision of the medical.

Team midwifery (in various forms), one-to-one services, birth centres, Domino (Domiciliary in and out) services and caseload midwifery have all attempted to promote continuity and humanity with regard to childbirth for some women. However, despite this, the essential elements of the institution remain, namely the hierarchy, the language, the technology and the doctors. There is a need for both patience and persistence. The self-proclaimed infallibility of health institutions and their vested interest in the status quo must be eroded and, as Achterberg (1990) aptly stated, only time alters the face of monoliths.

- Birth in the UK take place within a western medical scientific paradigm.
- The divide between natural and medical birth reflects the gendered divide between obstetrics/midwifery and midwifery/motherhood.
- Some women are choosing medical birth (e.g. elective Caesarean section and epidural analgesia) as a result of fear and as a reflection of a technological society.
- Medical technology has led to greater medical control of birth and the ability to diagnose fetal conditions, often resulting in the marginalisation of women.
- The media and information technologies reinforce birth as a medical event, dramatising and popularising hospital births, and conditioning women to expect similar interventions during their own labours. Natural birth does not have the same media impact.
- Women do not have true choice and control with regard to childbearing. Only a new paradigm of inclusion and equality could achieve this.

References

- Achterberg J (1990) *Woman as Healer.* Rider Books, London.
- Annandale E and Clark J (1996) What is gender? Feminist theory and the sociology of human reproduction. *Sociol Health Illness.* **18**: 17–44.
- Ball L, Curtis P and Kirkham M (2002) *Why Do Midwives Leave?* Royal College of Midwives, London.
- Basset KL, Lyer N and Kazanjian L (2000) Defensive medicine during hospital obstetrical care: a by-product of the technological age. *Soc Sci Med.* **51**: 523–37.
- Becker G and Nachtignall RD (1992) Eager for medicalisation: the social production of infertility as a disease. *Sociol Health Illness.* **14**: 456–71.
- Bjornsdottir K (2001) Language, research and nursing practice. *J Adv Nurs.* **33**: 159–66.
- Boyle M (2000) Childbirth in bed: the historical perspective. *Pract Midwife.* **3**: 21–4.
- Cahill HA (2001) Male appropriation and medicalisation of childbirth: an historical analysis. *J Adv Nurs.* **33**: 334–42.
- Campbell R and Porter S (1997) Feminist theory and the sociology of childbirth: a response to Ellen Annandale and Judith Clark. *Sociol Health Illness.* **19**: 348–58.
- Challoner J (1999) *The Baby Makers: the history of artificial conception.* Channel 4 Books, London.
- Davis-Floyd RE (1990) The role of obstetrical rituals in the resolution of cultural anomaly. *Soc Sci Med.* **31**: 175–89.
- Davis-Floyd RE and Sargent CF (1997) Introduction: the anthropology of birth. In: RE Davis-Floyd and CF Sargent (eds) *Childbirth and Authoritative Knowledge: cross-cultural perspectives.* University of California Press, Berkeley, CA.
- Department of Health (1993) *Changing Childbirth (the Cumberledge Report). The Report of the Expert Maternity Group.* HMSO, London.
- DeVries RG (1993) A cross-national view of the status of midwives. In: E Riska and K Wegar (eds) *Gender, Work and Medicine. Women and the medical division of labour.* Sage Publications, London.
- Fay T (2001) *Labour Ward Rules.* BMJ Books, London.
- Field PA (1990) Effectiveness and efficacy of antenatal care. *Midwifery.* **6**: 215–23.
- Foucault M (1976) *The Birth of the Clinic.* Routledge, London.
- Fox B (1999) Revisiting the critique of medicalized childbirth. *Gender Soc.* **13**: 326–47.
- Gable J and Calnan M (1989) The limits of medicine: women's perception of medical technology. *Soc Sci Med.* **28**: 223–31.
- Haralambos M and Holborn M (1995) *Sociology: themes and perspectives.* Collins Educational, London.
- Illich I (1976) *Limits to Medicine. Medical nemesis: the expropriation of health.* Penguin Books, Harmondsworth.
- Iphofen R and Poland F (1998) *Sociology in Practice for Health Care Professionals.* Macmillan, Basingstoke.
- Jordan B (1997) Authoritative knowledge and its construction. In: RE Davis-Floyd and CF Sargent (eds) *Childbirth and Authoritative Knowledge: cross-cultural perspectives.* University of California Press, Berkeley, CA.

- Kent J (2000) *Social Perspectives on Pregnancy and Childbirth for Midwives, Nurses and the Caring Professions.* Open University Press, Buckingham.
- Kirkham M (1989) Midwives and information giving in labour. In: S Robinson and A Thomson (eds) *Midwives, Research and Childbirth. Volume I.* Chapman & Hall, London.
- Kirkham M and Stapleton H (2000) Midwives support needs as childbirth changes. *J Adv Nurs.* **32**: 465–72.
- Kitzinger S (1992) Birth and violence against women. In: H Roberts (ed.) *Women's Health Matters.* Routledge, London.
- Kitzinger S (2001) The great childbirth blackmail. *Daily Mail.* **13 June**: 52.
- LoCicero AK (1993) Explaining excessive rates of Caesareans and other childbirth interventions: contributions from contemporary theories of gender and psychosocial development. *Soc Sci Med.* **37**: 1261–9.
- Marsh B (2001) The demise of natural childbirth. *Daily Mail.* **13 June**: 1.
- Mason J (2000) Defining midwifery practice. *J Assoc Improve Matern Serv.* **12**: 5–6.
- Oakley A (1979) *Becoming a Mother.* Martin Robinson, Oxford.
- Oakley A (1984) *The Captured Womb: a history of the medical care of pregnant women.* Basil Blackwell, Oxford.
- Oakley A (1990) Who's afraid of the randomised controlled trial? In: H Roberts (ed.) *Women's Health Counts.* Routledge, London.
- Oakley A (1993) *Essays on Women, Health and Medicine.* Edinburgh University Press, Edinburgh.
- Pike-Urlacher CL (1998) Middle-class beliefs – how they define normal birth. *Midwif Today.* **Autumn Issue**: 22–3.
- Rothwell H (1995) Medicalisation of childbearing. *Br J Midwif.* **3**: 318–31.
- Sandall J (1991) *Continuity of Care? Recent developments in maternity care in Britain: towards a sociological perspective.* University of London, Royal Holloway and Bedford New College, London.
- Sandall J (1995) Choice, continuity and control: changing midwifery, towards a sociological perspective. *Midwifery.* **11**: 201–9.
- Simkin P (1996) Labour support: where has it been and where is it going? *Int J Childbirth Educ.* **14**: 22–3.
- Towler J and Bramall J (1986) *Midwives in History and Society.* Croom Helm, London.
- Viisainen K (2001) Negotiating control and meaning: home-birth as a self-constructed choice in Finland. *Soc Sci Med.* **53**: 1109–21.

CHAPTER 12

Social support and childbirth

Christine McCourt

Social support has always been central to midwifery practice, but there is concern that its role in midwifery, although recognised, has diminished in the recent past due to continuing fragmentation and medicalisation of care. The meaning of social support is broad and diffuse, making it difficult to define and study. Nonetheless, there is considerable evidence that the level of social support has a major impact on health, and a number of theories and mechanisms have been proposed to explain this. This chapter discusses the meaning of social support and related concepts, and reviews the theoretical underpinnings and research evidence with regard to its effectiveness. It also discusses the balance between professional interventions and ordinary sources of support, noting that the evidence does not always suggest that health professionals are the best providers of support.

Introduction

She was much better in a way because if there was any small problem bothering you, you go to the hospital or the GP, you think oh, should I tell her? This is what was bothering me, whereas a midwife comes to you, you are friendly and you talk to them, you have no fears or anything, you can say to them, look, there is something bothering me, how small it is. They don't make you feel as if you are wasting their time.

I suppose when you are pregnant you want to be, I don't think they pampered me as much as I would have liked. Although you could have 5 children, you still want to be seen to ... maybe they felt I knew everything and it was OK, just to leave me to get on with it. I sensed that anyway. I don't think it is they didn't care, there just wasn't a great urgency. Making sense?

These quotes, which are taken from a study of women's experiences of maternity care (McCourt and Pearce, 2000; McCourt *et al.*, 2000), illustrate in a very direct way what is so important and so difficult to encapsulate about social support. They suggest that midwifery care is very important to women's feelings of being supported, and that this in turn is important to their experiences of pregnancy, birth and early motherhood. They also illustrate how diffuse the concept is and how difficult it is to define, and how easily overlooked social support may be in modern maternity care.

A recent advisory report on midwifery and nursing (Standing Nursing and Midwifery Advisory Committee and Department of Health, 1998) advocated extended roles for midwives, so that they could play a greater part in supporting the health of women and their families. Midwives were viewed as being in an ideal position to influence public health positively through their work with women before and around the time of birth. Pregnancy is acknowledged to be a time when women are receptive to (and indeed eager for) health information and advice and require particular support. The work of this Government Committee reflected a shift in policy during the 1990s towards the issue of health and social well-being. In 1992, the House of Commons Select Committee on Maternal and Infant Health (House of Commons, 1992) acknowledged some of the problems with regard to changes that had taken place in maternity care during previous decades (e.g. the shift to hospital-based services), and advocated a broader, more 'joined-up' approach to policy and service provision. It noted that the influences on maternal and infant health are wider in scope than the traditional remit of healthcare, including social and economic conditions of family life.

Much of the evidence to support this shift in policy thinking rests on concepts such as social support and social inequality, as well as more recently defined concepts, such as social capital. This chapter focuses on social support and its relationship to the health of mothers and their children. It explores the meanings and applications of the concept and the research evidence that supports its importance. Finally, it critically examines the historical and current relationship between the concept of social support and the practice of midwifery, and suggests some indications for the future of midwifery care.

What is social support?

Social support is a rather flexible concept, as it is so broad that its meaning can easily be assumed, or bent to different purposes, rather than explicitly attended to. This gives rise to problems in researching social support, since the underlying assumptions or theoretical frameworks of the work are not always spelt out. Midwives often describe social support as being essential to their role, and as being part of what distinguishes midwifery from obstetrics, beyond the traditional normal/abnormal division of labour that was instituted in the Midwives Act of 1902. The old English meaning of midwife (*mid wif*, meaning 'with woman') is regarded as a fundamental root of midwifery practice. Consequently, a large part of the midwifery literature in recent decades focused on the withdrawal of much of this supporting and 'presencing' role (Mander, 2001) as services became increasingly organised around a fragmented, production-line model of hospital-centred care (Robinson, 1990; Davis-Floyd, 1994).

Social support has been defined 'as an exchange of resources between at least two individuals perceived by the provider or recipient to be intended to enhance the well-being of the recipient' (Schumaker and Brownell, 1984: 13).

However, such definitions are so broad that it is difficult to pinpoint what social support is, or indeed what it is not. The problem with many definitions is that they may appear tautological, simply implying that social support is a relationship that is perceived to be supportive. It is therefore helpful to break down such general definitions into different attributes. The simplest distinction that is commonly made is to describe social support as either emotional or practical support. Key components of social support can be summarised as follows.

- *Emotional support*: the term implies a warm or caring relationship, but emotional support may be as simple as presence or companionship and willingness to listen. Some authors note the role of conveying esteem and providing security in emotional support.
- *Informational support*: being given good information and advice is widely perceived as being supportive. It underlies the ability to make positive choices, and increases confidence and a sense of security. It may also help by increasing an individual's personal sense of control.
- *Practical or tangible support*: the type of practical support may vary widely, and its importance should not be underestimated. It may include, for example, financial support for a pregnant woman, or physical comfort measures during labour and birth.

Perceived and received support

This distinction is useful because the effects of social support are likely to be strongly dependent on personal perception. Different people will view different things as supportive, influenced by their personal circumstances and preferences as well as by cultural and social factors that guide norms and expectations. For example, the needs of first- and second-time parents are likely to differ. Some people may have adequate personal sources of support, so they do not value professional support as highly, while others may regard offers of support from professionals as intrusive. In addition, if a means of support is to be experienced as positive, it should not incur possible costs (e.g. time, or demeaning the self) that would counter the intended benefits.

There is evidence from psychological research that support which is given but not perceived as such may be ineffective (Cohen and Wills, 1985) or may even have negative effects. It is the perceived adequacy of support that has been found in some studies to correlate positively with mental or physical health (Barrera, 1986; Hirsch and Rapkin, 1986). Indeed, a number of researchers have subsequently gone on to develop the theory that social support itself works particularly through people's perceptions – that feeling supported is a basic aspect of attachment which is fundamental to a person's sense of being esteemed or valued and their sense of agency or ability to control what happens to them.

Support that is offered is likely to be ineffective if it is perceived to be overprotective or lacking understanding. In many instances, health professionals may offer support or care which is not helpful (Oakley, 1992). For example, in discussing the value of trials to test the effects of health and social interventions, Oakley (1998) cites several examples of interventions that were intended to help but which had counter-productive effects. Such evidence is a useful reminder that social ties or relationships (personal or professional) cannot always be assumed to be beneficial. Similarly, offering interventions that may raise expectations without meeting them may also be unhelpful. Such considerations have particular resonance for maternity care, which often fails to deliver the type and level of support that it seems to promise, especially in postnatal services (Ball, 1994; Garcia *et al.*, 1998; Proctor, 1998).

Sources of social support

Sources of social support can be divided into two main categories, namely *formal* (professionals, paid helpers) and *informal* (family, friends, neighbours, community groups, etc.).

It is important to remember that professionals are not the main source of social support, except for very isolated individuals. Abrams, in his seminal study of neighbourhood care (Bulmer, 1986), argued that kin, friendships and neighbourhood relationships are of overwhelming importance in providing social support. Therefore public services should seek to facilitate such support networks where possible and avoid undermining or bypassing them, and they should consider focusing specific interventions on individuals who lack good support networks.

Related concepts

Care

The enduring importance of *care* in the provision of health services reflects the nature of health needs, including the need for social support. As Oakley (1993) has emphasised, the use of the placebo (from the Latin 'to please') in medical research highlights the importance to health of providing care and support and illuminates the enduring importance of care as an aspect of all healing. The ways in which placebo effects have been interpreted in biomedicine reflect an artificial dichotomy between pleasing the patient and benefiting him or her. Evidence that levels of social support influence health cuts across such a dichotomy. However, *care* is often distinguished from *cure* as a way of encapsulating perceived differences between the roles of medicine and of midwifery or nursing. Care is perceived as being more holistic and long term – an essential but undervalued aspect of healthcare, possibly due to its gendered nature.

Care has been described as having two key forms (Bulmer, 1987; Leininger, 1988)

- *caring for* – which may include physical tending or providing material and psychological resources, depending on the person's need
- *caring about* – which may not mean providing direct care, but which involves concern which is supportive at an individual or a more general level.

From these definitions we can see that the concept of care is closely related to that of social support, and such notions are often used interchangeably. However, *care* tends to imply something that is given to or provided for a person (used in the sense of *caring for*), wheras social support may be more indirect and diffuse.

Social capital

The term *social capital* refers to the types of resources that are essential underpinnings of social and community life. The use of the word *capital* draws on the notion that social relationships can be regarded as a type of resource, without which individuals and communities are unable to function effectively and achieve well-being. Although the growing use of the term in much recent social policy has been criticised (Morrow, 2001), it can be argued that it represents an attempt to move away from more individualised approaches to health. For example, although Government policy for health promotion during the 1980s and early 1990s tended to locate health problems within the individual (Department of Health, 1992), this approach was reformed in the late 1990s to focus more on the social conditions for health (Department of Health, 1997a,b).

This more structural focus is reflected in a number of recent policy initiatives that are relevant to health. For example, the New Deal for Communities funds regeneration schemes in deprived neighbourhoods that cut across institutional boundaries such as housing, leisure, employment, food, education and healthcare. Healthy Living Centres, although more specifically health focused, encompass a range of potentially health-promoting facilities and activities that could be described as forms of social support. Similarly, the Sure Start initiative is intended to promote the health and well-being of families with young children. All of these initiatives implicitly recognise the considerable evidence that the social networks and resources which people have available to them, not only personally but also within their local environment, can make a difference to health.

Social networks

The concept of social capital relies to some extent on earlier research conducted by anthropologists and sociologists on social networks, through the theory that the extent and quality of social networks are related to the health of individuals and populations.

Network analysis has also been useful for tackling the methodological problems of asking people to rate their levels of social support in a way that is not simply tautological – those with high levels of health and well-being being more likely to rate their social support more positively. It requires researchers and respondents to be more specific about the relationships involved. Social networks can be classified or measured in various ways, including the following:

- extent – the number of ties or relationships and how far-ranging they are
- density or interconnectedness – the degree to which individuals in the network are linked to each other
- quality – the nature and significance of relationships and whether they are close or distant
- types – that is, types of relationships involved (e.g. whether they are formal or personal)
- frequency – how often contacts are made
- duration or durability – how stable relationships are
- direction or symmetry – for example, whether relationships are mutual or involve dependency in one direction
- reciprocity – the extent to which relationships are reciprocal, acknowledging that a lack of balanced reciprocity can have negative effects on individuals' social status and self-esteem.

Individuals and groups can be asked to map their relationships as networks, using such principles to provide a detailed picture of the degree and type of social support that they may offer. Since the effectiveness of different interventions may depend on the extent to which support is appropriately targeted, network analysis may be a useful tool for researchers or practitioners to explore this aspect.

Theories of social support

Research on underpinning theory is important as a means of understanding the nature of social support and how its effects may operate. There are several key theoretical frameworks for understanding the potential mechanisms of effectiveness. Although they offer different and potentially conflicting theories, it is possible that in explaining such complex phenomena they are complementary.

The mechanisms whereby social support 'works' (e.g. by having a positive impact on health) are not clearly understood, but there is a great deal of evidence that social support works at a number of different levels. This should not be surprising, as health is multifaceted and influenced by a wide range of physiological, environmental and social factors. The approach of biomedicine has been rooted in a paradigm that tends to view such issues as separate. However, the findings of research into social support and health add weight to the alternative view that such factors are closely interrelated – what some commentators have described as an ecological view of health (Arney, 1982; Scheper-Hughes and Lock, 1987).

Psychological theories

Psychological theories tend to be individually oriented, focusing on the influence of various factors on the perceptions, feelings and behaviours of individuals. Key psychological theories include the *stress buffering*, *coping* and *effect on health behaviour* hypotheses:

- stress buffering hypothesis – that social support acts as a buffer against stress (Cobb, 1976)
- coping hypothesis – that social support assists the development of coping strategies that support health (Wheatley, 1998)
- effect on health behaviour hypothesis – that social support influences behaviours that impact on health (Culpepper and Jack, 1993)

Social support is therefore widely viewed as protective against the negative effects of psychosocial risk factors on health, and is often mediated through responses to stress. The 'buffering' hypothesis suggests that psychosocial supports can help to counter or decrease the impact of such negative effects (Wheatley, 1998). Some recent commentators have argued that the individual's sense of control is a key aspect of such buffering effects (Mander, 2001).

Stress is part of everyday life, and is increased during periods of considerable change, such as pregnancy, moving house, changing job, or bereavement (Murray-Parkes, 1971; Marris, 1974), even in cases where the change is viewed positively. Such psychological risk factors appear to play a role in reducing a person's ability to cope with stress, or they can encourage responses to stress that may not benefit health. For example, in a study of the influences on women's health behaviour during pregnancy, Aaronson (1989) found that both perceived and received support had independent positive effects on women's ability to modify behaviours such as drinking alcohol or smoking.

Another important theoretical strand comes from cognitive psychology – that is, the view that the beneficial effects of support are cognitively mediated. This theory proposes that perceptions of support may influence a person's interpretation of stressors, their knowledge of coping strategies and their self-concept (Cohen and McKay, 1983).

Sociological theories

Sociological theories place a greater emphasis on the influence of the social and cultural environment both on health and on the individual's capacity to cope with stressors and to maintain healthy behaviours. Such theories are supported by a large body of evidence on the negative health effects of inequality and poor social and environmental conditions, which are discussed in more depth in Chapter 3.

In a sense, sociological theories build on rather than contradict psychological theories, and they address some of the limitations of a more individually oriented approach. It is likely that psychological theories underpin sociological ones by exploring and explaining ways in which the effects of social conditions may operate on the individual, and by explaining why some people may cope better with difficult conditions than others.

Different sociological theories suggest that social support:

- has a protective effect on health by making the experience of stress less likely to occur in the first place
- can facilitate recovery from illness
- protects against the negative effects of psychosocial risk factors on health.

Again these factors are likely to be linked and iterative, and therefore self-confirming. Broadhead *et al.* (1983) argue that social support is both an outcome of healthy social competence and a contributing cause of good health. Individuals with good health or social resources are more likely to obtain social support, thus encouraging a cycle of positive health benefits. Conversely, those who lack such social resources are less likely to be able to obtain the support that they need. This view is supported by the findings of research on maternity care which suggest that socially disadvantaged women tend to receive a poorer quality of support from service providers (McCourt and Pearce, 2000). Similarly, Oakley's trial of social support for pregnant women suggested that women who were offered additional support were more likely to receive support from their partners (Oakley *et al.*, 1996).

Physiological theories

Physiological research is beginning to identify complex physiological mechanisms for the relationships that have been identified between social support and health. These have immense potential value in breaking down the dichotomous approach to natural and social sciences that has tended to prevail in health research – the disjuncture between 'mind' and 'body' and between the 'social' and the 'physical' body. They address the following question. Given the considerable evidence that social support (or stress) affects people's health, how does it work within the body? The growing body of evidence supports those psychological and socio-logical theories that propose direct as well as indirect effects on people's health.

Much of the relevant research is endocrinological, supporting the view that hormonal mechanisms play an important role in responses to stress or support, with direct long-term effects on health. Much of this work draws on the physi-ology of stress responses developed by Selye (1976). This research suggested that the physiological responses to stress, which involve the hypothalamic–pituitary–adrenal axis, are normally protective. Once the source of stress is removed, the body stress hormones return to their normal level. However, if stressors are pro-longed or chronic, the prolonged exposure to raised levels can be damaging (Selye, 1976). A full exploration of physiological theory is beyond the scope of this chapter. Instead, we shall focus on some key examples of research that can inform our thinking with regard to social support and pregnancy.

Anxiety and umbilical cord blood flow

Teixeira et al. (1999) investigated the relationship between anxiety and low birth weight physiologically by looking at the potential impact of raised anxiety levels on umbilical cord blood flow. Drawing on endocrinological evidence, they postulated that raised anxiety levels resulting in increased levels of stress hor-mones such as noradrenaline would restrict blood flow from the mother. Such a mechanism could account at least in part for low birth weight, since blood flow has a direct effect on fetal development. Such an effect would work in a similar way to smoking, which has been shown to have a clear negative effect on fetal blood supply and birth weight. Texeira et al. (1999) found significant associations between anxiety levels and umbilical cord blood flow, which supports the postu-lated relationship between stress, anxiety and low birth weight.

The authors noted in their discussion that it was unclear to what extent the associations were with current or long-term anxiety, since most women with raised anxiety levels had high scores on both trait (general) and state (current feel-ings) anxiety. This would have implications for considering social support inter-ventions, since if long-term anxiety is the key factor, the effects of short-term and time-limited interventions in pregnancy may be limited.

Possible hormonal factors: oxytocin

There is considerable indirect evidence to suggest that a complex relationship exists between stress, anxiety and the hormone oxytocin, which plays an important role in pregnancy and labour. The results of animal studies suggest that oxytocin itself may have an anxiety-reducing effect, but also that stress levels may affect the synthesis of oxytocin in the body (Uvnas-Moberg, 1998). Research on childbirth suggests that associations exist between anxiety, oxytocin synthesis and women's need for oxytocic augmentation of labour and pharmacological pain relief (Haddad, 1989). Such findings have led to increasing interest in the possible role of endogenous oxytocin in determining the anxiety and pain threshold during pregnancy and labour, and in specific interventions to enhance oxytocin synthesis during the latter half of pregnancy. The evidence of an association between anxiety levels and oxytocin suggests that such interventions would need to be directed towards reducing women's anxiety – through their responses to stress and the life events and problems that contribute to raised anxiety levels.

Research on massage

Physiological experiments have also shown that a variety of sensory stimuli, such as touch (including massage and baby holding), have endocrinological effects that decrease blood pressure and stress responses. Massage has been used by traditional birth attendants and a range of therapists both historically and across a wide range of cultures. Jordan (1993) cites the example of the Mayan traditional midwife who massages the woman's abdomen during pregnancy and in labour. Many midwives and mothers in the UK use massage to provide comfort, relaxation and pain relief during pregnancy and labour.

In addition, a number of massage specialists now teach infant massage techniques to mothers, and there is a growing body of research evidence to suggest that these have benefits for mother–infant interactions, especially for premature babies. The evidence for effects on pregnancy and childbirth is more limited, but some small trials have found beneficial effects of massage on pain in a range of groups (Field *et al.*, 1997). The studies also found differences in anxiety levels between groups that received massage and control groups. Although massage may have direct effects (e.g. via the synthesis of oxytocin), its influence may also be indirectly mediated through effects on stress and anxiety, which result in hormonal responses.

Research on consumers' views of social support

In researching perceptions of social support, Gottlieb (1978) found that what ordinary individuals valued most were:

- emotionally sustaining behaviours (e.g. listening, showing concern, conveying intimacy)
- problem-solving behaviours (e.g. material and financial help).

Similarly, the findings of studies of women's experiences and perceptions of pregnancy and birth are highly consistent in indicating what they view as supportive maternity care (Oakley, 1979, 1980; Green *et al.*, 1988; Brown and Lumley, 1994; McCourt *et al.*, 1998; Proctor, 1998; McCourt and Pearce, 2000). This can be summarised as follows:

- good communication – not only being given information, but also being listened to
- being treated as an individual, feeling known and understood
- a sense of choice and control with regard to what happens to them
- a sense of trust, and confidence both in themselves and in those caring for them
- a perception of professionals as being sensitive and caring.

Studies of women in different social classes and ethnic groups (MORI (Market and Opinion Research Institute), 1993; Handler *et al.*, 1996, Laslett *et al.*, 1997; Hirst *et al.*, 1998) suggest that such core principles are relevant to a wide range of women, rather than being confined to an articulate minority. However, women's specific concerns about support do vary, as do their specific experiences of healthcare. For example, many women in minority groups experience greater communication problems with service providers, and there is evidence that women in lower social class groups receive information of poorer quality from service providers (Cartwright, 1979; Reid and Garcia, 1989; Walker *et al.*, 1995).

In a survey of Finnish mothers' perceptions of maternity care, Tarkka and Paunonen (1996) found that, during pregnancy, women regarded partners, family and friends (respectively) rather than professionals as their main source of support. However, midwives were the most important source of support during birth. The support that was given by midwives during labour was valued most in the domain of affect (emotional support), and emotional support was also associated with positive birth experiences. Issues that were particularly important with regard to mothers' experiences included the following:

- their reception and treatment by staff
- encouragement
- a sense of security
- alleviation of pain
- individuality of treatment
- continuity.

In a study by Bryanton *et al.* (1994) in the USA of mothers' views about maternity support, the women viewed all of the categories of help as important, but behaviours that were categorised as 'emotional support' were perceived to be most helpful. The most helpful behaviours included the following:

- feeling cared about as an individual and being treated with respect
- receiving praise
- staff appearing calm and confident
- receiving assistance with breathing and relaxing.

A study of Hong Kong Chinese women's views of labour support by Yin-King (1998) highlights the extent to which the perceived supportiveness of particular behaviours may vary culturally. As in many other studies, information and emotional support were rated most highly, and tangible support was rated lowest. Consistent with Chinese cultural norms with regard to presentation of self, being praised was rated most highly, while being touched was rated as least helpful.

Effects of social support: the psychological evidence

In an overview of evidence for the health effects of social support, Cobb interpreted social support as information leading the subject to believe that 'he (*sic*) is cared for and loved, that he is esteemed and valued and that he belongs to a network of communication and mutual obligation' (Cobb, 1976: 300). Drawing on Nuckolls' research on pregnancy as a significant life event, Cobb suggests that the interaction between levels of social support and levels of stressful life events is crucial. In Nuckolls' study of 'army wives', it was the group with both high levels of 'life change' and low levels of social support who had an excessive level of pregnancy and birth complications (91%). Women with high levels of social support had significantly fewer complications (33%). For women with low levels of 'life change', levels of support appeared to matter less (Nuckolls et al., 1972). A study of asthma patients using a similar methodology showed comparable effects. Patients with high levels of 'life change' and low levels of social support required significantly higher doses of steroids to control their symptoms. Patients with high levels of 'life events' *and* high levels of social support did not require more medication than those with lower life event scores, suggesting a protective effect of social support (de Araujo et al., 1973).

In another study reviewed by Cobb (1976), Egbert et al. (1964) randomised surgical patients to two groups, providing additional supportive care from the anaesthetist for one group, in a way that was blinded to the surgeons involved. They found that patients in this group needed lower levels of pain relief and were discharged earlier than those in the control group. This replicated similar findings obtained for children undergoing tonsillectomy (Jessner et al., 1952). The findings of such early studies have been established in healthcare principles to the extent that not providing patients (including children) with appropriate information is now widely regarded as poor practice.

Effects of social support: the sociological evidence

A seminal sociological study pointing to the effects of social support was that by Brown and Harris (1978) of women and depression. The authors found a very high prevalence of depression among women, particularly those at home with young children and those not in paid work. On this basis, they postulated that much depression among women has social origins and is linked to social isolation and lack of support.

A series of qualitative studies by Oakley (1979, 1980) also highlighted the problems associated with women's gender roles and the impact of social isolation on many women as housewives and mothers. These studies led Oakley to investigate the issue of social support further with a trial of the effects of social support in pregnancy (see below).

In her account of this trial, Oakley (1992) reviewed a range of studies which provided evidence that social support influences physical and psychological health. Among these, a large-scale, community-based study of patterns of mortality in the USA (Cohen and Syme, 1987) showed that long-term survival was correlated with social support independently of other potentially related factors, such as initial physical health, social status, or habits such as smoking. In general, social involvement predicted better survival, although the types of involvement that mattered differed for men and women.

In an early qualitative study of 41 middle- and upper-class mothers, Abernethy (1973) examined the effects of a tight or loose social network in predicting a woman's attitude to her children and her response to the demands of the maternal role. She concluded that women in loose networks appeared to suffer from insufficient feedback and were therefore likely to be exposed to a confusing array of variance in childrearing theory. Women who were in a tight social network were more likely to have confidence in their maternal competence, while those in loose networks were more likely to be frustrated by motherhood and to feel unsure about how to relate to their children.

As will be seen in the following section, such studies highlight the fact that social support is far broader than the remit and power of health services – the most important sources of social support are likely to be in people's personal and community networks, and these vary greatly. Thus the findings of studies of the impact of maternity care may vary according to the nature of the support offered and the way in which it is targeted and received.

Effects of social support: the midwifery evidence

Pregnancy

An early overview of 14 trials of social support interventions in maternity care identified the following key features associated with increased levels of support:

- reduced anxiety (e.g. greater confidence, lack of nervousness, reduced fear, positive feelings with regard to birth)
- reduced psychological and physical morbidity
- in most cases, increased satisfaction with care and communication
- an increased sense of control (Elbourne et al., 1989).

There was no significant impact on labour interventions or outcomes, but the authors concluded that, given the positive impact of social support on women's feelings about pregnancy and birth, and the lack of negative effects found in these trials, such support should be regarded as integral to good maternity care, rather than being viewed as some kind of 'optional extra'. They highlighted the fact that increasing fragmentation of care and obstetric focus in the maternity services had made this more difficult.

Following this, a series of trials was conducted to assess the potential impact of social support in pregnancy on birth weight (Oakley et al., 1990, 1996; Oakley, 1992; Villar et al., 1992; Norbeck et al., 1996). Birth weight has been repeatedly selected for testing the effects of social support because it is considered to be a relatively reliable, valid and readily measurable indicator of maternal and infant health (Barker, 1998).

The intervention tested in the trial by Oakley et al. (1990) was a series of home visits by research midwives plus telephone support offered to women with a previous low-birth-weight baby (< 2500 g). The study also used a range of secondary outcome measures that were possible indicators of maternal and infant well-being, and gathered both quantitative and qualitative data.

Although the study did not find a statistically significant increase in birth weight, there were fewer very-low-birth-weight babies, fewer antenatal hospital admissions, a lower rate of use of epidural pain relief, more spontaneous labours and more spontaneous vaginal births. There was no significant difference in the number of babies that needed special care, but those in the support group required less invasive resuscitation methods and less intensive care. The mothers reported better physical health both of themselves and of their babies, and less use of health services, 6 weeks after the birth. Their views about the intervention were positive, highlighting the importance of the midwife listening to them.

In a long-term follow-up study (something which is unusual due to difficulties of finding and also maintaining contact with study participants), the mothers reported fewer health problems in their children, fewer concerns about their social well-being, a higher level of personal well-being and greater ability to obtain social support from others, particularly their partners (Oakley *et al.*, 1996).

The findings of this study were highly suggestive of certain benefits of social support. However, it also had a number of drawbacks that highlight the difficulty of conducting trials in order to test the effects of complex interventions, especially of concepts such as social support which may be poorly defined, as well as operating far beyond the reaches of healthcare. Not least, it did not establish a significant difference in the primary outcome measure chosen, namely the incidence of low birth weight.

In the Cochrane overview of trials of social support in pregnancy and birth weight, Hodnett (2002a) reported that the clinical benefits found in such trials were marginal, and the following cautionary points were noted.

- Such interventions may not be adequate to counter the well-researched effects of poverty and social disadvantage on health.
- The outcomes measured in such trials may not be the only ones which matter.
- Although receiving prenatal care is generally associated with better health outcomes, little is known about what components of such care are useful or effective.
- The trials covered a wide range of interventions, all of which were classed as social support.

These cautions are well illustrated by a large multi-centre South American trial of the effects of social support on birth weight (Villar *et al.*, 1992), which was included in the Cochrane review's meta-analysis. The support was home based, was provided by social workers, included an educational focus as well as social support, and was targeted at women who were at high 'psychological and social risk' (Langer *et al.*, 1996). This was conceived as an ecological model of social support in which health education and social support would function synergistically. No difference in birth weight was found. However, the women's views about the intervention were not specifically studied, and it was not clear that they perceived the intervention to be supportive.

The only trial that was included which *did* find a significant difference in birth weight, by Norbeck *et al.* (1996), was targeted at low-income African-American women who were identified during pregnancy as lacking the usual sources of social support from a mother or partner. This approach is subtly but perhaps importantly different to others that targeted women at 'high risk' defined in various ways (e.g. having had a previous low-birth-weight baby), but not by reference to their own sources of support. The intervention was also more clearly client-centred than some of the trials included in the review. The intervention was designed (using previous qualitative research) to be culturally appropriate and to model the type of support that a mother or partner might provide.

Hodnett's cautions are well illustrated by the difference in findings across these studies – apparently of the same phenomenon. In a commentary on the South American trial of Villar *et al.* (1992), Hodnett (1993) suggests that current research evidence may not be focusing on what is most important about social support. Like Sandall (1995), she also notes that social support interventions during pregnancy cannot be expected to compensate for social inequality and long-term, deep-seated problems that contribute to low birth weight. This view was echoed by Langer *et al.* (1996), who concluded from their trial that psychosocial interventions that were offered solely during pregnancy, and on a scale feasible within public services in poorer countries, would not counter the adverse effects of psychosocial distress.

In another overview, in this case of trials of home visitation programmes offering support to socially disadvantaged mothers, Hodnett and Roberts (2002) found differences in other outcomes relating to capacity to care for the child, although these differences were 'promising' rather than substantial. Several descriptive studies have also looked at the impact of peer support, with encouraging findings. Again, potentially effective approaches tended to model ordinary sources of support. The Mentoring Mothers Programme, which was studied by Navaie-Waliser *et al.* (1996), trained mature local women to be volunteer mentors to young socially disadvantaged pregnant women within a continuing caring one-to-one relationship. The programme targeted three communities that were known to have a high incidence of low birth weight, and recruited 42 volunteers. This was described as a community-empowering approach. Although this was not a trial, so had no formal comparisons, the outcomes for the mothers involved were positive by comparison with general outcomes for this community, and they reported a decreased sense of isolation. In addition, they reported positive responses from the volunteer women themselves, including enhanced self-esteem and motivation. Although the study was not designed to formally test the outcomes of an intervention, it provides an example of the way in which professionals can facilitate the provision of ordinary sources of social support within a community, in a way that may be more enduring than any health-service-based intervention.

Labour and birth

A number of trials have also tested the potential impact of support during labour on birth outcomes. The support investigated included continuous support by lay (doula) or professional companions during labour.

In the Cochrane review of trials of support in labour, Hodnett (1999) looked at the impact of *continuous* support by either trained or untrained individuals. The review included 11 trials in a wide range of cultural and medical settings, some of which excluded other companions. The meta-analysis showed reductions in the following:

- duration of labour
- likelihood of requiring medication for pain relief
- operative vaginal delivery
- 5-minute Apgar score of < 7
- where companions were not normally admitted, a reduced likelihood of birth by Caesarean section.

In addition, some trials found evidence of the following:

• greater satisfaction with birth
• longer duration of breastfeeding
• decreases in perineal trauma
• less postnatal depression and less difficulty in mothering.

The review included two early and influential trials in Guatemala in a busy public hospital where companions were not normally admitted and one-to-one professional support was not the norm (Sosa *et al.*, 1980, Klaus *et al.*, 1986).

The trial conducted by Klaus *et al.* (1986), which replicated the earlier study on a larger scale, included healthy women admitted without a companion, in early but established labour. Those women who were randomised to the intervention group were supported by a doula, while the women in the control group received standard care. Klaus and colleagues found significant reductions in the duration and augmentation of labour, Caesarean sections, admission to the neonatal unit and perinatal complications. In addition, regression analysis suggested that the effects were greater in women who were living alone. The study indicated that very large differences could be achieved with 'poor women who routinely undergo labour alone on a crowded ward' (Klaus *et al.*, 1986: 586).

The trial was then replicated in a North American (US) context, in a busy obstetrically oriented unit with high prevailing intervention rates but greater access to pain relief. As in the Guatemalan context, it included a large proportion of women who were socially disadvantaged and non-English-speaking. The labour supporters were bilingual local women with personal experience of a normal birth, who were given 3 weeks of preparation. Similar results were obtained (Kennell *et al.*, 1991).

This study included both an observed group (observed unobtrusively by a researcher) without support and a control group that was assessed by review of hospital notes after birth. Interestingly, similar differences, but of a smaller magnitude, were found between the control group with review of notes only and the group that was observed by a researcher. This unexpected finding suggested that even continuous presence – without active engagement or support – could have a protective effect. However, the authors noted that the reason for this difference was unclear, and that it could equally well be explained by the researcher's presence having an effect on hospital staff behaviour.

A similar trial in Canada by Hodnett and Osborn (1989) examined the impact of continuous support by a familiar, trained caregiver, using self-employed 'coaches' who were either lay or student midwives. This Canadian teaching hospital cared for mainly white, middle-class women, who were routinely allowed the companionship of their husband or partner. As in the US unit, there was a high level of routine intervention in labour, but good staff-to-patient ratios. The study found significant reductions in the use of pain relief medication and episiotomy, but not in major outcomes such as mode of birth. The authors noted the difficulty of conducting such a trial in a setting where actively managed and accelerated labour was the norm (only 8 out of 103 women included in the trial laboured with no intervention). It is also likely that since the women in this trial were able to have continuous support from a chosen birth companion, the difference made by a 'doula' might be reduced.

The limitations of such findings should alert us to the need to take context as well as type of intervention into account when studying the effects of social support. In this case, the women selected were not those likely to be in greatest need of social support from professionals, but the setting also placed limitations on the capacity of supportive care to influence interventions at the time of birth.

Models of midwifery and maternity care

The *Changing Childbirth* report (Department of Health, 1993) advocated a shift in the organisation of maternity care to enable a more woman-centred approach. Acknowledging the impact of fragmentation of care on women's experiences, a number of schemes to improve continuity of care and carer were piloted. A series of studies of such schemes suggests that continuity of care and carer are important to women's perceptions that care is supportive.

An overview of trials of continuity of carer indicated beneficial effects on the use of pain relief and episiotomies, and these women were more satisfied with their care (Hodnett, 2002b). Other studies indicate that greater continuity, and the relationships between mothers and midwives that this facilitates, increase the mothers' confidence both in the midwife and in themselves (McCourt *et al.*, 1998, 2000; Walsh, 1998; Sandall *et al.*, 2001). In interviews, mothers described the importance of a known midwife being with them throughout labour and birth in terms of feeling understood and respected, being relaxed and confident, and feeling comforted (McCourt *et al.*, 2000). Women who lacked such continuity of support were more likely to describe feelings of anxiety, fear and confusion in their accounts of pregnancy and birth. This was particularly the case for those who were socially disadvantaged or from ethnic minority groups, who tend to receive less information and less supportive care in the health services.

It could be argued that these mothers' accounts are primarily about feeling supported by their midwife carers – support which should be achievable by ensuring a consistent approach rather than needing known carers, or simply by 'good midwives'. However, the lack of such accounts (except for a very few cases), from women receiving shared or conventional consultant-led maternity care suggests that the supportive or caring qualities of midwives cannot be readily separated from the organisation and environment of their work. The manner in which services are organised and provided may have an important impact on the levels or forms of support that midwives are able to offer women.

Postnatal support

A number of studies have indicated the importance to women of postnatal social support, but also the lack of supportive care found in current health systems. Ball's major study highlighted the way in which hospital practices often worked *against* the provision of social support (Ball, 1994). These included the following:

- unnecessary separation of the mother and her baby soon after birth (then, once maternal–infant bonding was recognised as an issue, 'rooming in' coupled with loss of practical support)

- fragmentation of care
- task-based rather than person-based work and routines
- a didactic style when giving help or advice
- care focused mainly on physical examination of the mother and feeding of the baby
- inadequate support with regard to breastfeeding.

Compounding this, Ball (1994) found a mismatch between midwives' summing up of women's emotional states and their more specific comments (e.g. on the numbers of women who had been crying or showing sleep or appetite disturbances), suggesting that they either regard this as 'normal' or give low priority to emotional states.

Factor analysis in Ball's study showed that emotional well-being and satisfaction with motherhood were associated with the following:

- antecedent factors (e.g. in the woman's own background)
- other stress factors
- self-confidence on returning home.

The experience of 'other stress factors' was strongly influenced by postnatal care practices, the key factors being feelings at the time of birth, self-image when feeding the baby in hospital, and conflicting advice or lack of rest in hospital.

What is particularly disappointing is that studies conducted since then, despite *Changing Childbirth* policy (Department of Health, 1993), suggest that there has been little change in postnatal care (Garcia *et al.*, 1998).

A number of maternity interventions have been piloted to offer additional postnatal support to women. An overview of trials of home-based postnatal support for disadvantaged women (Hodnett and Roberts, 2002) found some evidence of beneficial effects (e.g. better take-up of immunisations and reduced hospitalisations), with no evidence of harmful effects. However, this evidence has very limited applicability, as most of the trials were in the USA, where there is no routine postnatal midwifery home care, and they tended to be geared towards prevention of child abuse and child health or service utilisation problems, only rarely focusing on psychosocial or physical health effects on the mother. Nonetheless, some schemes used the skills of experienced mothers living in local communities. This resource, as with antenatal support, may well provide less expensive and more culturally sensitive support than professional, hospital-based programmes.

A recent trial of community postnatal support in the UK (Morrell *et al.*, 2000) did not find any significant differences in women's psychological or general health, or in breastfeeding rates. Like the trials of antenatal care and low birth weight, this study highlights the need for caution in assuming that additional supportive maternity care will have a significant impact on women's health. However, like some of those trials, the intervention was not targeted at women who lacked ordinary sources of support. It might be argued that offering additional support to those who do not need it may decrease or at least delay their ability to take up the informal sources of help that are available to them. A similar need for caution may be suggested by the extent to which research on breastfeeding has indicated that professional support is not necessarily or always helpful or effective (Renfrew *et al.*, 2000).

Conclusion

This brief overview has indicated that social support is an important concept with clear implications for health and general well-being, and that it is therefore highly relevant to maternity care. Midwives' roles have traditionally focused on supportive care during the transition of childbirth, combining a number of roles. However, historical changes throughout the twentieth century have undermined the degree to which 'support' has been integral to the midwife's role (Tew, 1998; Mander, 2001).

This chapter has discussed how the concept of social support – despite the considerable evidence for its fundamental importance in health and healthcare – is very difficult to define or measure. However, it is the very flexibility and breadth of the concept that may be an undeniable aspect of its power. On the one hand, such concepts need to be unpicked so that they can be viewed critically and researched effectively, yet on the other they may work through their integration of a range of functions in a way that may be undermined by such unpicking. In addition, it must be recognised that the meaning of support for the receiver is highly subjective, which is also a crucial aspect of its effectiveness. What is supportive for one person may not be so for another, even though clear patterns can be discerned and have been demonstrated in the research on women's experiences of maternity and healthcare.

Related concepts, such as reciprocity, are highly relevant here because they show that being the receiver of a gift or service can mean loss of power or status, unless the form of reciprocity is appropriately balanced. This provides a warning to health professionals that giving (providing services) is not as straightforward a 'good' as it might appear. It may also explain the extent to which the evidence reviewed in this chapter suggests that 'lay' or 'peer' models of support may be as effective, if not more so, than professional models. This indicates that professional thinking about ways of providing support needs to change, and that it should be increasingly geared towards underpinning, facilitating and promoting non-professional sources of support. The concept of social capital (working to build the networks and social cohesion of local communities or other social groups) appears relevant here, but critical research on social capital also highlights the difficulties of aiming for community empowerment among people who are substantially deprived. High levels of deprivation undermine individuals' ability to form, sustain and participate in support networks.

The research on mechanisms of social support is building up a picture of ways in which social support may work to enhance health, or at least reduce the negative health effects of a range of stressors or threats. Such research also clearly demonstrates a traditional rationale of midwifery – that the mind and the body are not separate, and that care must address physiological, psychological and environmental factors in an integrated fashion (what is often called 'holistic care').

The varied and sometimes disappointing findings of research on the effectiveness of health professional interventions to offer social support highlight the need for caution in planning services. It is tempting for professionals and policy makers to regard social support interventions as solutions to what are often structural and deep-rooted problems, such as social inequality. Such interventions might instead be viewed as complementary to social policies to support good-quality housing, education, employment, nutrition and a range of community resources and facilities.

While planners are presented with the challenges of targeting and designing appropriate support interventions, and researchers continue to tease out and identify what seems to work best and for whom, it seems wise to echo Elbourne's sentiments (Elbourne *et al.*, 1989) – that support should be seen quite simply as part of providing good midwifery care. The fact that this is not always the case, and for all women, is the challenge to midwives in the twenty-first century.

- Appropriate social support has a positive impact on general health and well-being.
- Professionals should note that a high proportion of social support is provided by friends, family and community, rather than by professionals or formal interventions.
- Organising and providing midwifery care in different ways can have an important impact on the levels of supportive care.
- There is evidence that some maternal health interventions have a positive influence, especially if they are targeted towards mothers with low levels of social support and they are perceived as supportive by the mothers themselves.
- The concept of social support is broad and difficult to define, but careful attention needs to be given to definitions and meanings when researching the effects of interventions.

References

- Aaronson LS (1989) Perceived and received support: effects on health behavior during pregnancy. *Nurs Res.* **38**: 4–9.
- Abernethy VD (1973) Social network and response to the maternal role. *Int J Sociol Fam.* **3**: 86–92.
- Arney W (1982) *Power and the Profession of Obstetrics.* University of Chicago Press, Chicago, IL.
- Ball J (1994) *Reactions to Motherhood: the role of postnatal care.* Cambridge University Press, Cambridge.
- Barker DJP (1998) *Mothers, Babies and Health in Later Life.* Churchill Livingstone, Edinburgh.
- Barrera M (1986) Distinctions between social support concepts, measures, and models. *Am J Commun Psychol.* **14**: 413–45.
- Broadhead WT, Kaplan BH, James SA, Wagner EH and Schonbach VJ (1983) The epidemiological evidence for a relationship between social support and health. *Am J Epidemiol.* **117**: 521–37.
- Brown, GW and Harris T (1978) *Social Origins of Depression: a study of psychiatric disorder in women.* Tavistock, London.
- Brown S and Lumley J (1994) Satisfaction with care in labor and birth: a survey of 790 Australian women. *Birth.* **21**: 4–13.
- Bryanton J, Fraser-Davey H and Sullivan P (1994) Women's perceptions of nursing support during labor. *J Obstet Gynecol Neonatal Nurs.* **23**: 638–44.
- Bulmer M (1986) *Neighbours: the work of Philip Abrams.* Cambridge University Press, Cambridge.

- Bulmer M (1987) *The Social Basis of Community Care.* Allen and Unwin, London.
- Cartwright A (1979) *The Dignity of Labour? A study of childbearing and induction.* Tavistock, London.
- Cobb S (1976) Social support as a moderator of life stress. *Psychosom Med.* **38**: 300–14.
- Cohen S and McKay G (1983) Social support, stress and the buffering hypothesis: a theoretical analysis. In: A Baum, JE Singer and S Taylor (eds) *Handbook of Psychology and Health. Volume 4.* Erlbaum, Hillsdale, NJ.
- Cohen S and Wills TA (1985) Stress, social support and the buffering hypothesis. *Psychol Bull.* **98**: 310–57.
- Cohen S and Syme (1987) *Social Support and Health.* Academic Press, New York.
- Culpepper L and Jack B (1993) Psychosocial issues in pregnancy. *Prim Care.* **20**: 599–619.
- Davis-Floyd R (1994) The ritual of hospital birth in America. In: JP Spradley and DW McCurdey (eds) *Conformity and Conflict. Readings in cultural anthropology.* Harper-Collins, New York.
- de Araujo G, van Arsdel PP, Holmes TH and Dudley DL (1973) Life change, coping ability and chronic intrinsic asthma. *J Psychosom Res.* **17**: 359–63.
- Department of Health (1992) *The Health of the Nation.* HMSO, London.
- Department of Health (1993) *Changing Childbirth. The Report of the Expert Maternity Group. 1.* Department of Health, London.
- Department of Health (1997a) *The New NHS: modern, dependable.* Department of Health, London.
- Department of Health (1997b) *Our Healthier Nation. A contract for health.* The Stationery Office, London.
- Egbert LD, Battit GE, Welch CE and Bartlett MK (1964) Reduction of post-operative pain by encouragement and instruction of patients. *NEJM.* **270**: 825–7.
- Elbourne D, Oakley A and Chalmers I (1989) Social and psychological support during pregnancy. In: I Chalmers, M Enkin and M Keirse (eds) *Effective Care in Pregnancy and Childbirth.* Oxford University Press, Oxford.
- Field T, Hernandez-Raif M, Taylor S *et al.* (1997) Labour pain is reduced by massage therapy. *J Psychosom Obstet Gynaecol.* **18**: 286–91.
- Garcia J, Redshaw M, Fitzsimons B and Keene J (1998) *First-Class Delivery: a national survey of women's views of maternity care.* Audit Commission/National Perinatal Epidemiology Unit, Abingdon.
- Gottlieb BH (1978) Development and application of a classification scheme of informal helping behaviour. *Can J Behav Sci.* **10**: 105–15.
- Green J, Coupland V, Kitzinger J *et al.* (1988) *Great Expectations. A prospective study of women's expectations and experiences of childbirth.* Childcare and Development Group, Cambridge University, Cambridge.
- Haddad F (1989) Effect of anxiety in pregnancy. *Contemp Rev Obstet Gynaecol.* **1**: 123–32.
- Handler H, Raube K, Kelley M *et al.* (1996) Women's satisfaction with prenatal care settings: a focus group study. *Birth.* **23**: 31–7.
- Hirsch BJ and Rapkin BD (1986) Social networks and adult identities: profiles and correlates of support and rejection. *Am J Commun Psychol.* **14**: 395–412.
- Hirst J, Hewison J, Dowswell T, Baslington H and Warrilow J (1998) Antenatal care: what do women want? In: S Clement (ed.) *Psychological Perspectives on Pregnancy and Childbirth.* Churchill Livingstone, Edinburgh.

- Hodnett E (1993) Social support during high-risk pregnancy: does it help? *Birth.* **20**: 218–19.
- Hodnett ED (1999) *Support from Caregivers During Childbirth. The Cochrane Library.* Update Software, Oxford.
- Hodnett ED (2002a) *Support During Pregnancy for Mothers at Increased Risk of Low Birthweight Babies.* The Cochrane Library. Update Software, Oxford.
- Hodnett ED (2002b) *Continuity of Caregivers During Pregnancy and Birth.* The Cochrane Library. Update Software, Oxford.
- Hodnett ED and Osborn RW (1989) Effects of continuous intrapartum professional support on childbirth outcomes. *Res Nurs Health.* **12**: 289–97.
- Hodnett ED and Roberts I (2002) *Home-Based Social Support for Socially Disadvantaged Mothers.* The Cochrane Library. Update Software, Oxford.
- House of Commons (1992) *Maternity Services: Government response to the Second Report from the Health Committee, Session 1991–92.* HMSO, London.
- Jessner L, Blom GE and Waldfogel S (1952) Emotional implications of tonsillectomy and adenoidectomy on children. *Psychoanal Stud Childhood.* **7**: 126–69.
- Jordan B (1993) *Birth in Four Cultures. A cross-cultural investigation of childbirth in Yucatan, Holland, Sweden and the United States.* Waveland Press, Prospect Heights, IL.
- Kennell J, Klaus M, McGrath S *et al.* (1991) Continuous emotional support during labor in a US hospital: a randomised controlled trial. *JAMA.* **265**: 2197–201.
- Klaus MH, Kennell JH, Robertson SS *et al.* (1986) Effects of social support during parturition on maternal and infant morbidity. *BMJ.* **293**: 585–7.
- Langer A, Farnot U, Garcia C *et al.* (1996) The Latin-American trial of psychosocial support during pregnancy: effects on mothers' well-being and satisfaction. *Soc Sci Med.* **42**: 1589–97.
- Laslett A, Brown S and Lumley J (1997) Women's views of different models of antenatal care in Victoria, Australia. *Birth.* **24**: 81–9.
- Leininger M (1988) *Caring: an essential human need.* Wayne State University Press, Detroit, MI.
- McCourt C and Pearce A (2000) Does continuity of carer matter to women from minority ethnic groups? *Midwifery.* **16**: 145–54.
- McCourt C, Page L, Hewison J and Vail A (1998) Evaluation of one-to-one midwifery: women's responses to care. *Birth.* **25**: 73–80.
- McCourt C, Hirst J and Page L (2000) Dimensions and attributes of caring: women's perceptions. In: L Page (ed.) *The New Midwifery: science and sensitivity in practice.* Churchill Livingstone, Edinburgh.
- Mander R (2001) *Supportive Care and Midwifery.* Blackwell Science, Oxford.
- Marris P (1974) *Loss and Change.* Routledge and Kegan Paul, London.
- MORI (Market and Opinion Research Institute) (1993) *A Survey of Women's Views of the Maternity Services. Maternity services research study.* Department of Health, London.
- Morrell CJ, Spiby H, Stewart P and Walters S (2000) *Costs and Benefits of Community Postnatal Support Workers: a randomised controlled trial.* Health Technology Assessment Programme, Department of Health, London.
- Morrow G (ed.) (2000) *An Appropriate Capital-Isation? Questioning social capital.* London School of Economics, London.

- Murray-Parkes C (1971) Psychosocial transitions. A field for study. *Soc Sci Med.* **5**: 101–15.
- Navaie-Waliser M, Gordon SK and Hibberd ME (1996) The mentoring mothers program: a community-empowering approach to reducing infant mortality. *J Perinatal Educ.* **5**: 47–58.
- Norbeck JS, Dejoseph JF and Smith RT (1996) A randomized trial of an empirically derived social support intervention to prevent low birth weight among African-American women. *Soc Sci Med.* **43**: 947–54.
- Nuckolls KB, Cassel JC and Kaplan BH (1972) Psychosocial assets, life crisis and the prognosis of pregnancy. *Am J Epidemiol.* **95**: 431–41.
- Oakley A (1979) *Becoming a Mother*. Martin Robertson, Oxford.
- Oakley A (1980) *Women Confined: towards a sociology of childbirth*. Martin Robertson, Oxford.
- Oakley A (1992) *Social Support and Motherhood. The natural history of a research project*. Blackwell, Oxford.
- Oakley A (1993) *Essays on Women, Medicine and Health*. Edinburgh University Press, Edinburgh.
- Oakley A (1998) Experimentation in social science: the case of health promotion. *Soc Sci Health.* **4**: 73–88.
- Oakley A, Rajan L and Grant A (1990) Social support and pregnancy outcome: report of a randomised controlled trial. *Br J Obstet Gynaecol.* **97**: 155–62.
- Oakley A, Hickey D, Rajan L *et al.* (1996) Social support in pregnancy: does it have long-term effects? *J Reprod Infant Psychol.* **14**: 7–22.
- Proctor S (1998) What determines quality in maternity care? Comparing the perceptions of childbearing women and midwives. *Birth.* **25**: 85–93.
- Reid M and Garcia J (1989) Women's views of care during pregnancy and childbirth. In: I Chalmers, M Enkin and M Keirse (eds) *Effective Care in Pregnancy and Childbirth*. Oxford University Press, Oxford.
- Renfrew M, Woolridge MW and Ross McGill H (2000) *Enabling Women to Breastfeed: a structured review with evidence-based guidance for practice*. The Stationery Office, London.
- Robinson S (1990) Maintaining the role of the midwife. In: J Garcia, R Kilpatrick and M Richards (eds) *The Politics of Maternity Care*. Clarendon Press, Oxford.
- Sandall J (1995) Choice, continuity and control: changing midwifery, towards a sociological perspective. *Midwifery.* **11**: 201–9.
- Sandall J, Davies J and Warwick C (2001) *Evaluation of the Albany Midwifery Practice*. King's College, London.
- Scheper-Hughes N and Lock M (1987) The mindful body. A prolegomenon to future work in medical anthropology. *Med Anthropol Q.* **1**: 6–41.
- Schumaker S and Brownell A (1984) Towards a theory of social support: closing conceptual gaps. *J Soc Issues.* **40**: 11–36.
- Selye H (1976) *Stress in Health and Disease*. Butterworth, London.
- Sosa R, Kennell J, Klaus M *et al.* (1980) The effect of a supportive companion on perinatal problems, length of labour, and mother–infant interaction. *NEJM.* **303**: 597–600.
- Standing Nursing and Midwifery Advisory Committee and Department of Health (1998) *Delivering our Future. Report by the Standing Nursing and Midwifery Advisory Committee*. The Stationery Office, London.

- Tarkka MT and Paunonen M (1996) Social support and its impact on mothers' experiences of childbirth. *J Adv Nurs.* **23**: 70–75.
- Teixeira J, Fisk N and Glover V (1999) Association between maternal anxiety in pregnancy and increased uterine artery resistance index: cohort-based study. *BMJ.* **318**: 153–7.
- Tew M (1998) *Safer Childbirth? A critical history of maternity care* (3e). Chapman and Hall, London.
- Uvnas-Moberg K (1998) Anti-stress pattern induced by oxytocin. *News Physiol Sci.* **13**: 22–6.
- Villar J, Farnot U, Barros F *et al.* (1992) A randomized trial of psychosocial support during high-risk pregnancies. *NEJM.* **327**: 1266–71.
- Walker J, Hall S and Thomas M (1995) The experience of labour: a perspective from those receiving care in a midwife-led unit. *Midwifery.* **11**: 120–29.
- Walsh D (1998) *An Ethnographic Study of Women's Experience of Partnership Caseload Midwifery Practice (the BUMPS) Scheme.* Masters Dissertation, De Montfort University, Leicester.
- Wheatley S (1998) Psychosocial support in pregnancy. In: S Clement (ed.) *Psychological Perspectives on Pregnancy and Childbirth.* Churchill Livingstone, Edinburgh.
- Yin-King L (1998) Hong Kong Chinese women in labour. Implications for midwives. *Pract Midwife.* **1**: 26–8.

CHAPTER 13

Fathers and childbirth

Tim Blackshaw

At present, fathers attend the birth of their children in unprecedented numbers. Historically, fathers have always played a role in the birth and aftercare of their children to varying degrees. This chapter describes how industrialisation and the hospitalisation of birth contributed to both the absence and the subsequent attendance of fathers at births. Socio-cultural and historic contexts and discourses that have contributed to the present levels of attendance are explored. In critically examining the *how* and *why* of fathers' birth attendance, emphasis is placed on the possible consequences that may accrue from attendance. These include the impact that attendance may have on the parents' sexuality and well-being, the possibility of a relationship between fathers' attendance and the increased incidence of instrumental deliveries, and what parents and healthcare professionals think about fathers attending the birth. Finally, a brief discussion will examine how fathers feel that midwives can best help them in supporting their partner.

Introduction

Not so long ago, the majority of fathers-to-be would have spent the hours preceding their child's birth in a state of banishment. They might have been found pacing the well-worn carpet of some maternity unit waiting-room, striding up and down a hospital corridor chain-smoking, or down the 'local', waiting for a telephone call, protected from the perceived gruesome reality of childbirth. Indeed, where 'Dad' was and what he was doing when you were born passed into family folklore, as may have been the case for some readers of this chapter.

However, for those younger readers with children, it is far more likely that the father was present at the birth. Furthermore, the younger the reader, the greater the likelihood that the father was both present and actively involved throughout the pregnancy (Smith, 1999). This could be dismissed as a vaguely interesting anecdote were it not for the fact that the increase in the number of fathers attending and participating at the birth of their children has been meteoric over the last 40 years. Furthermore, it is globally and historically unprecedented (Burgess, 1997a). In the past, fathers who wanted to attend the birth were regarded as potentially deviant, and only 5% of fathers attended hospital births in the 1950s (Smith, 1999a). Today, attendance is seen as de rigueur (Newburn, 2000), with 97% of fathers attending hospital births in the 1990s (Smith, 1999). Watts goes so far as to describe this as a 'badge of manhood' (Watts, 1995: 59).

This transformation has been supported by a number of interested parties, including Maternity Alliance, Fathers Direct and the National Childbirth Trust (NCT), and it has the New Labour Government seal of approval. In demonstrating its backing for a more 'hands-on' approach to fatherhood, the Government has funded both free distribution of *The Bounty Guide to Fatherhood* to new fathers (Fathers Direct, 1999) and the largest ever survey of first-time fathers in the UK – *Becoming a Father* (National Childbirth Trust, 2000). The survey portrays some fathers as feeling poorly informed, unsupported and ignored by health professionals, despite their desire to be involved from the beginning of the pregnancy. The Government has responded by announcing that its proposed £100 million improvement and refurbishment of maternity units will include facilities for fathers and families (Carlowe, 2001).

The absentee father is now a rarity – a 'statistical deviant'. In the present consumer-orientated health service, healthcare professionals would want to be certain that they could justify the exclusion of a father from the birth of his child. Although the changing professional and societal attitudes are clear, the transformation has not gone unopposed. Childbirth has been regarded by some as one of life's great mysterious experiences from which fathers since the beginning of time should be excluded. For others, concern is expressed in terms of stereotypes which rest upon the propensity for fathers to faint, panic, behave inappropriately (e.g. wielding a camera/camcorder) (Thomas, 2000) or require support from the midwife that should be going to the woman in labour.

The leading polemicist of the 'anti-fathers-at-the-birth movement' is a French obstetrician, Dr Michel Odent. He believes that men are emotionally unintuitive and too rational during the labour, thereby impeding women from getting on with the primal business of giving birth. Fathers, he posits, distract their partners, which leads to a delay in the birth, resulting in women requiring more analgesia, more interventions such as epidurals, and more Caesarean sections (Boseley, 2000).

In order to gain a balanced perspective it is necessary to examine the interplay between cultural and social change in the attitudes of men and women with regard to men's involvement at the birth. The beliefs, values and attitudes of fathers, their partners, midwives and other health professionals are critically examined. In contextualising the father's birth experience, a range of social science perspectives is used with a view to addressing what is said to be the important question. Is the presence of fathers at the birth a good thing, and if so, for whom? However, what will best enable readers to draw their own conclusions are the *how* and the *why* of fathers' birth attendance.

The chapter begins with a social historical account and a comparative cultural overview of fatherhood, fathers and birth attendance prior to the twentieth century. It then examines how the rise of the biomedical model in obstetric practices and new social movements and discourses transformed the birth process and fathers' birth attendance throughout the twentieth century to the present time. Finally, the consequences of the new orthodoxy of fathers' attendance are examined.

Fatherhood and the social contexts of birth

For thousands of years, women in the majority of cultures have facilitated the birth process (Turner, 1995). Fathers have been absent for two key reasons, namely the manner in which gender and parental roles have been socially constructed, and specific cultural taboos relating to women, pregnancy and birth within particular social contexts. However, fathers' absence from the birth does not mean that they were not in the vicinity of the birth or actively involved both physically and emotionally.

Anthropologists have documented the diversity of inherited beliefs that exist among differing cultures about conception, pregnancy and birth. Hahn and Muecke (1987) call such belief systems the *birth culture*. This birth culture informs a society's members about the nature of conception, the proper conditions of procreation and childbearing, the nature of pregnancy and labour, and the rules and rituals of pre- and postnatal behaviour.

Globally, the presence or absence of fathers at the birth can be partly explained by reference to the birth culture of a particular social group. Anthropological work has largely focused on the differences between fathers in industrialised and low- or non-industrialised societies. In so doing, anthropologists and historians have demonstrated that birth cultures in non- or low-industrialised contexts are predominantly derived from lay and/or theological bodies of knowledge (Helman, 1993). Kitzinger (2000) notes that the core cultural values of societies are revealed in the beliefs and rituals surrounding birth and death. The more technologically orientated a society is, the more technological the birth culture will be.

For fathers in western society (with the exception, to this day, of The Netherlands), it was the onset of modernity in the late eighteenth century, with the advent of industrialisation, that heralded the demise of the home and its environs as the place of work and living. Fathers' (and later mothers') workplaces were increasingly geographically distinct from the home. Furthermore, salaried work was more and more a contributory factor in the gendering of social roles, relationships and identities (Burgess, 1997a). This, together with an increase in cultural secularity, facilitated the rise of a medicalised scientific discourse concerning conception, pregnancy and specifically the place and process of birth (Mishler, 1981).

As such, it marks the beginning of the absent father. As late as the 1960s, fathers were commonly refused admission to hospital births, and in 1975 one in three obstetricians still excluded fathers (Burgess, 1997a). However, this does not mean that British fathers had not wished to or had not attended births prior to this time. Nor indeed was it necessarily the case that they had limited parental input, contrary to the popular image of the father in times past.

Fathers, fatherhood and birth attendance: pre-modernity

In order to explain why birth was primarily a 'women-only' business until the mid-eighteenth century, it is necessary to understand the ways in which the roles of men and fathers have been socially constructed, and to identify the ideologies and belief systems that underpin these constructions.

The ways in which masculinity and fatherhood have been constructed by differing discourses and ideologies have shaped men's perceptions and behaviour during pregnancy, birth and subsequent paternal activity in terms of childcare and domestic labour. Burgess (1997a) describes images of the father and fatherhood that were prevalent during the last few centuries, from the distant, godly patriarch of pre-enlightenment times to the distant, rational patriarch of the enlightenment. There is also the gradual emergence (post industrialisation) of the 'new dad', from the playful post-war father to the so-called co-parent of the 1990s.

Although there is a lack of hard data on what fathers in past times did with regard to birth, labour and child-rearing, the diaries, journals and writings of just a few hundred fathers offer us what Burgess (1997a) describes as a tantalising glimpse into their lives. She suggests that general trends emerge, and specifically the patterns of paternal involvement. At present there are no official central UK Government records documenting fathers' birth attendance (Draper, 1997).

For example, Ralph Josselin, a seventeenth-century English country vicar, noted in his diary all manner of details about the progress of his babies. He specified the dates, time and circumstances of their births, even noting when he and his wife had decided to wean their babies, and his feelings about the death of his young son (MacFarlane, 1970).

In his novel *Amelia* (published in 1751), the English novelist/dramatist Henry Fielding describes conflicting ideas as to what men should be doing during the labour:

> I thought the best husbands looked on their wives lying-in as a time of festival and jollity. 'What! Did you not even get drunk in the time of your wife's delivery? Tell me honestly, how did you employ yourself at this time?' 'Why then honestly', replied he, 'and in defiance of your laughter, I lay behind her bolster and supported her in my arms.'
>
> (Kitzinger, 1987: 150)

The writings of Josselin and Fielding would appear to challenge some of the stereotypical images of the father of past times. From these and other historical texts, several observations can be made as to how social and working life prior to industrialisation impacted broadly on fathers as parents, and more specifically their availability and location during labour and birth.

The most striking observation is the day-to-day availability of the father. This, at different periods in time, occurred for several reasons. From the time of the Tudors most families' incomes were partly derived from piecework, with only a minority of parents working away from the home. This symbiotic relationship between domestic and economic organisation required the presence of the parent(s) to create and maintain the family and home as an economic unit.

The late seventeenth century saw the rise of retailing occupations as a source of income. Once again the family was the agency of training, with the home and business being either geographically close to each other or one and the same. It is reasonable to assume that younger children, given the lack of formal schooling, would play or work around their fathers for most of the day: 'Playing in the village street and fields ... hanging around the farmyards ... thronging the churches ... crowding around the cottage fires'. Laslett (1983) notes that 'the perpetual distraction of childish noise and talk must have affected everyone almost all of the time'.

Even a well-to-do household with servants did not prohibit paternal involvement. In 1668, the Earl of Lauderdale offered a graphic description of the night his daughter gave birth, his wife being ill in bed. He notes that he was in:

troublesome governance going to and from one sick to another [At this point his newly born grandson] took convulsions and the smallpox. ... Sure I slept little [because] my babe Charles slept ill all night, was most impatient for the breast, and was in cruel heat [and] all this while the mother and grandmother knew nothing, for the physician positively forbade it. ... I sent my excuse to the King, compelled by my wife's sickness and my daughter's lying-in to stay here.

(Pollock, 1983)

Lewis-Stempel (2001) has documented the existence of childcare manuals that were written in the sixteenth and seventeenth century specifically for fathers. This is not surprising given that between 1599 and 1811, a quarter of children under 16 years of age lived in lone-father households, and one-third of the fathers managed without any live-in female help (Burgess, 1997b).

Furthermore, architectural evidence does not support the myth that prior to the late nineteenth century all children of the rich were raised in a nursery wing, separate from their parents (Hardyment, 1982). The worlds of work and social interactions were family focused, with the nature of the built environment creating close proximity between fathers and children. In most homes there was no separation between adult and child space, or for that matter between working, eating and sleeping space. This is significant, given that until the earlier part of the twentieth century the home was the place of birth.

Although it should be emphasised that these examples in no way represent what all men were doing, they do indicate that social life prior to industrialisation was such that men were likely to be involved in family life, domestic labour and, to varying degrees, the birth of their children. By the 1920s, male obstetricians were increasingly controlling of the mother through the medicalisation of birth, excluding the father and prescriptive with regard to the place of birth and the dynamics of the parents' relationship and roles, specifically during labour.

Rites and rituals: birth culture and the transition to fatherhood

Although in most western birth cultures the contemporary trend is increasingly one of fathers regarding it as their 'right' to attend the birth, in other cultures this is not the case, and childbirth and pregnancy remain both physically and socially female events. However, as in the case of pre-industrial Britain, the exclusion of the father does not mean the absence of physical or emotional involvement for him.

In many birth cultures the father's involvement takes the form of enacting specific ritual tasks during the pregnancy, birth and postpartum period. Such tasks are performed in order to protect the mother and child and facilitate an easier delivery. Heggenhougan (1980) calls these tasks *ritual couvade* (*couvade* is derived from the Basque-Spanish word *couver*, meaning to brood or hatch) (Helman, 1993). The father is required to observe certain taboos. In some societies the parents follow similar taboos, with the father often supporting the mother during labour. In other societies he may take to his bed during labour, but subsequently take care of and 'mother' the baby.

In societies where the father is present at the birth, his role is invariably functional, with the ritual tasks being viewed as integral to the birth process. For example, tasks may take the form of rituals designed to distract or lure away evil spirits until the baby is safely delivered. Linguistically, in societies where child-bearing is regarded as involving both parents, the phrase 'to bear a child' is applied to men as well as women (Helman, 1993).

Within examples of 'ritual couvade' is the belief that by enacting specific rituals the father is creating his child's spirit/soul. Rivière (1974) cites an extreme example in which the mother is perceived as a mere vessel or conduit for the baby, whereas the father is considered to be the sole creator of the baby. In addition, rituals have protective functions and also facilitate the expression of empathy for the mother and baby.

Rituals exist in all societies, and are a means by which humans structure, maintain and reproduce social life. Furthermore, they facilitate the management of potentially dangerous and polluting phenomena, and in essence allow for the creation of order in the presence of 'chaotic nature' (Douglas, 1966). Okely (1983) states that for British traveller-gypsy men and fathers, birth is viewed as a major source of potential 'pollution'. Therefore it is common practice that if the birth takes place in obstetric units (which are regarded as already polluted), the father does not attend or participate, even to the extent of not subsequently discussing the birth with the mother.

Some rituals are specific to social transitions, such as becoming a father. Van Gennep (1960) called these rituals 'rites of passage'. Such rituals connect the changes in the human life cycle to the attendant change in the social hierarchy, thus uniting the physical and social aspects of the individual's biography. Rites of passage have three stages, namely rituals of separation, transition and incorporation. In essence, 'ritual couvade' can be regarded as 'rites of passage', facilitating/celebrating the transitional journey into fatherhood (Lester and Moorsom, 1997). This transition begins in pregnancy, moving through birth and into new fatherhood

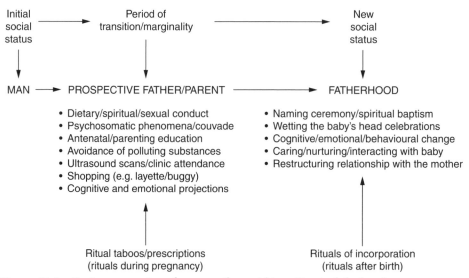

Figure 13.1   Contemporary rites of passage: the social transition to fatherhood.

(Goldberg, 1988). Utilising Van Gennep's concepts, these rituals are illustrated in relation to contemporary fatherhood in Figure 13.1.

Seel (1987) has suggested that fathers' attendance in western birth cultures is a modern *couvade* ritual. As social and family structures have changed during the last 50 years, there has been a decline in 'traditional' ritual practices, a proliferation of divorce, and the reconstitution of families. The father's presence at the birth is now seen as an official way of announcing paternity (Hearn, 1984).

In 1968, the anthropologist Mary Douglas forecast that these changes in family structure would lead to fathers increasingly being present at the birth of their children. Although this theory had a pertinence at the time, she could not have foreseen the impact that DNA analysis would have in effectively establishing paternity, nor could she have predicted the widespread acceptance of cohabitation. However, neither of the above has deterred fathers from attending births. An interesting exception to this trend is to be found in Japan, where most women leave their partner and return to their mother's home before the birth (Boseley, 2000).

Fathers in the UK and other western societies are increasingly participating in antenatal classes as well as breastfeeding and natural childbirth workshops. While some regard these activities as appropriate manifestations of western ritual couvade behaviour (National Childbirth Trust, 2000), for others they are merely 'fashion' statements (Heiney, 1986; Eagle, 1988). During the last 20 years, research into an age-old phenomenon called *couvade syndrome* has suggested that such rituals, whether old or new, have significance for the well-being of the father-to-be. Couvade syndrome is more commonly known as *sympathetic pregnancy*. In the UK it has been constructed as a humorous eccentricity, as exemplified by Charles Hawtrey in the 1968 cinematic gem *Carry On Doctor*. Researchers have described cultures in which ritual couvade is not practised or conducted 'appropriately', with some prospective fathers reporting physical and psychological symptoms during the mother's pregnancy, birth and postpartum period (Helman, 1993).

In Lipkin and Lamb's study of couvade syndrome, 22.5% of the 267 partners of expectant mothers suffered from the syndrome (Lipkin and Lamb, 1982). Many of their symptoms had characteristic vagueness and non-specificity (e.g. feeling 'low', 'run down', 'weakness') and there were also more 'pregnant' symptoms (e.g. backache, fluid retention, genital/retrosternal burning, abdominal cramps and dizziness). Klein (1991) describes expectant fathers who presented with a range of bodily symptoms, such as indigestion, altered appetite, weight gain, altered bowel function, headache and toothache. Masoni *et al.* (1994) also noted nausea and insomnia. Such symptoms typically appear during the third month of the pregnancy, with increasing symptomatology in the last two months of the pregnancy. The symptoms typically resolve at the time of the birth. Khanobdee *et al.* (1993) also reported identical findings in Thai fathers.

Significantly, researchers noted that the symptoms had no obvious physiological basis. However, a range of psychological explanations have been offered, including the somatisation of anxiety arising from concern about the mother, the baby and role transition, ambivalence about fatherhood, and a statement of paternity. Less flatteringly, pseudo-sibling rivalry and parturition envy have also been suggested (Klein, 1991). Masoni and colleagues concluded that although there is a lack of data to support a physiological explanation for couvade syndrome, 'we think that some male experiences, which constitute a peculiar imaginary and behavioural reality of the father-to-be, do exist' (Masoni *et al.*, 1994: 130).

An interesting caveat to the purported lack of a physiological explanation for couvade syndrome is to be found in an intriguing study conducted in 2001. It suggests that fathers experience dramatic hormone changes after the birth. The author, Dr Wynne-Edwards from Ontario, Canada, claims to have demonstrated a reduction in testosterone and cortisol levels but also, crucially, increased levels of oestradiol, as measured in the saliva samples of a group of men attending pre- and postnatal classes, and a control group. Although multiple studies have demonstrated that women's hormones are altered during and after pregnancy, only two studies have explored the biochemical effects of parenthood on the father. Wynne-Edwards' study confirms and expands the results of the only previous study (Lewis-Stempel, 2001). She states that the finding of raised levels of oestradiol, which were detected in a larger proportion of the samples from fathers than in those from a control group, is 'ground breaking' (cited in McVeigh, 2001).

Although she was unable to offer an explanatory mechanism for the changes, Wynne-Edwards suggests that it could occur as a result of fathers experiencing increased exposure to the hormone from the mother. Both the tabloids and the broadsheets have been quick to suggest that such hormonal changes 'transform the toughest unreconstituted fathers into big softies' (McVeigh, 2001), thereby explaining the behaviour of so-called 'celebrity dads' such as DJ 'Fat Boy Slim', the Gallagher Brothers (Oasis), the Prime Minister Tony Blair, the film director Guy Ritchie, the footballer David Beckham, and the rap-star and film actor Will Smith (Stevenson, 2001).

On a more academic note, Dr Malcolm Carruthers, who treats men who experience the menopause, suggests that oestradiol, which makes women 'broody', could exert a similar effect on men. Further research is needed, and although oestradiol has long been known to be significant in mammalian maternal behaviour, no animal research has found changes in male mammals. It could be that the human father is unique (McVeigh, 2001).

Fathers' birth attendance in the twentieth century

By the 1930s, birth in the USA was streamlined and mechanistic, incorporating a range of surgical and pharmacological interventions (Mishler, 1981). Britain was not slow in replicating this approach to birth management. Such interventions required hospitalisation, and this process occurred rapidly in this country. Between 1927 and 1946 the rate of hospital births increased from 15% to 54%. After the war, a succession of Government publications, namely the *Guilleband Report* (published in 1955), the *Cranbrook Report* (published in 1959) and the *Peel Report* (published in 1970) promoted hospital births (Tew, 1998). Since then hospitalisation has continued unabated, the rate increasing from 64.4% in 1957 to 99% in 1984 (Open University, 1992), with little decline thereafter.

Throughout this period the dominant obstetric discourse maintained that the presence of the father at the birth:

- was an increased infection risk
- was perverse and sadistic

- would inhibit future sexual relations between the couple
- created a nuisance due to the father interfering or fainting (Bedford and John-son, 1988).

These ideologies embodied a pseudoscientific rationale for denying admission to fathers, and offered a practical mechanism for avoiding the complex psychody-namics involved in having to relate to both parents (Henslin and Biggs, 1971). Complexities arising from the increasingly invasive 'clinical intimacy' during the birth process, and subsequent concerns about complaint or litigation, arguably also had an influence.

It therefore came to be regarded as normal and 'appropriate' professional practice to exclude fathers, and subsequently this was integrated into both lay and professional health beliefs and behaviours, albeit with regional variations. The 1959 British Medical Association (BMA) publication *You and Your Baby* is a good example of public exposure to medical beliefs about fathers and the birth:

> The last requirement of all for a successful delivery at home is the husband — the poor father. If he is of the right mentality, and very few are, he may sustain his wife's morale during the first part of her labour. Otherwise he is best employed making tea, keeping the kettles boiling, and answering the front doorbell.
>
> (Kitzinger, 1987: 150)

The fact that a father might wish to be present on his own account alone was not considered reason enough. Even the most progressive obstetricians assumed that the father had to be of use. In the late 1940s and early 1950s, the American obstetrician Robert Bradley agreed that husbands should be involved in the birth experience. He therefore developed the *Bradley Method* or *Husband-Coached Childbirth*. This focused on educating the couple so that the husband could serve as a 'coach' during labour. In 1947, American fathers were first allowed to attend the birth, on the condition that they acted as labour coaches (Burgess, 1997a).

Despite the efforts of some obstetricians and midwives to create a more 'natural' approach to childbirth, which was inclusive of the father, the vast majority of practitioners adopted and reinforced the ideology of excluding fathers, and not just for the reasons cited above. Increasingly, the dire structural and material constraints under which the maternity services were operating created additional reasons for excluding fathers.

Before World War Two (1939–45), women in the higher socio-economic groups in Britain had given birth at home or in a nursing home. After the war, young middle-class couples found themselves with less space and domestic help. Home birth became inconvenient and was regarded less favourably as hospitals offered women analgesia in labour, as well as a period of recuperation after the birth (Squire, 2000). As the numbers of women experiencing hospital births increased, so did the diversity of the parents, reflecting the changing socio-economic, cultural and ethnic context and their different expectations. This stimulated the re-attendance of fathers at the birth of their children.

A new 'breed' of mother, unused to the routine condescension, minor humiliations and poor physical surroundings endured by the public patients, now sought hospital care. Cohen observed that 'This type of woman, informed, articulate, and perhaps of a higher social grade than the midwives, did not take kindly to regimentation; she was a "difficult patient", and she wrote to the papers or joined a mysterious league to reform the whole maternity service' (Cohen, 1964: 93). In the maternity services, these influential women and their husbands/ partners experienced the common touch and did not like it. What they disliked was the inability of the service to cope with two problems, namely waiting in antenatal clinics and 'frightened loneliness in labour' (Cohen, 1964: 95). The former problem objectified women in the time-squandering humiliations of the clinic with its 'batch management' ethos (Goffman, 1961). The latter problem was a direct consequence of the prohibitive visitation and attendance policies operated by labour wards, particularly those relating to fathers.

The idea of expectant fathers partnering the midwifery team evoked strong emotions. Many midwives 'felt there was no place for husbands during the second stage of labour'. Some hospitals conceded that 'if there was a specific request, each case would be considered on its merits' (Cohen, 1964: 97). This begs the question of what constituted 'merit'. Unsurprisingly, there were few 'specific requests'. Some London hospitals (Queen Charlottes' Hospital, Charing Cross Hospital and University College Hospital) began to encourage husbands to support their wives during birth. At the latter two hospitals about 50% of all fathers attended (Cohen, 1964).

In 1961, Mrs Groves wrote:

> I have recently returned home from having my second child within two years at Queen Charlotte's. ... When my elder daughter was born, my husband visited me in the labour ward during official visiting hours 7–8 p.m. I was in labour 55 hours and recall it as a time of great loneliness and tedium. This time, however, my husband was admitted without preamble to the labour ward and remained with me until I requested him to leave.
>
> (Beech and Thomas, 2000: 7)

Not all obstetricians were convinced of the benefits of fathers attending. When asked what he thought, a distinguished obstetrician at Queen Charlotte's Hospital responded 'What do I feel about this?', paused for a moment, and then with the grim hesitation adopted by someone describing an atrocity, he asked 'Have *you* ever seen a woman give birth?' (Cohen, 1964: 97).

The trend of allowing fathers to attend births snowballed during the 1960s, mirroring the social changes that were occurring in work patterns and traditional social roles and identities. Such changes, underpinned and augmented by the 'political' gains of second-wave feminist groups, challenged the assumptions that men held about women, and men's own social roles.

By the late 1970s a clear culture of fathers' birth attendance had emerged, as had the term 'birthing rooms'. Increasingly, hospitals had made pragmatic changes. Recognising that labouring mothers required psychological support, while tacitly acknowledging that midwives and nurses had little time to give it, they allowed and encouraged men to assume active roles in the care of their partners (Enkin *et al.*, 1995). Thus they acknowledged the importance of parent and baby bonding and the father's support of the mother during the birth. The old 'rationales' which had justified excluding fathers from the birth were being challenged both academically and politically (Summersgill, 1993), and a new 'rationale/discourse' emerged that championed the fathers' presence. The obstetrician Peter Huntingford typifies this new thinking:

> Why should he not share responsibility with his partner, and her medical attendants, for her care? Why should he be sent out of the room when treatment is given and examinations made during labour? These symbols of the barrier that is erected to male participation in childbearing mean that there is less chance for fathers to share the sensations and emotions of birth.
>
> (Huntingford, 1978)

Women were enthusiastic about the 'natural birthing' campaigns that were promoted in the 1970s and 1980s by obstetricians such as Fredrique Leboyer and Michel Odent. Maternity departments responded further by providing a less institutional experience for the mother, that was inclusive of the father. However, although they were beginning to give parents what they wanted, the hospitals did not relinquish power over the major procedures used in birth (Porter, 1999). By the 1980s, the majority of fathers were attending births. It had been the response of the public and of parents to these ideologies, set against changing social contexts and material constraints, that transformed fathers' birth attendance.

The new orthodoxy of attendance: is the participation of the father at the birth dangerous?

From the few atypical parents of the 1950s, fathers' birth attendance has become normative, and a new 'negotiated order' (Strauss *et al.*, 1963) between practitioners, fathers and parents has emerged. However, as fathers' attendance has become widely accepted, questions have arisen.

Michel Odent speculates that fathers' birth attendance may be 'dangerous' (Odent, 1999: 23). He believes that the dawn of the twenty-first century signifies a new phase in the history of childbirth, the current turning point being the fast development of evidence-based obstetrics and midwifery. This new phase represents a unique opportunity to reconsider many theories and preconceived ideas, and to make an inventory of the questions that we must raise.

> Where the participation of the father at birth is concerned, we must raise at least three questions. Can the participation of the father at the birth influence the sex life of the couple afterwards? Can all men cope with the strong emotional reactions that they may have while participating in the birth? Does the participation of the father aid or hinder the birth?
>
> (Odent, 1999: 24)

In addition, one could ask what benefits might occur as a result of the father's presence, or why most fathers want to attend. These questions, arising from the lived experience of practitioners and fathers attending births, will now be addressed.

Sexuality and birth attendance

From the earliest times sexuality and gender constructs have influenced the exclusion of fathers from the birth. In many cultures the locating of birth in a specific place, administered by women, could be interpreted as overtly desexualising the birth process. However, it is possible that there is a covert assumption that men's sexuality and 'gaze' inherently threaten the birth process, based on the notion that men regard birth as a potentially erotic situation, and only conceptualise women's secondary sexual characteristics as sites of (male) pleasure, as opposed to 'functional organs'. This underpins a popular but unsubstantiated belief that couples primarily experience problems with their subsequent sexual relationship as a result of the father being present at the birth. It thus ignores possible previous sexual difficulties.

Although changing notions about sexuality, gender roles and relationships contributed to fathers' presence in the delivery room in the 1960s and 1970s, it would be incorrect to assume that sexuality is no longer a pertinent issue. As one tabloid subtly observed, 'Is it good for the rest of us (fathers) to see much industry taking place in an area once laced with Janet Reger?' (Young, 1994: 43).

Indeed, this is one of the central tenets of those who would like to reverse the trend of attending fathers. According to Michel Odent:

> There are issues about the future sex life of the couple. ... Older women who gave birth when men were expected to stay in the pub are often appalled at the idea of their partner witnessing the physical spectacle of delivery. ... Sexual attraction is mysterious. ... Perhaps it needs a bit of mystery. ... I have seen so many couples who had wonderful births according to present criteria, yet several years later they divorced. They have remained good friends, but not sexual partners any more.
>
> (Boseley, 2000)

Seel (1994) notes that sex therapists working with 'sexually dysfunctional' couples have observed that the man's experience of what was for him a traumatic labour/birth can subsequently stifle any sexual feelings for his partner. As one man described it:

> Suddenly this part of Angela that had been terribly private was being stared at by five other men. She didn't mind ... in fact, she said that while it was going on the whole world could have watched and she wouldn't have given a damn ... but I did. I felt it was a grotesque intrusion into our lives. And there was so much blood it shocked me, it was like seeing the person you love most on a battlefield. I had nightmares about it for weeks afterwards, and that affected the way I saw her as a sexual being.
>
> (Craig, 1993: 131)

Jackson (1997) calls this 'post-traumatic parturition syndrome', and reasons that it can occur in men as the onlookers as well as in women as the receivers. She likens this to the well-documented feelings of violation that are experienced after rape (Raphael-Leff, 1991; Walton, 1994).

On the surface this appears to be a hard case to answer. However, closer analysis suggests that although there is little doubt that witnessing a birth can be traumatic for some men, this is not the case for the majority of them. People experience problems with their sexual relationships for a multiplicity of reasons which can be grouped as being linked to biological factors (Hulme, 1993) and physical and psychological factors (Walton, 1994).

Given the significant social role transformations that occur on becoming a parent and which require immediate adaptation, it is not surprising that problems occur within a relationship. As Walton has observed:

> Sexuality is a fundamental aspect of life and so must be involved in the momentous adjustments that are made by men and women on becoming parents, and that change which started with the pregnancy continues in the postnatal period onwards.
>
> (Walton, 1994)

Problems can therefore occur as a consequence of roles adopted by the parents and the socio-cultural context of the relationship. For example, the division of domestic and salaried labour, and the relationship between the father, the mother and the baby are other significant factors.

Riley (1989) claims that, following the birth of their first child, two-thirds of couples have not resumed sexual intercourse within six weeks. The evidence suggests that for many men and women their experience of sexuality is not related solely to sexual activity, and therefore a narrow focus on sexuality as sexual activity is misleading, as it ignores the totality of human sexuality, as well as the impact of roles and societal values on the couple's sexuality. Given the diverse and complex reasons that people give to explain difficulties in their sexual relationships after birth, it is untenable to suggest, given the lack of supporting data, that the father's presence at the birth is the main source of such problems. Sexuality during early parenthood is only *one* factor in the ongoing process of negotiating relationships and roles after the birth (Curtis and Dunn, 1994).

Michel Odent further speculates on the existence of male postnatal depression:

> Are we sure all men can cope with the strong emotional reaction they can have when their wife is in labour?. ... Most cultures have rituals for keeping a man busy while his partner is in labour ... modern birthing practice makes little allowance for this.
>
> (Boseley, 2000)

A National Opinion Poll stated that 4% of men in the UK and 10% of men in London believe that they suffer from 'postnatal depression'. Although some of the physical symptoms could be attributed to altered hormone levels, as discussed earlier, Steve Jamieson of Men's Health Forum believes that this recently recognised phenomenon has a variety of contributory 'causes', including the sudden extra responsibility and financial burden, a lack of preparation for the role change, and acute/chronic tiredness. Many fathers who believed that they were depressed had witnessed the birth and found it 'offputting' (BBC, 1999).

Although the presence of the father at the birth would appear to impact on sexual relationships and contribute to depressive feelings in some fathers, this is not the case for the majority of them. However, this suggests that some fathers may want or seek support from midwives.

Attending fathers: help or hindrance?

Perhaps the most serious concern that has been raised with regard to fathers' attendance at births is that in some way their presence has contributed to the sharp increase in the number of Caesarean sections and medically assisted births. Odent believes that this has occurred in part because fathers become anxious and distressed at seeing their partners in pain, and they therefore try to talk to them, asking rational questions about what is happening. This requires the mother to respond using the intellectual as opposed to emotional side of the brain. This, he argues, inhibits the woman's ability to manage labour emotionally, and leads her to opt for analgesia and more interventionist approaches in the management of her labour (Boseley, 2000).

In aiming to protect his partner, a father might request that she have an epidural or even a Caesarean birth in order to avoid experiencing too much pain. Odent attributes this to men's respect for technology and gadgets to solve the 'problems' of natural childbirth: 'men feel happier knowing that their wives are getting as much medical attention as possible' (Walters, 2000). Indeed, he speculates that this may be responsible for the upsurge in Caesarean sections, and that fathers are sometimes inclined to celebrate the birth too soon, distracting the woman before the vital delivery of the placenta.

The sixfold increase in the number of Caesarean sections in parts of England, Wales and Northern Ireland during the last 30 years means that one in five of all births (21.5%) is via Caesarean section. In London and Wales the figure is as high as one in four (24.2%) (Department of Health, 2001). These data require some unravelling. Is it possible that the father's presence at the birth could have contributed to the increase in medical interventions?

The two periods of greatest increase were the 1970s and the 1990s. Although the 1970s represent the period during which fathers started to attend births in significant numbers, Odent's hypothesis does not stand up to scrutiny. In the National Sentinel Caesarean Section Audit 2001, the main reasons offered by clinicians for performing Caesarean sections were fetal distress, failure to progress in labour, breech presentation, previous Caesarean section and the mother's specific request. However, these reasons need to be viewed in the light of the audit's key findings, which are summarised below (Boseley, 2001).

1   Women are still restricted in their movements during labour because they are attached to oversensitive and inaccurate fetal heart monitors.
2   Drugs are too frequently used to induce labour when the pregnancy has run to term.
3   Labouring women do not receive continuous attention, with one-third of all units unable to offer one-to-one care, and midwives in 5% of units could be caring for two to three women at any one time.
4   There is an increase in the age of women who are having babies.
5   There is a high rate of hospital births.

6 There is lack of agreement between the World Health Organization (WHO) and the Royal College of Obstetricians and Gynaecologists (RCOG) as to what constitutes 'a high rate of Caesarean sections'.

7 There is an increased number of 'defensive' Caesarean sections arising from fear of litigation.

8 There is an increased number of elective procedures (most notably in private practice) at the mother's request, in the absence of clinical indications.

The presence of fathers is noticeably absent as a contributory factor (although it may not have been considered). Odent is aware that he is challenging what has become an orthodoxy, and he does publicly acknowledge that 'there is little scientific evidence for his view that men can be a hindrance rather than a help' (Boseley, 2000).

Here to stay: why do fathers want to attend?

Although the majority of fathers willingly attend the birth, some do so reluctantly for a variety of reasons, including squeamishness, uncertainty about their role, previous life experiences and personal beliefs (Robertson, 1993). Is it possible that a minority of men are being 'forced' into the labour room? Seel (1994) believes that this new orthodoxy puts enormous pressure on fathers who are reluctant — from women, partners, staff or other men. One prospective father commented on how he was finding it particularly difficult to receive support from his colleagues: 'My mates keep skitting me about it ... it does make me feel a bit guilty' (Lavender, 1997: 94). For some men this creates a 'Catch 22' situation: 'There are so many people expecting you to be at the birth, yet nobody really asks you if you want to be' (Lavender, 1997: 94).

In essence, the father's attendance has come to be construed as part of the expression of the ideal closeness and mutual dependence of contemporary relationships, and his intention to be a 'father' to the child. Therefore it is not uncommon for the father who does not witness the birth to be viewed as an incompetent father and an inadequate man who has shirked his duty to the child and denied the mutuality that is so necessary for relationships. Worse still, his partner is to be pitied.

The literature suggests that only a few men encounter this dilemma, and given that high levels of attendance have persisted for over 20 years, this not a passing fad, but one which is likely to be continued by the future generation of fathers (O'Brien and Jones, 1995). It would appear that fathers are here to stay. Therefore it is pertinent at this stage to examine why men want to attend the birth, the expectations and experiences of the couple, and what fathers have felt enabled them to be supportive of their partners during the birth.

Although fathers have different reasons for wanting to attend the birth, Richman (1982) describes them collectively as having a 'kaleidoscopic pattern of motives'. Birth attendance is the culmination of months of preparation for fatherhood. A study of new fathers showed that 93% of them wanted and had planned to be present at the birth (Royal College of Midwives, 1995). Fathers want to be close to and supporting of their labouring partner, and to witness the birth of a new life (Draper, 1997). They equate attendance with developing a close relationship with the baby, which enables them to express loving feelings towards him or her. Attendance at the birth also facilitates their involvement in the daily care of the baby, and makes it clear that they are parents with the associated responsibilities (Palkovitz, 1987). Some fathers were aware that their presence served to remind healthcare workers that childbirth could not be viewed entirely as a medical event (Beail and McGuire, 1982).

Expectations and experiences of attendance

Despite having differing expectations of childbirth, fathers generally reported that labour and birth were stressful events for them, with anxiety arising from their concern about the physical and emotional well-being of their labouring partner (May and Perrin, 1985). Doubts about their ability to be supportive of their partner while trying to hide their own feelings (Berry, 1988), and uncertainty about their roles during the labour and birth (Bothamley, 1990) were additional stressors. Chandler and Field (1997) have illustrated how these stressors and the consequent anxiety had different foci, duration and intensity, which were determined by where the couple was on the 'labour path'.

Consistent with the unique motives and expectations that fathers have for attending the birth, they also adopt different roles during labour and the birth. From the behaviours that fathers display, Chapman (1991) identified three commonly adopted roles, namely coach, team mate and witness.

'Coaches' actively assisted their partner, and had a strong need to feel in control of themselves and the labour experience. Their partners wanted them to be physically involved in the labour, regarding this as crucial to their own ability to maintain control.

'Team mates' assisted their partner in response to requests for physical or emotional support, occasionally leading. These fathers saw themselves as a member of the birth team, and were less concerned with issues of control. They focused on the needs of their partner, who wanted them there both for their presence and for their willingness to follow directions.

'Witnesses' described their primary role as being a companion who provided emotional and moral support. These fathers witnessed the birth of the baby, but believed that there was little they could do to help their partner. Therefore they looked to others to take charge of the situation, and were often seen reading or watching television. This role was viewed as creating 'togetherness without the pressures of having to be in control' (Chapman, 1992).

Irrespective of the roles adopted during the labour and birth, the most important role for the partner of a labouring mother is just 'being there' (Flint, 1986). Many mothers benefit from the supportive presence of the father – the very fact of him being there meant that the mother had access to physical and emotional support as required. Although some fathers may have been of little practical help, their mere presence was supportive (Stolte, 1987), even if fathers did not get it right all of the time. As one mother commented, 'I wasn't particularly amused at being offered fish and chips. ... That's just trying to help' (Somers-Smith, 1999: 106).

However, many mothers stated that the presence of their partner could alleviate the loneliness, pain and uncertainty during the delivery, and gave them strength to endure their suffering as well as share their joy. The presence of the father meant 'communion' to the mother, and this communion emanates from the partners caring for each other and their baby. For the mothers, their partner was not only a support person, but also above all the father-to-be – a double and sometimes paradoxical role (Bondas-Salonen, 1998).

Further studies have described an enhanced positive emotional experience of the birth for the mother (Entwhistle and Doering, 1988). May (1982) noted that the shared experience of the birth had a positive impact on the couple's relationship, and more recently it was reported that 80% of couples did not anticipate any adverse effects on their future personal relationship (Szevérenyi *et al.*, 1998). Mothers experienced less pain and required less analgesia (Henneborn and Cogan, 1975; Niven, 1985), while Chopstick *et al.* (1986) identified a reduction in the frequency of epidurals for mothers who had the father's support.

In being present at the birth, fathers felt that they were valuing, caring for and appreciating their partners, and were pleased with the support that they had given (Somers-Smith, 1999). Fathers experienced immense joy, relief and overwhelming emotions both during and after the birth of the child, and what Hall (1995) describes as 'love at first sight'. Many fathers complete the experience with an enhanced respect for their partner, and feel that they have introduced themselves personally to the child (Chandler and Field, 1997). Furthermore, fathers who have involved themselves in the pregnancy, birth and subsequent care of the child often describe feelings of elation and enhanced self-esteem (Lewis, 1986; Bedford and Johnson, 1988).

Enabling fathers to be supportive at birth

Midwives have been known to complain that fathers are 'useless' in the labour ward (Robertson, 1999: 21). While stereotypes may contain a grain of truth, the majority of fathers want to help their partners during the birth, and to bond with the child. If the father is to provide practical help and emotional support, and to make the most of the opportunity, he will need insight, information and support from the midwife.

In antenatal classes, fathers valued an emphasis being placed on the 'whole birth thing'. The 'whole birth thing' was an awareness that just learning the medical facts and having a technical knowledge of labour was not enough, and implied that those leading the classes saw birth as a series of biological processes and medical procedures – a literal lack of wholeness. What was of most help to fathers was a clear acknowledgement of the father's supportive role, clear guidance on what he could do, practical tips and balanced insights into life with a baby. The 'whole birth thing' emphasises that labour and birth are part of the transition to parenthood, but does not assume that all fathers will be present at the labour, or that they will adopt similar roles.

This suggests a need to allow fathers to explore what being present at the birth means, in 'men only' forums (Smith, 1999b). Midwives need to be aware of the need to avoid stigmatising non-attendees, as this can lead to inappropriate care (May, 1982), and to avoid focusing solely on the father's perceived role as a 'labour coach', which could mean neglecting his psychological or other needs – antenatally or during the birth (Draper, 1997). Lester and Moorsom (1997) consider this to be a 'golden opportunity' for midwives to provide information and emotional support for fathers throughout the pregnancy, birth and postnatal period. Midwives should permit emotional catharsis, acknowledge 'couvade syndrome', and be as flexible as possible with regard to their working hours to allow for fathers' work commitments. In terms of obtaining information, the consensus of opinion among fathers was that midwives are the people to ask (Lavender, 1997). This is not surprising. Bothamley (1990) observed that some fathers felt inhibited in the hospital environment, even with regard to performing simple tasks such as moving a chair. She maintains that fathers need to be informed about what is happening, and about the hospital setting itself. It is through the 'presencing' and 'being there' that the father is enabled to feel that he is welcome, valued and integral to the birth team.

This can be exemplified as follows:

> We decided to have Ricky at home, and initially I didn't like the idea ... had all logical reasons why I didn't want to do it, about being safe in hospital. ... But once we embarked upon it, it was a brilliant experience. We had this wonderful midwife. I think she really liked me. She did something she said she had never done, and she has delivered over 1000 children, but she got me to get hold of his head and pull him out. And then she let me cut the cord! (Ralph, 37-year-old father of three)
> (Burgess, 1997a: 123–4)

Conclusion

Enabling fathers to be supportive of their partners through the births of their children is important and rewarding for both the couple and the midwife. Contrary to popular perceptions, fathers have historically been active in birth and childcare, prior to industrialisation and the hospitalisation of childbirth. Therefore the present trend of fathers attending births is not a totally new phenomenon, but rather the re-emergence of an old one – 'reconstructed'. The forces that have shaped and moulded this transition, and the subsequent outcomes, have been described and critically examined. Given that the high levels of attendance are set to continue, it is hoped that these insights into to the *how* and *why* of fathers attending the birth will enable midwives and other healthcare workers in their practice with the mother, the baby and the father.

- The present high numbers of fathers attending the birth of their child represent a relatively recent phenomenon. However, historically fathers have been involved in the birth of their children and their subsequent care.
- Although for western fathers the norm is one of attendance at the birth, globally this is not the case. In other societies, birth is administered by women, while the transition to fatherhood is enacted through *couvade rituals.*
- The hospitalisation of birth in the latter half of the twentieth century first prevented and then encouraged the attendance of fathers at the birth. However, concerns have been expressed about the merits and demerits of this phenomenon.

- The majority of fathers wish to attend the birth. Collectively, they have diverse motives for attending and different experiences and expectations of themselves, their partner and the birth.
- Midwives can enable fathers to be supportive of their labouring partner by acknowledging the significance of the father's role at the birth for the couple, and through antenatal education that is practically orientated and allows the father to be emotionally expressive.

Dedication

For Sharon, Jake and Poppy, without whom I would not have had the privilege of being a father.

References

- BBC (1999) Men suffer from baby blues. BBC News (online) 4th May; http// news.bbc.co.uk/hi/english/health/newsid (accessed on 17 March 2001).
- Beail N and McGuire J (1982) *Fathers: psychological perspectives.* Junction Books, London.
- Bedford V and Johnson N (1988) The role of the father. *Midwifery.* **4**: 190–5.
- Beech B and Thomas P (2000) Forty years ago: men in the labour wards. *Adv Midwif Sci J.* **12**: 7–8.
- Berry L (1988) Realistic expectations of the labor coach. *J Obstet Gynecol Neonatal Nurs.* **17**: 354–5.
- Bondas-Salonen T (1998) How women experience the presence of their partners at the births of their babies. *Qual Health Res.* **8**: 784–801.
- Boseley S (2000) Anxious fathers may be bad for the birth: 'Keep them away from the delivery room', advises childbirth guru. *Guardian.* **17 January**: 5.
- Boseley S (2001) Caesarean births soar to one in five: survey puts UK way above WHO limits. *Guardian.* **26 October**: 13.
- Bothamley J (1990) Are fathers getting a fair deal? *Nursing Times.* **86**: 68–9.
- Burgess A (1997a) *Fatherhood Reclaimed: the making of the modern father.* Vermilion, London.
- Burgess A (1997b) *Carlton Parenting Campaign: fathers' booklet.* Carlton Television, London.
- Carlowe J (2001) Birth control. *Observer Magazine.* **2 December**: 49.
- Chandler S and Field P (1997) Becoming a father: first-time fathers' experience of labour and delivery. *J Nurse Midwifery.* **42**: 17–24.
- Chapman L (1991) Searching: expectant fathers' experiences during labor and delivery. *J Perinat Neonat Nurs.* **44**: 21–9.
- Chapman L (1992) Expectant fathers' role during labor and birth. *J Obstet Gynecol Neonatal Nurs.* **21**: 114–20.
- Chopstick S, Taylor K, Hayes R and Morris N (1986) Partner support and the use of coping techniques in labour. *J Psychosom Res.* **30**: 497–503.
- Cohen GL (1964) *What's Wrong with Hospitals?* Penguin, Harmondsworth.
- Craig A (1993) Sex after stitches. Will your love life ever be the same? *She.* **September issue**: 130–32.

- Curtis P and Dunn K (1994) *How's the love life? Sexuality and early mother-hood.* Paper presented to the Annual Conference of the British Sociological Society, Sexualities in Social Context, at the University of Central Lancashire, March 1994.
- Department of Health (2001) *National Sentinel Caesarean Section Audit.* The Stationery Office, London.
- Douglas M (1966) *Purity and Danger.* Penguin, Harmondsworth..
- Draper J (1997) Whose welfare in the labour room? A discussion of the increasing trend of fathers' birth attendance. *Midwifery.* **13**: 132–8.
- Eagle R (1988) Bedside man. *Vogue.* **March issue**: 330–31.
- Enkin M, Keirse MJNC, Renfrew M *et al.* (1995) *A Guide to Effective Care in Pregnancy and Childbirth.* Oxford University Press, Oxford.
- Entwhistle D and Doering S (1988) The emergent father role. *Sex Roles.* **18**: 119–41.
- Fathers Direct (1999) (online); http://www.europrofem.org/02.info (accessed 17 January 2001).
- Flint C (1986) *Sensitive Midwifery.* Heinemann, London.
- Goffman E (1961) *Asylums: essays on the social situation of mental patients and other inmates.* Pelican Books, Harmondsworth.
- Goldberg WA (1988) *Introduction: perspectives on the transition to parenthood.* In: GY Michaels and WA Goldberg (eds) *The Transition to Parenthood.* Cambridge University Press, Cambridge.
- Hahn RA and Muecke MA (1987) The anthropology of birth in five US ethnic populations: implications for obstetrical practice. *Curr Prob Obstet Gynecol Fertil.* **10**: 131–71.
- Hall EO (1995) From fun and excitement to joy and trouble. An explorative study of three Danish fathers' experiences around birth. *Scand J Caring Sci.* **9**: 171–9.
- Hardyment C (1982) *Dream Babies: childcare from Locke to Spock.* Jonathan Cape, London.
- Hearn J (1984) Childbirth, men and the problem of fatherhood. *Rad Commun Med.* **17**: 9–19.
- Heggenhougan HK (1980) Fathers and childbirth: an anthropological perspective. *J Nurse Midwifery.* **25**: 21–6.
- Heiney P (1986) Fathers voting against forced labour. *The Times.* **21 July**: 11.
- Helman CG (1993) *Culture, Health and Illness.* Butterworth-Heinemann, Oxford.
- Henneborn WJ and Cogan R (1975) The effect of husband participation on reported and probability of medication during labour and birth. *J Psychosom Res.* **19**: 215–22.
- Henslin JM and Biggs MA (1971) The sociology of the vaginal examination. In: M Henslin (ed.) *Down to Earth Sociology: introductory readings.* Free Press, New York.
- Hulme H (1993) Grin and bear it. *Nursing Times.* **89**: 66.
- Huntingford P (1978) *The Baby Book for Fathers.* Fenwick and Fenwick, London.
- Jackson KB (1977) Paternal presence at delivery. *Br J Midwifery.* **25**: 682–4.
- Khanobdee C, Sukratanachaiyakul V and Gay JT (1993) Couvade syndrome in expectant Thai fathers. *Int J Nurs Stud.* **30**: 125–31.
- Kitzinger S (1987) *The Experience of Childbirth.* Penguin, Harmondsworth.
- Kitzinger S (2000) Some cultural perspectives on birth. *Br J Midwifery.* **8**: 746–50.

- Klein H (1991) Couvade syndrome: male counterpart to pregnancy. *Int J Psychiatr Med.* **21**: 57–69.
- Laslett P (1983) *The World We Have Lost: further explored.* Routledge, London.
- Lavender T (1997) Can midwives respond to the needs of fathers? *Br J Midwifery.* **5**: 92–6.
- Lester A and Moorsom S (1997) Do men need midwives? Facilitating a greater involvement in parenting. *Br J Midwifery.* **5**: 678–81.
- Lewis C (1986) *Becoming a Father.* Oxford University Press, Oxford.
- Lewis-Stempel J (2001) *Fatherhood: an anthology.* Simon & Schuster, London.
- Lipkin M and Lamb GS (1982) The couvade syndrome: an epidemiological study. *Ann Int Med.* **96**: 509–11.
- MacFarlane A (1970) *The Family Life of Ralph Josselin.* Cambridge University Press, Cambridge.
- McVeigh T (2001) Tough guys get the baby blues, too. *Observer.* **24 June**: 7.
- Masoni S, Maio A, Trimarchi G, de Punzio C and Fioretti P (1994) The couvade syndrome. *J Psychosom Obstet Gynaecol.* **15**: 125–31.
- May K (1982) Three phases of father involvement in pregnancy. *Nurs Res.* **51**: 337–42.
- May K and Perrin S (1985) Prelude: pregnancy and birth. In: S Hanson and F Bozzet (eds) *Dimensions of Fatherhood.* Sage Publications, Beverly Hills, CA.
- Ministry of Health (1959) *Report of Maternity Services Committee: Cranbrook Report.* HMSO, London.
- Mishler EG (1981) *Social Contexts of Health, Illness and Patient Care.* Cambridge University Press, Cambridge.
- National Childbirth Trust (2000) Press release. *Government-Funded Study of 'Blair Fathers' Demands Better Support for New Dads*; http://www.midirs.org/midirs/midweb (accessed on 22 May 2001).
- Newburn M (2000) *Head to Head: fathers and childbirth.* BBC News Online; http://news.bbc.co.uk/hi/english/health/newsid (accessed on 17 January 2001).
- Niven C (1985) How helpful is the presence of the husband at childbirth? *J Reprod Infant Psychol.* **3**: 45–53.
- O'Brien M and Jones D (1995) Young people's attitudes to fatherhood. In: P Moss (ed.) *Father Figures: fathers in the 1990s.* HMSO, London.
- Odent M (1999) Is the participation of the father at birth dangerous? *Midwifery Today.* **51**: 23–5.
- Okely J (1983) *The Traveller-Gypsies.* Cambridge University Press, Cambridge.
- Open University (1992) *Health and Well-Being.* Open University, Milton Keynes.
- Palkovitz R (1987) Fathers' motives for birth attendance. *Matern Child Nurs J.* **16**: 123–9.
- Pollock LA (1983) *Forgotten Children: parent–child relations from 1500–1900.* Cambridge University Press, Cambridge.
- Porter R (1999) *The Greatest Benefit to Mankind: a medical history of humanity from antiquity to the present.* Fontana Press, London.
- Raphael-Leff J (1991) *Psychological Processes of Childbearing.* Chapman and Hall, London.
- Richman J (1982) Men's experience of pregnancy and childbirth. In: L McKee and M O'Brien (eds) *The Father Figure.* Tavistock Publications, New York.
- Riley AJ (1989) Sex after childbirth. *Br J Sexual Med.* **16**: 185–7.
- Rivière PG (1974) The couvade: a problem reborn. *Man.* **9**: 423–35.

- Robertson A (1999) Get the fathers involved! The needs of men in pregnancy classes. *Pract Midwife.* **2**: 21–2.
- Robertson I (1993) Birth pains. *BMJ.* **307**: 687.
- Royal College of Midwives (1995) RCM survey (summary): men at birth. *Midwives.* **108**: 18.
- Seel R (1987) *The Uncertain Father.* Gateway Books, Bath.
- Seel R (1994) Men at the birth. *New Generation.* **13**: 16–17.
- Smith J (1999a) Antenatal classes and the transition to fatherhood: a study of some fathers' views. *MIDIRS Midwif. Digest.* **9**: 327–30.
- Smith N (1999b) Men in antenatal classes: teaching 'the whole birth thing'. *Pract Midwife.* **2**: 23–6.
- Somers-Smith MJ (1999) A place for the partner? Expectations and experiences of support during childbirth. *Midwifery.* **15**: 101–8.
- Squire C (2000) Pain relief: past and present. In: M Yerby (ed.) *Pain in Childbearing. Key issues in management.* Baillière Tindall, London.
- Stevenson S (2001) Why new fathers are such softies. *Metro.* **25 June**: 14.
- Stolte K (1987) A comparison of women's expectations of labour with the actual event. *Birth.* **14**: 99–103.
- Strauss A, Schatzman L, Ehrlich D, Bucher R and Sabshin M (1963) The hospital and its negotiated order. In: E Freidson (ed.) *The Hospital and Modern Society.* Free Press, London.
- Summersgill P (1993) Couvade – the retaliation of the marginalised fathers. In: J Alexander, V Levy and S Roch (eds) *Midwifery Practice. A research-based approach.* Macmillan, Basingstoke.
- Szevérenyi P, Póka R, Hetey M and Török Z (1998) Contents of childbirth-related fear among couples wishing the partner's presence at delivery. *J Psychosom Obstet Gynecol.* **19**: 38–43.
- Tew M (1998) *Safer Childbirth?* Chapman and Hall, London.
- Thomas C (2000) *Childbirth Scares Men Too.* BBC News Online; http://news.bbc.co.uk/hi/english/health/newsid (accessed on 15 March 2001).
- Turner BS (1995) *Medical Power and Social Knowledge.* Sage Publications, London.
- Van Gennep A (1960) *The Rites of Passage.* Routledge and Kegan Paul, London.
- Walters C (2000) *Millennium Babies: current research on the health of the unborn generation.* Families Magazine (online); http://www.familiesmagazine.co.uk/topics/babies/babies-father-birth (accessed on 15 March 2001).
- Walton I (1994) *Sexuality and Motherhood.* Books for Midwifes Press, Hale.
- Watts J (1995) *Gendering One, Gendering Two.* Unpublished paper.
- Young J (1994) Birth day blues of a dad. *Daily Mail.* **28 April**: 43.

CHAPTER 14

Unhappiness after childbirth

Christine Grabowska

This chapter critically appraises the circumstances of women's transition into motherhood, based on social norms and cultural expectations. It is proposed that some women find the transition difficult because of the value and status attached to earning an income. The imagery to which women are exposed prior to having their first child is romanticised and often unrealistic. The social need for competition and why that skill is inappropriate for all intimate relationships and is thus the cause of unhappiness is discussed. The effects of overworking when a woman is trying to take on the roles of mother, lover, housewife and career woman can leave her feeling out of control, particularly if she does not feel satisfied with her involvement in any of these areas. Post-traumatic stress syndrome following childbirth has now been recognised. The incidence of the condition appears to be increasing in mothers, manifested as a form of extreme anxiety. Women with the syndrome will find every area of their lives affected. They often cannot function effectively, and this results in the disruption of their lives and those of their family. Consideration of women during the maternity experience needs to be prioritised by service provision and Government policy. The chapter concludes by asking for political solutions in the short term, but ultimately a radical change in behaviour and social expectations is needed in order to support the mothering role.

Introduction

Women have often been made to feel personally responsible for their own suffering. They are told by knowledgeable others that their feelings are caused by their hormones, unrealistic expectations of childbirth, having an idealised image of motherhood, listening to too many stories, and so on. This blaming culture increases the woman's internalisation of her own unhappiness and she is left with no other recourse but the knowledge that if she created it, she must deal with it. Society is thus absolved of any responsibility for the creation of each woman's unhappiness, so no social or political resolution needs to be instituted. Society does not need to support motherhood – mothers are left to do this themselves.

The aim of this chapter is to propose that mothers are integral to the functioning of society, and that therefore society has a responsibility to support the mothering role. It will be suggested that unhappiness, for some mothers, is socially created (Gilbert, 1992; Pilgrim and Bentall, 1999).

Women are surviving traumas of their everyday life and coping. Motherhood changes their whole being and the way in which they see themselves as well as the way in which they are viewed by others. It is a birth into a new social role, a transition from a woman's former self into what could be seen as a personally fulfilling experience in the development of a person. Many women go through this transition and emerge excited and fulfilled at being mothers. However, for some it is one trauma that they will not survive or be able to cope with. It may be viewed with such feelings as contempt, bewilderment, sadness, anger and resentment. It may be a transition that was neither anticipated nor wanted. These feelings are not dependent on the decision to have a baby (Nicolson, 1998), but rather they result from the outcome of childbearing (Ussher, 1992). The explanation of the reasons why some women have reached such a place in their lives will often depend on their history and their present cultural surroundings. All women need to find some form of contentment or even happiness in becoming a mother, which will aid their confidence and abilities.

History

Women who have felt loved throughout their lives have the greatest chance of experiencing happiness when they become mothers. However, Gilbert (1992) points out that historically societies have been more concerned about success in promoting the social ideal than about individual happiness. Odent (1999) agrees that in the past love was put on the back burner and mothers were positively discouraged from openly displaying love for their children in order to produce aggression and competitiveness, particularly among male children. This creates the initial conflict of interests for women entering motherhood. Social success is defined through the capitalist economy for all western societies, and people are defined by the amount of money that they are able to generate. Motherhood does not create wealth, and may therefore be regarded as a low-status activity.

Many authors (Sheppard, 1997; Hope *et al.*, 1999; Reading and Reynolds, 2001; Nicolson and Ussher, 1992) refer to the classic study by Brown and Harris (1978) of depression in order to highlight the circumstances of women's lives that may have contributed to their unhappiness. Brown and Harris (1978) identified four vulnerability factors that predispose women to the onset of unhappiness:

1   lack of a confiding relationship with their partner
2   the presence at home of three or more children under the age of 14 years
3   the loss of their own mother before the age of 11 years
4   the absence of outside employment.

Lack of a confiding relationship with their partner

The sharing of daily experiences, regardless of their worth and value, is a way of debriefing and thus coping with the next onslaught of experiences with greater calm and ease. It enables an individual to move through life with courage. Courage is enhanced by encouragement (Smail, 2001), which people have a greater chance of receiving when relating to others. For many people it is difficult to be this relaxed about themselves, and thus it is difficult for them to be open and vulnerable, because generally speaking people have been taught as children to present 'a good image' or 'not to wash their dirty linen in public'. Equally, as individuals interact with each other they may have seen others take advantage of this vulnerability, including their partners, and therefore to allow vulnerability involves being confident in oneself. Confidence develops when someone else is confident in you (Smail, 2001). The confiding relationships that a woman has involve trust and love. It is where others see the woman's worth and value that will determine the woman's confidence in herself as a mother. Being able to confide in someone on a regular basis is nurturing to the mother, who will in turn be able to nurture her young. However, some women have no such confiding relationships.

People often embark on relationships that are based on lust, and sometimes friendship has no place in those relationships. The latter can become competitive, with each partner feeling that they constantly have to prove their own worth and value in order to be liked. This leaves no room for vulnerability and truth-telling, and may be the source of breakdown of relationships due to lack of communication. Romito *et al.* (1999) believe that unless the relationship is considered to be good or even better, it is preferable to be a single parent.

Why do people behave competitively in relationships? It is because this is the nature of the world in which they live. In order for business to function, profit has to be made, and thus competition is created to vie for profit. People are exposed to this on a daily basis, and it is considered to be normal behaviour. Often people find that they cannot change their behaviour easily, especially if competition is the socially preferable way of behaving (Ussher, 1991; Smail, 2001).

People may have been children in families where this behaviour was seen and encouraged, and therefore being open and vulnerable will cause fear and thus avoidance. Inter-collegial socialising and networking are often interpreted as developing friendships. However, these tend to be competitive gatherings where much mutual evaluation, resourcing and 'taking what you can get from it' is going on. People often form relationships from such gatherings. Behavioural changes away from these interactions then become difficult, as they are frightened of loving, mutual dependency, sharing, caring and availability when competition, independence and teamwork are valued. Teamwork here means that everyone is assigned a specific area of responsibility which will link with the whole, not spending the working day making time available to listen to colleagues. Often people will be 'advised' to take time off 'sick' with stress, when all they want to do is debrief.

The way in which individuals behave in relationships will have been determined by the way in which they were socialised through life experiences. In motherhood, the woman has a baby who is open and vulnerable. The mother will experience basic human nature for which she may have had no training or preparation. She may turn to the relationship with her partner for support. However, her partner may well have had no training in supporting others up to this point. He may deal with this situation by withdrawing from the relationship, trying to give practical help or trying to find practical solutions, such as the employment of domestic help. On the other hand, he may start to listen to his partner and develop their relationship, leading to total acceptance of each other.

The presence at home of three or more children under the age of 14 years

The demands of children are relentless. For many parents this may feel like a one-way system in which they give to the children but receive very little. The younger the children are, the more demanding they tend to be, and needless to say the more of them there are, the more likely it is that their demands may become insurmountable.

What help does a family have to enable it to cope with these demands? Sometimes there are relatives living nearby who are willing to help out, but generally the culture in the UK promotes the nuclear family. Geographical mobility exists in order to provide a workforce for the capitalist market economy. People make themselves available to this market in order to earn an income, and because this is seen as a priority, being available to the family takes a back seat. This leaves the children with a limited number of adult carers. Some of those adult carers will be paid to care for the children. Thus again priority is given to the exchange of money, and according to Raphael-Leff (1991) this is instead of a genuine regard for other human beings and caring for each other. However, many families require two incomes in order to have an adequate standard of living, and some women choose to work in order to maintain their mental health.

This attitude of viewing caring as a job and not as a social need will also have been observed from the provision of 'caring' social organisations. These are organisations specifically created to take caring out of the home, and virtually all of them charge a fee for their services. Consider old people's homes, nurseries, respite care, child-minding, and so on. There are very few voluntary or Government-funded organisations. The cultural norm is therefore an expectation of the exchange of money for services rendered. However, perhaps the meaning of the word 'caring' needs to be considered. It involves more than physical minding, and it is usually women who put the love into caring for others. Consequently, a woman might very well be unhappy that her services to her child go unrecognised – not just in monetary terms but also in emotional terms – by the other people in her life as well as the children.

There is a social expectation that mothers will behave favourably and respond to their children's needs with total disregard for their own needs (Hochschild, 1983). This expectation is inconsistent with all of a woman's learning about social behaviour and the satisfaction of personal needs as a priority (Ussher, 1992). The larger the family, the less likely it is that the mother will have time for other interests, and therefore her life choices will be reduced. This includes employment outside the home, as the costs of childcare can be prohibitive (Rachman, 1998). The materialist culture promotes choice. Through advertisements, the public are urged on a daily basis to choose between products in order to boost consumerism. The mother has to live with another conflict in that she is admonished for reducing her consumer capacity (largely due to financial circumstances) and finding little support to make choices in her own life (Price, 1988).

The loss of their own mother before the age of 11 years

A woman often gains a greater understanding of her own mother when she takes on this role herself, and often their relationship changes at this point. Loss of her own mother and the grief that may have resulted may resurface at the time when she becomes a mother herself. The social attitude of 'life goes on' following a death may mean that grieving was inhibited or disturbed. Role modelling by a mother will have been limited to the potential mother as she developed but, more importantly, a loving and nurturing relationship may also have been missing (Deaves, 2001). Showing love towards a child enables the growth of that person. It allows them to develop the confidence to fulfil a full range of social roles. When children feel supported, they can 'test out' the environment from a safe place and know that the security of their relationship with their mother exists and she will protect them. Children know that they can find approval and acknowledgement in this relationship, and their exploration of and learning about the world is done from a safe base (Smith and Cowie, 1998). However, if this is missing from a child's life, they may be afraid to take risks in life and possibly lack confidence. The mother may also re-experience the pain of grieving for her own mother, followed by a potential lack of support for her mothering role. Motherhood — one of the greatest journeys in life — may not be safe for this child, who is now the mother, and she may hit the crash barrier. She may have been unprepared for taking this risk, but now there are no buffers in sight.

The absence of outside employment

Outside employment is familiar to those who worked outside the home prior to motherhood. It is a place where people feel valued, if only in the sense that they receive a monetary reward (Warner *et al.*, 1996). Many people value monetary reward highly because of the goods and services that they can buy with it. People may feel powerful when they can control what they want in life through money. This view is supported by the economy and capitalism in which mothers are living their lives (Smail, 2001). The interpretation that is often made of wanting the best for their baby is in materialist terms — the 'best' pram, the 'best' cot, the 'best' clothes and the 'best' milk — these commodities are usually costly and enforce the culture of separatism between the mother and her child. For example, a pram or cot will take the baby out of his or her mother's arms, and by giving the baby formula milk the mother is allowing others to feed the child, thus depriving him or her of the 'best' food. Employment separates the mother from her baby for many hours, yet the social expectation is to support working women. It may be inconsistent, but it is here that she regains her esteem based on the high value that is attached to earning an income — motherhood has no such rewards.

One of the advantages of employment is that it can prevent loneliness, in that people socialise and debrief at work. Outside employment can also raise self-esteem because personal identity exists in employment. For example, 'Sally the midwife' has a different meaning to 'Sally the mother'. In other words, greater social value is attached to career status than to family position (Hope *et al.*, 1999). Interestingly, the value changes depending on the total amount of personal income, with higher values being accorded to those who receive higher salaries. Children are socialised into seeing the value of different careers, and they are often encouraged to choose a career on the basis of the status and power attached to it, rather than because of a personal preference for a particular job.

Motherhood as a loss

Most women have no awareness of the factors in society that mitigate against their role as mothers. What they do know, however, is that they can be feeling a deep sense of loss. Ussher (1992) considers that unhappiness at the start of motherhood is a normal state and will aid the transition to this new role. The beginning of motherhood can be a form of bereavement (Nicolson, 1998) in that the woman is grieving the loss of her former self and the lifestyle to which she had become accustomed. Hochschild (1983) refers to motherhood as 'hurting an illusion' (the public image of motherhood that does not match the reality). As the mother begins to yearn for the 'illusion' and her previous lifestyle, she thus begins to feel unhappy with the reality. The constant tiredness during the first 3 months after the birth may seem to make the losses insurmountable.

Dalton (1980) describes the mother as having lost not only happiness and sleep but also her interests, enthusiasm, energy, security, pleasure, adequacy, insight, clear thinking, pleasure, libido, memory, concentration, bowel movement, weight and appetite. By analysing just one of these areas, namely loss of libido, it is possible to see many new areas of difficulty and conflict that the mother now has to deal with. Larme (1998) has postulated that extramarital affairs increase during the postnatal period. It is easy to blame the woman's loss of libido, which could be the direct result of exhaustion, but equally there is the question of the basis of the relationship. This is a time when the woman needs love, support and nurturing, and what she in fact faces is rejection. Love in the relationship may have been interpreted as sex. Sex created a time of closeness, and the meaning that may have been attached to this physical act could have been about caring for each other. When one partner is unable (for whatever reason) to take part in this physical act, may the other take this to mean that he is not cared about any more?

These meanings are not individual, but are taken from the culture. For example, advertising aims to persuade individuals to spend their money. Sex, in the form of barely clad people, is often used to sell products – the message is about satisfying personal needs by buying the product (Jenkins *et al.*, 1990). Films are made that depict sex as being the only expression of love, and magazines and books are full of stories about the priority that sex has in loving. It is questionable whether the majority of couples spend most of their time together making love, yet the media imagery is very powerful.

If people depend on society to guide the way towards the creation of a loving relationship, they will be left with the media images whose priority is profit, not the enhancement of loving relationships. Even the definition of what is a sexual 'turn on' is socially mediated. In western culture the breast is often depicted as a sexual organ, whereas in other cultures, where women's bodies are rarely seen, an ankle could fulfil the same function. The capitalist culture makes use of this socially constructed knowledge.

Many people lose 'friends' at the time of having their first baby because their interests change dramatically. People (including the mother's partner) get bored with listening to what colour the nappies are, although this may very well be the mother's current concern. Some interpret this conversation as being somewhat shallow when they would prefer to discuss the economy, for instance. Visiting friends may involve arranging babysitting and having a disposable income in order to be able to enjoy a 'night out'. Having subsequent babies, when one is already part of a network of friends who have children, may now involve having parties in the middle of the day that involve the children. So the mother's whole way of socializing has now changed. However, if the couple previously used to enjoy an evening out together, followed by lovemaking, and this routine is broken by the baby, then the nature of the relationship will change and some partners may find this adaptation difficult, or refuse to accept that a baby can alter one's life so dramatically. For the mother, caring for her children takes priority over most other matters, as it is here that she may feel that she can make a difference.

Having a baby is exhausting, and being exhausted can impair mind and body functions (Huang and Mathers, 2001). The mother will sense these changes (Ussher, 1992), which include a loss of concentration, loss of memory, loss of a quick response time, loss of regular bowel movements, loss of appetite and loss of motivation, among other things (Tisdall, 1997). How does this state of existence fit in with having sex? It seems obvious that one way for the mother to reduce her exhaustion is to have help. The help that is often chosen is dependent on family and friends, but their availability may be limited by, for example, geographical distance or daily employment. Society does make provision here if one is wealthy, in which case a nanny or childminder can be employed. The idea is to maintain some degree of 'normality' — that is, to try to achieve the lifestyle one had prior to motherhood.

Superwomen

Women are expected to manage not only their families, but also their careers and domestic chores. Many women, due to the limited number of hours that are available in a day, may feel anxious and guilty because they are not managing any of these areas to the best of their ability (Finn *et al.*, 1985; Nicolson, 1998). This situation is often exacerbated by such factors as poor housing, poor financial resources, poor relationships, poor social support and low income. Women even take on self-blame for living in poor social circumstances (Smail, 2001). The risk of becoming unhappy is now increasing (Sheppard, 1997; Romito *et al.*, 1999; Saurel-Cubizolles *et al.*, 2000; Reading and Reynolds, 2001).

The woman risks becoming overworked when there is an unequal distribution of domestic tasks (Finn *et al.*, 1985) and childcare (Um and Dancy, 1999). Yet in a patriarchal society there is a social expectation that women will take on the bulk of the domestic chores and childcare (Brown and Siegal, 1988). Men are often described as 'helping' women and do not see the inequality in their relationship. The role is often modelled from the family of origin, or is taken for granted as the role ascribed within a heterosexual partnership in a patriarchal society (Nicolson and Ussher, 1992).

Men receive much in return for entering into personal relationships with women. They often have their housework, ironing, washing, childcare, cooking and washing up done for them. They will expect and often receive help with their work and entertaining of colleagues, and their biological urge to reproduce is satisfied. This is one area of the social order in which money is not exchanged for services. Many women feel that they need to have sex because it is part of 'earning their keep', while on the other hand they feel that they would like to or need to care for their partner because, after all, that is their role. The paternalistic structure of society means that women often subordinate their own needs to those of their male partners (Gilbert, 1992).

Nicolson states that motherhood is 'the key means of women's oppression in patriarchal societies' (Nicholson, 1998: 7). Many mothers will feel dissatisfied, but often they do not realise why this is so. The family needs then add an extra burden to the mother's ability to provide services. The lack of material and verbal recognition for the provision of services, most of which are repetitive and boring, can generate either great frustration and unhappiness in a woman's life, or the opposite.

What is a good mother?

Mothers may thus have to cope with feelings of anxiety and guilt (Finn *et al.*, 1985). Most mothers have conflicting feelings about returning to work because they fear for their child. When they are away from their child, at work, they can only hope that he or she is being cared for adequately, and therefore they become anxious and feel guilty (Nahas and Amasheh, 1999). Many of the sentences that they will use in relation to their child will be punctuated by 'if only', and thus the feeling of guilt arises (Smail, 2001). Feelings of anxiety and guilt are caused by the social image of a good mother (Gilbert, 1992).

A good mother is portrayed as being self-sacrificing, with no needs or wants of her own (Finn *et al.*, 1985). She is totally available to her children, and this availability is often extended to her partner as well. The image of martyrdom does not in general reflect people who are not mothers, especially in view of the way in which people have been socialised into being selfish, competitive and resourceful within the capitalist economy. This makes no allowance for working alongside anyone, let alone giving up the self completely with no material reward for working for the family. Perhaps, as Price (1988) suggests, mothers should aim no higher than being 'good enough', and that still requires a considerable degree of self-sacrifice.

Unconditional love is something that many people resist. The expectation is to receive as well as to give. How many people talk about a relationship as being 50/50? Does this mean that people are willing to give only 50% of themselves, their time and their energy, or that they are only in the relationship for 50% of the time? Yet motherhood requires 100% of the mother to be available to the child. If adults cannot give to each other (as well as receive), where will they learn to do this for their children? There are so many conflicts that women face during their development as mothers. For some women the conflicts are unbearable, their resources are limited and they cannot adapt to motherhood with ease, but only with dis-ease. Ussher believes that 'it is the society which is sick, not the woman' (Ussher, 1991: 20).

Post-traumatic stress disorder (PTSD)

The possibility of PTSD should now be considered following a traumatic birth (Welford, 1998). PTSD is included in this chapter because it is thought that those who care for women throughout their pregnancy and birth experience may have a part in its creation (Creedy *et al.*, 2000). It is an area where action can be taken by professionals in order to prevent the occurrence of PTSD. Women's narratives are widely available to read in journals such as *Association for Improvements in the Maternity Services (AIMS)* or *New Generation,* and these narratives indicate those areas about which women feel aggrieved. The action that is required is often to consider and be respectful of the woman and her individuality, rather than following routines and procedures.

Woods states that PTSD 'may be a normal adaptive reaction to abnormal, extreme stress' (Woods, 2000: 311). However, the trauma will be personally interpreted, as it will affect the way in which the mother feels about and within herself. Previously, PTSD was defined as being applicable to veterans and survivors of torture, assault and rape (Michaels *et al.*, 1999). However, it is now recognised that as some women narrate their labour story they will use the same or similar words to rape survivors.

PTSD has been recognised for about 20 years (Rogers and Liness, 2000) as a classification of anxiety that will cause major 'changes in behaviour, cognitions (thoughts, and the way that we think) and physiology (physical feelings of anxiety). It can also affect a person's daily life, including work, relationships, hobbies and interests' (Rogers and Liness, 2000: 48). This is a step further than unhappiness, and while depression may be the result of unresolved anxiety, Rachman tells us that anxiety is 'a feeling of uneasy suspense ... tense anticipation of a threatening but "vague event"' (Rachman, 1998: 25). This cannot be labelled depression. It has to be recognised that treating a woman for clinical depression when the latter is not present will not resolve the initial trigger for her anxiety.

Rogers and Liness (2000) explain that the first 4 weeks following the trauma will be classified as acute stress disorder, and if there is no resolution, then the classification of PTSD is applied. It is easy to see how the postpartum woman is likely to be labelled as depressed at this time, because giving the label of PTSD takes the onus of responsibility for the cause away from the woman and passes it on to the professionals. So if it is not the woman's hormones that are causing the way she feels, is it the way in which she was treated during labour?

The factors that contribute to PTSD include a violent birth, fear for the baby, postpartum pain, low energy levels, disturbed sleep, worry, being sexually abused while pregnant, excessive vomiting during pregnancy, ectopic pregnancy, hospital treatment for miscarriage, macrosomia, and episodes of preterm labour throughout the pregnancy, although the mother gave birth at term (Seng *et al.*, 2001). Laing (2001) considers that PTSD can result from loss of control and a sense of powerlessness during labour, but adds that women view that as not being treated with respect or given adequate information. Laing (2001) suggests that there are other factors that will predispose a woman to PTSD, such as the following:

- a pre-existing personality disorder or emotional disorder
- a family history of psychiatric disorders
- a poor adaptive coping style
- the severity of the actual event
- the nature of the outside support.

It is difficult to evaluate these factors because some individuals will cope better, despite having a cruel history, compared with others who appear to have had fewer life stresses. Therefore, whilst recognising risk factors for PTSD in the antenatal period, it is important to make an individual assessment of the woman who is presenting as a totality.

Ayers and Pickering (2001) suggest that 3% of women may develop PTSD as a result of childbirth. However, we do not know whether the 10–15% who are diagnosed as having postnatal depression in fact have PTSD (Robinson, 1999). Creedy *et al.* (2000) mention that the classification of PTSD comes from the *Diagnostic and Statistical Manual of Mental Disorders*, and they describe the condition as follows.

1   The stress involves an event (i.e. labour) that could entail actual or threatened death or serious injury, or damage to the self or others. It is well known that pregnant women often think about dying during childbirth and in labour, and each intervention is capable of restimulating those thoughts. It is possible to read narratives of women's experiences in books and journals where the horror of the labour is recalled, together with the emotional context, only to realise that these women often wonder how they survived.
2   The woman's response involves intense fear, helplessness or horror. LeMarquand (2000) provides a narrative to demonstrate this. Loss of control is a recurring feature (Laing, 2001). Axe (2000) acknowledges that women experience physical damage, stigmatisation, betrayal and powerlessness during labour.
3   There is persistent re-experiencing of the labour, with intrusive thoughts, persistent memories, nightmares and flashbacks (Bracken, 2001). Michaels *et al.* (1998) state that there will be recurring memories, which will be felt physically and visually, and even acted out. There will be no information processing in the memory storage, so no processing will have taken place.
4   There will be persistent avoidance of any stimuli associated with the labour. These women may avoid other pregnant or postnatal women, hospitals or health professionals. They succeed in achieving an emotional numbing.
5   The woman will experience symptoms of increased physiological arousal that involve the fight/flight hormones, and therefore she will be in a state of heightened awareness, with extreme vigilance, insomnia and resultant irritability. The sympathetic nervous system is thus called into action in the extreme, leaving little room for parasympathetic function. The physiological results of this could be manifested as irritable bowel syndrome, heartburn, digestive difficulties, bladder problems and sexual dysfunction, among other symptoms.

Creedy *et al.* (2000) have pointed out that as the level of intervention increases, satisfaction with care decreases, and that is when the care is perceived to be inadequate. The risk of PTSD will increase at this point.

Conclusion

This chapter has discussed the realities of life, which impinge upon the way that women feel on becoming mothers. Social factors cannot be ignored, as they are integral to the aetiology of unhappiness. However, once they are recognised, the solution becomes obvious. Motherhood needs to be socially and politically supported. The evolving culture needs to recognise the value of motherhood to society, and to reward mothers' contribution to this. Radical policy changes from the Government would have to be instituted so that women felt valued within the cultural norm. This would include acceptance of fathers performing the traditional mothering role, and remunerating women (or men), while also allowing respite breaks from childcare.

Maternity services are partly responsible for the creation of PTSD, and therefore need to select staff carefully and then support them so that they are able to give the best care possible. However, children grow up and life moves on. Therefore there is a chance of the unhappiness passing even if nothing is done. The time that is spent being unhappy, and its effects on the baby and others with whom the mother is in contact, are worthy of consideration. The long-term effects have been shown to have a negative impact on children both behaviourally and intellectually, with an increase in the incidence of non-accidental injury (Almond, 1996). There is an urgent need to radically modify behaviour towards mothers and increase the support that is given to them in order to produce a world in which people are more likely to share in each other's happiness, and thereby create happiness in the future.

- Unhappiness can be a rational process of adaptation to motherhood.
- Mothering can reduce life choices.
- Normality can exist in the procurement of a lifestyle that was maintained prior to motherhood.
- Mothers may grieve for their former lifestyle.
- Motherhood is regarded as a low-status activity within a capitalist economy.

Useful addresses

The Association of Postnatal Illness
145 Dawes Road
London SW6 7EB
Helpline: 0207 386 0868
Fax: 0207 386 8885
Email: Info@APNI.org
Website: www.APNI.org

Meet a Mum
77 Westbury View
Peasedown St John
Bath
Avon BA2 8TZ
Tel: 01761 433 598
Helpline: 0208 768 0123

National Childbirth Trust (Postnatal Depression Co-ordination)
Alexandra House
Oldham Terrace
Acton
London W3 6NH
Tel: 0870 444 8707

Crysis Helpline
BCM Cry-sis
London WC1N 3XX
Tel: 0207 404 5011

Parent Advice Line
Unit 520
Highgate Studios
53–57 Highgate Road
London NW5 1TL
Tel: 0808 800 222

References

- Almond P (1996) How health visitors assess the health of postnatal women. *Health Visitor.* **69**: 12 495–8.
- Axe S (2000) Women's issues. Labour debriefing is crucial for good psychological care. *Br J Midwifery.* **8**: 630–1.
- Ayers S and Pickering AD (2001) Do women get post-traumatic stress disorder as a result of childbirth? *Birth.* **28**: 111–18.
- Bracken PJ (2001) Post-modernity and post-traumatic stress disorder. *Soc Sci Med.* **53**: 733–43.
- Brown GW and Harris T (1978) *The Social Origins of Depression.* Tavistock Publications, London.
- Brown JD and Siegal JM (1988) Attribution for negative life events and depression: the role of perceived control. *J Pers Soc Psychol.* **54**: 316–22.
- Creedy DK, Spochet IM and Horsfall J (2000) Childbirth and the development of acute trauma symptoms. *Birth.* **27**: 104–11.
- Dalton K (1980) *Depression after Childbirth.* Oxford University Press, Oxford.
- Deaves D (2001) Prevention and management of postnatal depression. *Commun Practitioner.* **74**: 263–7.
- Finn WF, Tallmer M, Seeland IB, Kutscher AH and Clark EJ (1985) *Women and Loss.* Praeger Scientific, New York.
- Gilbert P (1992) *Depression: the evolution of powerlessness.* Lawrence Erlbaum Associates, Hove.
- Hochschild AR (1983) *The Managed Heart: commercialization of human feeling.* University of California Press, Berkeley, CA.
- Hope S, Power C and Rodgers B (1999) Does financial hardship account for elevated psychological distress in lone mothers? *Soc Sci Med.* **49**: 1637–49.
- Huang Y and Mathers N (2001) Postnatal depression – biological or cultural? A comparative study of postnatal women in the UK and Taiwan. *J Adv Nurs.* **33**: 279–87.
- Jenkins A, Sweeney N and Potrykus C (1990) The shock of motherhood. *Health Visitor.* **63**: 154–5.
- Laing KG (2001) Post-traumatic stress disorder: myth or reality? *Br J Midwif.* **9**: 447–51.
- Larme AC (1998) Environment, vulnerability and gender in Andean ethnomedicine. *Soc Sci Med.* **47**: 1005–15.
- LeMarquand J (2000) 'Normal' birth in Jersey. *Assoc Improve Matern Serv.* **12**: 13–15.

- Michaels AJ, Michaels CE, Moon CH, Zimmermann MA, Peterson C and Rodriguez JL (1998) Psychosocial factors limit outcomes after trauma. *J Trauma Injury Infect Crit Care*. **44**: 644–8.
- Michaels AJ, Michaels CE, Moon CH *et al*. (1999) Post-traumatic stress disorders after injury. *J Trauma Injury Infect Crit Care*. **47**: 460–7.
- Nahas V and Amasheh N (1999) Culture care meanings and experiences of postpartum depression among Jordanian Australian women. *J Transcult Nurs* **10**: 37–45.
- Nicolson P (1998) *Postnatal Depression*. Routledge, London.
- Nicolson P and Ussher J (1992) *The Psychology of Women's Health and Health Care*. Macmillan, Basingstoke.
- Odent M (1999) *The Scientification of Love*. Free Association Books, London.
- Pilgrim D and Bentall R (1999) The medicalization of misery. *J Ment Health*. **8**: 261–74.
- Price J (1988) *Motherhood: what it does to your mind*. Pandora, London.
- Rachman S (1998) *Anxiety*. Psychology Press, Hove.
- Raphael-Leff J (1991) *Psychological Processes of Childbearing*. Chapman and Hall, London.
- Reading R and Reynolds S (2001) Debt, social disadvantage and maternal depression. *Soc Sci Med*. **53**: 441–53.
- Robinson J (1999) When delivery is torture. *Br J Midwif*. **7**: 684.
- Rogers P and Liness S (2000) Post-traumatic stress disorder. *Nurs Standard*. **14**: 47–54.
- Romito P, Cubizolles-Saurel MJ and Lelong N (1999) What makes new mothers unhappy: psychological distress one year after birth in Italy and France. *Soc Sci Med*. **49**: 1651–61.
- Saurel-Cubizolles MJ, Romito P, Ancel PY and Lelong N (2000) Unemployment and psychological distress one year after childbirth in France. *J Epidemiol Commun Health*. **54**: 185–91.
- Seng JS, Oakley DJ, Sampselle CM *et al*. (2001) Post-traumatic stress disorder and pregnancy complications. *Obstet Gynaecol*. **97**: 17–22.
- Sheppard M (1997) Depression in female health visitor consulters. *J Adv Nurs*. **26**: 921–29.
- Smail D (2001) *The Nature of Unhappiness*. Constable Publishers, London.
- Smith PK and Cowie H (1998) *Understanding Children's Development* (3e). Blackwell Science, Oxford.
- Tisdall N (1997) *Psychology of Childbearing*. Books for Midwives Press, Hale.
- Um CC and Dancy BL (1999) Relationship between coping strategies and depression among employed Korean immigrant wives. *Issues Ment Health Nurs*. **20**: 485–94.
- Ussher J (1991) *Women's Madness*. Harvester Wheatsheaf, Hemel Hempstead.
- Ussher J (1992) Reproductive rhetoric and the blaming of the body. In: P Nicolson and J Ussher (eds) *The Psychology of Women's Health and Health Care*. Macmillan, Basingstoke.
- Warner R, Appleby L, Whitton A and Faragher B (1996) Demographic and obstetric risk factors for postnatal psychiatric morbidity. *Br J Psychiatry*. **168**: 607–11.
- Welford H (1998) *Book of Postnatal Depression*. Thorsons, London.
- Woods SJ (2000) Prevalence and patterns of post-traumatic stress disorder in abused and postabused women. *Issues Ment Health Nurs*. **21**: 309–24.

CHAPTER 15

Childbirth and sexual abuse during childhood

Caroline Squire

Childhood sexual abuse is an important area that midwives and healthcare workers need to confront and understand. Many women survivors will make use of the maternity services, and midwives and healthcare workers need to be fully prepared and aware of the difficulties these women may face. This chapter provides background information about the definition and prevalence of childhood sexual abuse, but the main focus is on the long-term effects and the specific issues related to pregnancy and childbirth. The relationship between childhood sexual abuse and adolescent pregnancy, preterm labour, labour and birth, language, breastfeeding, and unhappiness after birth is considered. Finally, there is a brief consideration of clinicians who have been sexually abused as children, with particular reference to the effects on their clinical judgement.

Introduction

> I was sexually abused by my grandfather and other family members from the age of two until I was approximately 12 years old .... In the delivery room, whenever a contraction would come, I simply 'stepped out', looking right through whoever was there until the contraction subsided. My daughter was posterior and the doctor turned her .... Finally, my baby was pulled from my body. I laid back on the bed and felt totally, utterly violated.
>
> (Christensen, 1992: 34)

Childbirth can be a traumatic experience for any woman, but for women who have been sexually abused as children, the likelihood of experiencing birth as violence is increased. It is a significant trauma that is likely to have a lifelong impact on survivors. Despite the high prevalence of child sexual abuse, lack of knowledge and understanding still exists among many healthcare professionals, including midwives. This lack of understanding of the complex difficulties that survivors face during childbirth may lead to insensitive care and subsequent further emotional and psychological trauma. Many midwives will have assisted women during their births unaware that these women were sexually abused as children. On other occasions, women will disclose their tragic histories, and it is important that midwives feel as confident as they can that they have background knowledge and understanding to support these survivors. This chapter will consider definitions and the prevalence of childhood sexual abuse and, in particular, issues related to childbirth, including adolescent pregnancy, preterm labour, language and power, unhappiness after birth, and breastfeeding. It is hoped that such knowledge will help midwives to empower women who are survivors of childhood sexual abuse and prevent further emotional trauma.

Definition

Defining childhood sexual abuse is problematic for healthcare professionals and researchers. The definitions in the literature vary according to the types of activities that are considered to be 'sexual' and the age at which a child is considered competent to give 'informed consent'. Clearly, childhood sexual abuse is part of the wider issue of child abuse in general, and the official definitions that are used when children's names are placed on local child protection registers have widened. These registers, which are maintained by local authority social services departments, are lists of all children in the area for whom there are unresolved child protection issues and who are currently the subject of an inter-agency protection plan (Home Office, Department of Health, Department of Education and Science and Welsh Office, 1991). There are currently four categories in use in England and Wales, defined as follows (Home Office, Department of Health, Department of Education and Science and Welsh Office, 1991).

1 *Physical injury:* actual or likely physical injury to a child, or failure to prevent physical injury (or suffering) to a child, including deliberate poisoning, suffocating and Munchausen's syndrome by proxy.
2 *Neglect:* the persistent or severe neglect of a child, or the failure to protect a child from exposure to any kind of danger, including cold or starvation, or extreme failure to carry out important aspects of care, resulting in the significant impairment of the child's health or development, including non-organic failure to thrive.
3 *Sexual abuse:* actual or likely sexual exploitation of a child or adolescent. The child may be dependent and/or developmentally immature.
4 *Emotional abuse:* actual or likely severe adverse effect on the emotional and behavioural development of a child caused by persistent or severe emotional ill-treatment or rejection. All abuse involves some emotional ill-treatment. This category should be used where it is the main or sole form of abuse.

The problems inherent in the above general definitions are that they omit some forms of harm to children, such as child labour and the consequences of war and civil unrest, and they also require a degree of subjective judgement about the presence or absence of abuse. For example, perspectives on child abuse are culture specific, and child labour may be regarded as child abuse in one country but not in another (Hallett, 1995).

In their feasibility study for a national prevalence study, Ghate and Spencer (1995) found that definitions of sexual abuse vary in terms of the following factors.

- Type of activity (usually distinguishing between contact and non-contact).
- Age of victim/survivor (in most studies the top limit is set at 16 years).
- Age differential between abuser and abused (usually 5 years, with some studies specifying 5 years for children under 12 years, 8–10 years for children over 12 years, or 5-year differential for total sample, but perpetrator over 16 years of age). Definitions which set an age differential are attempting to operationalise a distinction between abusive sexual experiences and cases of sexual exploration among peers.
- Nature of the relationship between the abuser and the abused. In previous studies, distinctions have been made between relatives (intra-familial) and people who are not related (extra-familial). Ghate and Spencer suggest that finer distinctions are required with regard to extra-familial perpetrators, which differentiate between people in a position of trust (e.g. peers, family friends, acquaintances, babysitters) and strangers.
- Issue of consent/responsibility/legality. Some studies probe consent, while others argue that children do not have the maturity to withhold consent.

It is clear that the different definitions that are employed in different studies will alter the prevalence rates and interpretations of the data.

In the UK, Creighton and Russell (1995) have used the following definition:

> the involvement of dependent children under the age of 16 in a sexual activity which they do not fully understand and to which they are not in a position to give informed consent − the activity being intended to gratify or satisfy the needs of the other person.

This definition does not include peer sexual experimentation, but it does include the issue of informed consent.

In the USA, childhood sexual abuse has been defined as any activity that engages a child in sexual activities that are developmentally inappropriate, with or without threatened or actual violence or injury. Sexual abuse does not always involve sexual intercourse or physical force. Rather, it is usually characterised by deception and coercion. Activities may include genital or anal contact, oral–genital contact and insertion of objects, and can encompass incest or sexual assault by a relative or stranger. Childhood sexual abuse is often a chronic violation rather than a single incident (Petersen, 1993). This lengthy definition is useful in that it makes explicit the fact that perpetrators may be family members or strangers, contact and non-contact activities are included, and it addresses the exploitation of adult authority (and maturity) over the child.

Finkelhor (1997) suggests the following definition as being consistent with most legal and research definitions of child sexual abuse. It was formulated by the National Center on Child Abuse and Neglect (1978: 2), and it has many of the advantages of the previous definition. This definition also makes it clear that the perpetrator may be under 18 years of age.

> Contacts or interactions between a child and an adult when the child is being used for the sexual stimulation of the perpetrator or another person. Sexual abuse may also be committed by a person under the age of 18, when that person is significantly older than the victim or when the perpetrator is in a position of power or control over another child.

Cawson *et al.* (2000) made a distinction between abuse involving physical contact (e.g. intercourse, oral sex, touching and fondling, sexual hugging or kissing) and 'non-contact' abuse (e.g. using the child to make pornographic photographs or videos, showing the child pornography, forcing or encouraging the child to watch live sexual acts, exposing sex organs to excite themselves or shock the child). Again it is easy to see how other studies may not make the same distinction, and may therefore produce different prevalence rates and interpretations.

Scott (1996) argues that where definitions become more restrictive, prevalence rates fall, and this would partially explain the wide variations in the data on the prevalence of sexual abuse. It may be that too narrow a definition of abuse works against children's rights, while the capacity to construe almost any situation as abusive could result in the statistics being ignored and/or the issue not being taken seriously (Fitzsimons, 1999).

Prevalence

Childhood sexual abuse occurs much more frequently than was originally believed but, as mentioned above, the prevalence rates are affected by the way in which sexual abuse is defined (Burke Draucker, 2000). The reported prevalence of childhood sexual abuse is highest in studies that include subjects seeking psychiatric treatment for depression, substance abuse, suicide, post-traumatic stress disorder, eating disorders and multiple personality disorder (Herman *et al.*, 1986; Courtois, 1993). The National Society for the Prevention of Cruelty to Children (NSPCC) recently reported the findings of a survey of the childhood experiences of 2869 young people aged 18–24 years (Cawson *et al.*, 2000). The main findings are listed below. The rates of physical and emotional abuse are included here because children who are sexually abused suffer physical and emotional abuse as well.

- 7% suffered serious physical abuse as children at the hands of parents or carers, including being hit with a fist or implement, beaten up, burned or scalded.
- 6% suffered serious physical neglect at home, including being left regularly without food as a young child, not being looked after or taken to the doctor when they were ill, or being left to fend for themselves because the parents were absent or had drug- or alcohol-related problems. In total, 5% had been placed at risk by being left alone at home overnight or out overnight (their whereabouts unknown) at young ages.
- 6% suffered multiple attacks on their emotional well-being and self-confidence, including living with frequent violence between their parents, being 'really afraid' of their parents, being regularly humiliated, being threatened with being sent away or thrown out, or being told that their parents wished they were dead or had never been born.
- 1% had been sexually abused by a parent, and 3% had been sexually abused by another relative (ranging from penetrative or oral sex to taking pornographic photographs of them).
- 1% (mainly girls, under the age of 16 years) had been forced or threatened by people known to them into taking part in sexual acts against their will.
- 25% said that there were things that had happened to them during their childhood which they found difficult to talk about. For example, only just over

25% of respondents who had been sexually abused or coerced into sexual activity had told anyone at the time that it happened.

Epidemiological reports from the USA estimate that as many as one in four American women have been victims of sexual abuse during childhood. The number of sexually abused children during 1994 was estimated to be over 300 000, and girls were found to have been sexually abused three times more frequently than boys (Sedlack and Broadhurst, 1996).

Finkelhor (1994) reviewed 21 international population studies of child sexual abuse, primarily from English-speaking and northern European countries. The prevalence rates ranged from 7% to 36% for women and from 3% to 29% for men. Despite the variation in rates, it appears that the number of people with a history of abuse is significant, with a higher prevalence for women.

Similarly, in Australia a retrospective study of 710 women randomly selected from Australian federal electoral rolls (Fleming, 1997) revealed that 20% had experienced childhood sexual abuse, and that among this 20%:

- 10% had experienced either vaginal or anal intercourse
- the mean age at the first episode was 10 years (71% were under 12 years)
- 98% of the perpetrators were male; they were usually known to the child, and 41% were relatives
- the mean age of abusers was 34 years, with a median age difference of 24 years older than that of the abused child.
- only 10% reported their experiences to the police, a doctor or a helping agency.

From the above listing of some of the available prevalence rates for childhood sexual abuse, it would appear that more women than men are sexually abused as children, and that only a fraction disclose their experiences to anyone. This is of great significance for midwives and healthcare professionals who work with women during pregnancy and childbirth, since most survivors will be unknown to them, rendering the notion of being 'with woman' and 'woman-centred' even more difficult.

Background characteristics associated with sexual abuse of children

Jehu (1988) has described the following as characteristics of the family with incestuous sexual relationships:

- high levels of marital conflict, often with physical abuse of the mother
- the father may select children as sexual objects when his sexual and emotional needs are not met within the marriage
- high levels of mobility, with passing of the child to one relative or another, leading to a lack of consistent stable care from the parents
- such families often lack social skills and are isolated from others
- confusion with regard to family roles and responsibilities for tasks at home.

Furthermore, Araji and Finkelor (1986) proposed four conditions which they considered to be necessary before sexual abuse could occur.

1   The perpetrator needs to desire the child, and this may occur as a result of disinhibition due to alcohol or drugs. Yet arousal may also be partly due to a need to dominate or because of low self-esteem or immaturity.
2   Perpetrators can often make children feel guilty and responsible for the abuse. They are sometimes able to persuade themselves that children desire sex within situations of step-parenting, because there are no biological ties and therefore the taboo is less strong.
3   Constraints from outside need to be considered by the perpetrator. The abuser has more opportunity when the mother is out and when the child is unsupervised. Most abuse occurs when children are alone.
4   The perpetrator needs to deal with the child's resistance, usually by threatening violence. Other adults and peers are kept away from the child in order to reduce the likelihood of discovery, and this adds to the child's isolation.

Cawson *et al.* (2000) found that socio-economic background made no difference to the prevalence of childhood sexual abuse. This contrasted with physical abuse, which was more likely in low-income groups. In truth, there are no clear reasons why adults sexually abuse children, and offenders may commit these acts for a variety of reasons. It is likely that both pathopsychological forces and the social structures of society form a complex mesh that may have a part in determining why some individuals engage in sexual activities with young children (Wallace, 1999).

To date, it would seem that the male has been regarded as the sole possible abuser, but it is recognised that women do sexually abuse children. It could be said that socialisation of males in society tends to reinforce sexually aggressive behaviour, but that socialisation of women inhibits it, so that for women to offend against children sexually, they have to deviate greatly from the accepted schema of the qualities that are considered to be female. Therefore it is extremely unlikely that as many women as men will be found to be perpetrators of child sexual abuse (Saradjian, 1996).

However, the under-reporting of sexual abuse by females, especially in intrafamilial situations, might be due to society's tendency to view males as aggressors and females as victims, or to possible differences in the types of offence that are committed by female offenders. Mothers in particular are construed as a special and 'purer' form of womanhood, being virtually 'asexual' (Saradjian, 1996). Offences by women may be less overt and embedded in typical parenting behaviours, such as caressing the child while bathing him or her, or becoming sexual with a child while 'cuddling' in bed (Burke Draucker, 2000). Therefore it needs to be recognised that women have been the offenders in a sizeable minority of cases of children who have been sexually abused, and that the notion that the perpetrators are always men and the victims are always female is incorrect.

Long-term effects

Relatively recent research has revealed that experiences of child sexual abuse are associated with numerous and varied long-term psychological, behavioural, interpersonal and physical effects (Bohn and Holz, 1996; Burke Draucker, 2000). Specific long-term effects with regard to pregnancy and childbirth will be discussed in more detail later in the chapter.

Psychological effects have been identified in several comprehensive reviews of the literature on long-term consequences of child sexual abuse (Finkelhor, 1990; Polusny and Follette, 1995; Young, 1992). They include increased levels of depression, multiple personality disorder, suicidal ideation and suicide, as well as anxiety disorders such as phobias, panic attacks and obsessive behaviours (Bifulco et al., 1991; Yellowlees and Kaushik, 1994).

A key psychological effect is dissociation, which is postulated to be a coping mechanism used by many incest survivors that allows the child to endure the pain, humiliation and rage engendered by the abuse. The child mentally leaves his or her body during the abuse and escapes to a safe place, often watching the abuse as if it were happening to someone else (Bala, 1994), or else they may be able to numb body parts at will (Kendall-Tackett, 1998). As adults they may later use the technique to cope with any stressful, intimate or dangerous situation. Medically intrusive procedures such as vaginal examinations or events related to previously traumatised body parts, such as childbirth or breastfeeding, may cause abuse survivors to dissociate. They may appear 'far away', may not respond to questions appropriately or may not remember parts of a discussion.

Sexual and relationship difficulties have also been reported (Mullen et al., 1993), which may include promiscuity, prostitution, sexual deviance, sexual dysfunction and engaging in sexual behaviour that is not of their choosing or for the purposes of obtaining drugs or a place to stay (Bachman et al., 1988; Courtois, 1993; Hendricks-Matthews, 1993). Behavioural and sexual problems that are experienced by abuse survivors may change over time and vary with the age of the survivor. For example, the abused child may display self-destructive behaviour by frequently darting into streets, climbing and playing in unsafe areas, and taking physical risks, whereas the abused adolescent may run away or give sex in exchange for money or drugs.

Cohen (1995) published a preliminary report of an investigation of the maternal functioning of woman survivors of child sexual abuse. A study group of 26 mothers who were adult survivors was compared with a control group of 28 mothers with no such history of abuse. Cohen studied seven areas of parenting skills, namely role image, objectivity, expectations, rapport, communication, limit-setting and role support. She found significant differences on all seven scales, characterised by a tendency of the study group to be less skilful with regard to maternal functioning than the control group. Particularly large differences were found on the scales of role support, communication and role image. Cohen (1995) suggests that secrecy, shame and self-blame may provide a partial explanation for the study group's generally undeveloped social skills, as well as other factors such as age of onset, severity and age at termination of the abuse.

Female abuse survivors most frequently present for healthcare with physical complaints. They may make repeated visits with the same or varied and often vague symptoms. These complaints are often stress or anxiety related, or symptoms of post-traumatic stress syndrome. They include sleep disorders (with repetitive dreams and nightmares), gastrointestinal problems (e.g. nausea, vomiting, diarrhoea, constipation, irritable bowel syndrome), muscle tension, headaches, palpitations or choking sensations, and chronic pelvic pain (Hendricks-Matthews, 1993; Walling et al., 1994).

The adult survivor may chain-smoke, overeat (causing bulimia and/or obesity), drink excessively or ignore basic health needs and problems (Bushnell et al., 1992;

Koss and Heslet, 1992; Courtois, 1993; Bohn and Holz, 1996). Other self-destructive behaviours may include self-mutilation, suicide attempts, substance abuse and unprotected sex with multiple partners (Bohn and Holz, 1996). Childhood abuse survivors are also 33–66% more likely to be assaulted and raped as adults both by strangers and by people known to them (Bohn and Holz, 1996). Low self-esteem, self-hatred, guilt, a sense of unworthiness and an inability to trust their own senses and set safe boundaries may cause adult survivors to be perceived by abusers as vulnerable or easy targets.

Issues specific to pregnancy and childbirth

Research into pregnancy-related consequences of childhood sexual abuse is still in the early stages of development, and is for the most part anecdotal (Bohn and Holz, 1996). However, there are a number of problems that are more likely to occur in survivors of childhood sexual abuse. They include unplanned, frequent and teenage pregnancy, spontaneous miscarriage, termination of pregnancy, hyperemesis, infertility, preterm labour, increased need for medical intervention and/or operative delivery, postpartum depression and breastfeeding difficulties (Courtois, 1993; Holz, 1994). Buist and Barnett (1995) and Buist (1998) found that the mother–infant relationship was impaired in women who had been sexually, physically and/or emotionally abused as children, and they were more likely to suffer from postnatal depression. Infertile women with histories of abuse may consider that they are being punished for early sexual experiences. During pregnancy, abuse survivors may report a fear of becoming fat, especially if an eating disorder is also present. Many women fear labour or are afraid that they will be unable to protect their child from abuse once it has been born, so they may require induction of labour and have to undergo the interventions which that entails (Bohn and Holz, 1996). Some of these key issues will be addressed further below:

Preterm labour

Horan *et al.* (2000) have postulated that early events of abuse, perhaps via stimulation of gene expression of corticotropin-releasing hormone (CRH) in the brain, may increase vulnerability to later experiences of unusual stress (e.g. pregnancy/childbirth). These experiences increase the production of CRH in the brain, and elevated CRH levels have been associated with preterm labour. Stevens-Simon *et al.* (1993) have postulated a connection between preterm labour and stress, and they have also described associations with depression, social isolation and substance abuse. Stevens-Simon and McAnarney (1994) published a study of the pregnancies of 127 poor black 12 to 18-year-old women, 33% of whom reported that they had been physically or sexually abused prior to conception. They found that these abused adolescents scored significantly higher on stress and depression scales, and they also rated their families as less supportive than did non-abused adolescents. They were more likely to report substance use during pregnancy, and they gave birth to significantly smaller and more preterm infants. However, the possible biological connection between stress and preterm labour requires further elucidation.

Adolescent pregnancy

It is postulated that childhood sexual abuse may disrupt psychosexual development in some adolescent women, and that some of them may react by voluntarily initiating sexual intercourse at a young age and becoming sexually promiscuous (Stevens-Simon and Reichert, 1994). As a result, a disproportionately large number of young women who become pregnant during adolescence have been found to be victims of childhood sexual abuse (Boyer and Fine, 1992; Stevens-Simon and McAnarney, 1994; Nagy *et al.*, 1995). Furthermore, adolescent women who have been sexually abused are more likely not to use contraception, so their risk of unintended pregnancy will be increased (Boyer and Fine, 1992; Nagy *et al.*, 1995; Esparza and Esperat, 1996; Dietz *et al.*, 1999).

Boyer and Fine (1992) reported that two-thirds of a sample of 535 women from the state of Washington who had become pregnant as adolescents had been sexually abused. They also found that these sexually victimised teenagers started intercourse a year earlier, were more likely to have used drugs and alcohol and were less likely to practise contraception. In addition, they were more likely to have been hit, slapped or beaten by a partner or to have exchanged sex for money, drugs or a place to stay. Furthermore, they were more likely to report that their own children had been abused or had been taken from them by the Child Protective Services.

Bayatpour *et al.* (1992) analysed data from a sample of 352 pregnant adolescent women in California, whose average age was 15 years. They found that 82% of the women were of ethnic-minority descent, 23% had been sexually or physically abused, and all of them were receiving public assistance. When they compared adolescents who had been sexually or physically abused with those who had not, their results revealed significant differences with regard to marijuana and cocaine use, as well as self-destructive behaviours such as suicidal thoughts and actions.

Labour and birth

Labour and birth can be frightening for any woman, but for those with a history of childhood sexual abuse the experience of childbirth may remind them of the times when they were attacked as children. They may feel out of control, be immobilised on a bed, experience pain and be subjected to intrusive procedures such as vaginal examinations which make them feel objectified and depersonalised. The list of procedures that many women undergo in these days of institutionalised birth is endless. They may include abdominal palpations, vaginal examinations during pregnancy and labour, ultrasound scanning, induction of labour by rupture of the amniotic membranes or by pharmacological methods, monitoring of uterine contractions and fetal heart rate, insertion of intravenous/urinary catheters, immobilisation in lithotomy stirrups, epidural or other pharmacological analgesia, episiotomy, forceps/ventouse and Caesarean section delivery. Although these procedures may be of value for some women, they may make the woman who has been sexually abused as a child (or raped at any age) feel tied up and powerless. The use of lithotomy is something that many midwives and healthcare professionals take for granted, but which may induce particularly violent memories for women who have been sexually abused. Wet pads and sheets may bring flashbacks of ejaculated semen. Touching women in certain ways, such as helping to move their legs into the lithotomy poles or opening their legs in preparation for a vaginal examination or birth, may also bring back memories.

Kitzinger (1992) explored and compared the language used by women who were survivors of sexual violence with that of 345 women who had experienced traumatic births. She found that their descriptions were very similar. One woman said that the obstetrician 'hauled me around like a slab of meat', while others felt 'skewered, trussed up like an oven-ready turkey' or like 'a fish on a slab' or 'a carcass'. Both groups used the language of waste disposal, such as 'trash', 'rubbish', 'shit' and 'a bloody mess' (Kitzinger, 1992: 74). It is important to note that the midwife or healthcare professional may not always realise what the woman perceives to be traumatic, especially if the outcome is a healthy baby.

As mentioned previously, one of the ways in which women survivors of sexual abuse may cope with the overwhelming feelings they encounter during labour and birth is to dissociate themselves from the experiences as a means of having some control over the situation. This means that there is a separation of body and mind as a survival technique. In order to cope with their experiences of sexual abuse, women may have repressed memories of the abuse, but the invasive methods described above can reproduce overwhelming flashbacks of that abuse (Smith, 1998). Dissociation provided a way to gain some control for some participants in a study by Parratt (1994). Susan felt that her births were 'easy' and that dissociation helped:

> I think I always would have given birth fairly easily, but I think that being able to dissociate ... and to have sort of accepted interference as a matter of course might have meant that in some ways it was less traumatic.
>
> (Parratt, 1994: 33)

In a very informative article, Gutteridge (2001) relates her experiences of being a survivor of childhood sexual abuse to her experiences of being a midwife who has given birth in the current maternity services. She describes dissociation as a method that she has perfected throughout her life, and how she may slip into it when faced with problems. Those around her do not understand what is happening, and she is perceived as being impassive or submissive. Midwives and healthcare professionals may congratulate a mother who has dissociated herself from her labour, and may tell her how brave she was because she was so quiet and good with her breathing. This happened to Margaret, who had a long labour:

> It was a long time and I just kept quiet and I just did my breathing. I just got on with what I had to do and I breathed away every contraction. And then when it came to the second stage, when I actually wasn't allowed to push but wanted to, I panted away like mad ... I got it right. I do remember being told, 'Wow, you did well with your breathing!'
>
> (Smith, 1993: 95)

Alternatively, Rhodes and Hutchinson (1994) describe retreating as taking the form of reliving the sexual abuse. During the course of labour, some women may become confused and disoriented with regard to place and time. Some assume a childlike voice and protective body postures, such as curling into a fetal position or hiding under the bedcovers. Rhodes and Hutchinson (1994) quote the recollection of one nurse-midwife about a 16-year-old survivor who was unresponsive to those around her:

> In active labour she assumed a childlike voice, threw her head up to the ceiling, clearly was not in the same room with the rest of us in her mind, and pleaded quietly but hysterically: 'Don't hurt me there. If you'll stop hurting me I'll be good. I promise I'll be good. I promise I won't tell anybody!'.
>
> (Rhodes and Hutchinson, 1994: 218)

This reliving of sexual abuse is consistent with post-traumatic stress disorder (PTSD), since the 16-year-old survivor re-experienced her abuse because the dynamics of her birth had similarities with her past trauma. Crompton (1996) considers PTSD and postulates that women may come to childbirth with or without a history of previous trauma. They may or may not be traumatised or further traumatised during the event. However, their experience of childbirth may on the one hand be a healing event which allows them to integrate their past trauma, or it may cause them to develop PTSD. This is clearly food for thought for midwives and healthcare professionals. The key aims are to prevent women from feeling traumatised during childbirth, and to keep women with a history of sexual abuse 'grounded' so that they do not dissociate or relive their past experiences. In this way, childbirth could be a healing experience for them. Maintaining control is also very important to survivors of childhood sexual abuse. Rhodes and Hutchinson (1994) quote the following words from a woman speaking of her feelings during childbirth:

> The birth terrified me. I thought I was going to die. I felt like that during the sexual abuse. When you get in a situation where you feel like you've been violated or you feel like your life is in danger, or someone has so much power over you they can do anything, you're out of control. ... That's terrifying, and that's the feeling I remember when I was giving birth. I was going to die and there were no two ways about it.
>
> (Rhodes and Hutchinson, 1994: 219)

For a woman to feel in control, it may be easier if she has as few midwives as possible during her pregnancy and birth, and this is best achieved through caseload practice or in a small team.

Language

Women tend to give birth in institutions which are hierarchical, paternalistic and scientific, and which have their own language which the public is unable to understand. Such a power base may alienate women, and there is also a tendency to infantilise them. Below is a short list of phrases that the midwife and healthcare professional will have heard before.

- Lie still dear, this won't hurt (it always does, and the woman knows it).
- Just open your legs a little bit wider. THAT'S GOOD! WELL DONE!
- Lift your bottom up for me. THAT'S GOOD! WELL DONE!
- Just popping a little finger inside.
- 'You'll feel me touching you, sweetie' (Bergstrom *et al.*, 1992: 10).
- Good girl, you're doing very well.

It is not difficult to see that survivors may find such language reminiscent of the way in which the abusers spoke to them during the abuse when they were children.

Language is power, and underlying this is the way in which midwives control and manipulate women in a hierarchical, institutionalised setting, according to policies and procedures which could be said to control midwives as well as other women. Although it is difficult in such a culture, it would be beneficial for midwives to take the time to listen carefully to every woman's story and then carefully and individually formulate responses (Tilley, 2000).

Unhappiness after birth

As was mentioned earlier in this chapter, a number of studies have highlighted the association between childhood sexual abuse and later adult mental health problems (Bifulco *et al.*, 1991; Yellowlees and Kaushik, 1994). However, there is a paucity of research into the possible relationship between childhood sexual abuse and unhappiness after birth.

Buist and Barnett (1995) reviewed voluntary admissions to a mother-and-baby unit and found that 40% of mothers reported a history of sexual abuse, with the figure rising to 54% when a broader definition of abuse (to include physical and/or sexual abuse) was used. For all of these women this was their first psychiatric admission, and all of them displayed symptoms of high levels of anxiety and low levels of self-confidence which were also related to their infant care. The researchers found an unusually low tolerance of frustration, which is of particular concern when survivors need to cope with the many and unpredictable demands and stresses of caring for babies and children. They may also be bringing up their children in families that are experiencing poverty, with alcohol and physical abuse prevalent as added stressors (Mullen *et al.*, 1993). Buist and Barnett (1995) postulated that a history of childhood sexual abuse may be a risk factor not only for the occurrence of postnatal depression but also for its severity, duration and outcome. Clearly there are long-term issues to be addressed for these women with regard to their becoming mothers, when they may have only a poor role model at their disposal, and also with regard to maintaining relationships with their partner and raising their children.

Buist (1998) has reported the first stage of a 3-year follow-up study of 56 women who were admitted with postpartum depressive disorders. They were assessed with regard to their well-being, relationships and infant interaction. In total, 28 women had a history of sexual abuse before the age of 16 years, 9 women had a history of physical/emotional abuse and 19 women had no history of abuse. It was found that the effects of childhood sexual abuse were indistinguishable from those of childhood physical and emotional abuse. These results support previous research findings, such as those of Mullen *et al.* (1993). The most significant finding was a detrimental effect on the mother–infant relationship in those women who had a history of abuse. This finding has clear long-term implications, and further research into this area is clearly required.

Breastfeeding

It is of interest that a literature search which was undertaken for this chapter revealed very little about childhood sexual abuse and breastfeeding. Article after article finishes after the birth, yet the action of the baby suckling on the breast and the release of fluid (which may remind the woman of ejaculation) might be considered to be obvious areas of concern. Some survivors will have no difficulties with breastfeeding, others will not even tolerate the thought of it, some may find it a healing experience and others will have neutral feelings about it and wish to breastfeed their babies because they want what is best for them.

Kendall-Tackett (1998) has written an extensive and useful article in which she describes what is known about the effects of childhood sexual abuse and how they might relate to breastfeeding. For example, she describes what she calls 'cognitive distortions', whereby a survivor who has felt so powerless and out of control in the past may feel the same as a mother and may underestimate her ability to protect and provide for her baby. She may also experience postnatal depression. If she experiences breastfeeding difficulties, she may feel that there is little she can do to remedy the situation and that yet another part of her body is letting her down.

Kendall-Tackett (1998) also provides some interesting practical information which may not otherwise be considered, and suggests that night feeding, the early postpartum period and playful older infants are three key problem areas. For example, she discusses the issue of night-time breastfeeding in relation to the fact that it may be a particularly stressful time for the survivor if her abuse used to occur at that time. She suggests that some survivors may prefer to express their breast milk and use a bottle or ask for someone else to take on the night feeds.

Simkin (1996) considers that some women have an aversion to breastfeeding because the breasts must be available to the baby 'on demand'. This implies a kind of ownership, and therefore a loss of control over her body by the mother. She has also described how breastfeeding can be a source of difficulty if the abuse was associated with the developing breasts (Simkin, 1994). It may be useful here to consider the midwife or healthcare professional who holds a survivor's breast in order to help her to suckle her baby. There are other ways of helping women to breastfeed their babies.

Effects of childhood abuse on clinicians' personal and professional lives

A number of informative and courageous articles have been published about midwives and healthcare professionals who have been sexually abused (Rouf, 1999; Tilley, 2000; Gutteridge, 2001).

Jackson and Nuttall (1997) investigated whether the experience of childhood abuse actually affected the clinical judgements of various different clinicians. In their initial survey, they drew a random stratified sample of 1635 clinicians from the national directories of clinical social workers, paediatricians, psychiatrists and clinical psychologists (who all worked with children) in the USA. These clinicians were then given 16 vignettes of case histories of sexual abuse and asked whether they believed the victim's story.

Importantly, their findings seem to demonstrate that interpretations of sexual abuse allegations can be highly subjective and that, despite the fact that all of the respondents were experienced in working with cases of child abuse, factors had been taken into account which were beyond the boundaries of clinical relevance. Clearly this is an area in need of further research involving healthcare professionals who work with women in childbirth.

Conclusion

Supporting survivors of childhood sexual abuse through their pregnancies, births and afterwards is both challenging and rewarding for midwives and all those involved. Midwives may of course be with women and not know that they have suffered sexual abuse during their childhood, or the survivor herself may occasionally be unaware of her past tragic history. Having a positive pregnancy and birth can be a powerful and healing experience for a survivor and may help her to come to terms with the pain and betrayal of the past. On the other hand, insensitive care during pregnancy and a traumatic birth may re-enact the pain that the woman endured as a child, with devastating long-term effects. Midwives who listen and practise sensitively and with insight are in a key position to help the survivor in her transition to being a mother, and to help her achieve this with strength and confidence.

- Many women are survivors of sexual abuse, and some will not have disclosed their experiences.
- Many women who have haphazard pregnancies, self-destructive behaviour or miss antenatal appointments may well have a history of sexual abuse.
- Procedures and practices associated with birth have real potential to make survivors re-enact their experiences of childhood sexual abuse.
- Language is power, and the use of childlike phrases may make the survivor relive her childhood experiences.
- Childhood sexual abuse is a real problem, and society needs to acknowledge this in order to help to prevent it and enable a change in attitude to the survivor.

Useful addresses

Childline
Studd Street
London N1 0QW
Free telephone number for young people and children to ring in emergencies:
0800 1111
Tel: 0207 239 1000
Fax: 0207 239 1001

Kidscape
2 Grosvenor Gardens
London SW1 0DH
Tel: 0207 730 3300
Fax: 0207 730 7081

National Children's Bureau
8 Wakeley Street
London EC1V 7QE
Tel: 0207 843 6000
Fax: 0207 278 9512

National Society for the Prevention of Cruelty to Children (NSPCC)
42 Curtain Road
London EC2A 3NH
Tel: 0207 825 2763
Fax: 0207 825 2763
Email: infounit@nspcc.org.uk

National Childbirth Trust
Alexandra House
Oldham Terrace
London W3 6NH
Tel: 0870 444 8707

The Association of Postnatal Illness
145 Dawes Road
London SW6 7EB
Telephone helpline: 0207 386 0868
Fax: 0207 386 8885
Email: info@APNI.org
Website: www.APNI.org

References

- Araji S and Finkelhor D (1986) Abusers: a review of the research. In: D Finkelhor (ed.) *Sourcebook on Child Sexual Abuse*. Sage Publications, London.
- Bachman G, Moeller T and Bennet J (1988) Childhood sexual abuse and the consequences in adult women. *Obstet Gynecol*. **71**: 631–41.
- Bala M (1994) Caring for adult survivors of child sexual abuse: issues for family physicians. *Can Fam Physician*. **40**: 924–31.
- Bayatpour M, Wells RD and Holford S (1992) Physical and sexual abuse as predictors of substance use and suicide among pregnant teenagers. *Soc Adolesc Med*. **13**: 128–33.
- Bergstrom L, Roberts J, Skillman L and Seidel J (1992) 'You'll feel me touching you, sweetie': vaginal examinations during the second stage of labor. *Birth*. **19**: 10–18.
- Bifulco A, Brown G and Adler Z (1991) Early sexual abuse and clinical depression in adult life. *Br J Psychiatry*. **159**: 115–22

- Bohn DK and Holz KA (1996) Sequelae of abuse: health effects of childhood sexual abuse, domestic battering and rape. *J Nurse Midwifery.* **41**: 442–56.
- Boyer D and Fine D (1992) Sexual abuse as a factor in adolescent pregnancy and child maltreatment. *Fam Plann Perspect.* **24**: 4–19.
- Buist A (1998) Childhood abuse, parenting and postpartum depression. *Aust NZ J Psychiatry.* **32**: 479–87.
- Buist A and Barnett B (1995) Childhood sexual abuse: a risk factor for post-partum depression? *Aust NZ J Psychiatry.* **29**: 604–8.
- Burke Draucker C (2000) *Counselling Survivors of Childhood Sexual Abuse* (2e). Sage Publications, London.
- Bushnell JA, Wells JE and Oakley-Browne MA (1992) Long-term effects of intra-familial sexual abuse in childhood. *Acta Psychiatr Scand.* **85**: 136–42.
- Cawson P, Wattam C, Brooker S and Kelly G (2000) *Child Maltreatment in the United Kingdom. A study of the prevalence of child abuse and neglect.* NSPCC Publications, London.
- Christensen M (1992) Birth rape. *Midwifery Today.* **Summer Issue**: 34.
- Cohen T (1995) Motherhood among incest survivors. *Child Abuse Neglect.* **19**: 1423–9.
- Courtois CA (1993) Adult survivors of sexual abuse. *Primary Care.* **20**: 433–47.
- Creighton S and Russell N (1995) *Voices from Childhood: a survey of childhood experiences and attitudes to childbearing among adults in the United Kingdom.* Policy Practice Research Series. National Society for the Prevention of Cruelty to Children, London.
- Crompton J (1996) Post-traumatic stress disorder and childbirth. *Br J Midwif.* **4**: 290–4.
- Dietz PM, Spitz AM, Anda RF *et al.* (1999) Unintended pregnancy among adult women exposed to abuse or household dysfunction during their childhood. *JAMA.* **282**: 1359–64.
- Esparza DV and Esperat MCR (1996) The effects of childhood sexual abuse on minority adolescent mothers. *J Obstet Gynecol Neonatal Nurs.* **25**: 321–8.
- Finkelhor D (1990) Early and long-term effects of child sexual abuse: an update. *Prof Psychol Res Pract.* **21**: 325–30.
- Finkelhor D (1994) The international epidemiology of child sexual abuse. *Child Abuse Neglect.* **18**: 409–17.
- Finkelhor D (1997) Child sexual abuse. In: OW Barnett, CL Miller-Perrin and RD Perrin (eds) *Family Violence Across the Lifespan.* Sage, Thousand Oaks, CA.
- Fitzsimons P (1999) Michel Foucault: regimes of punishment and the question of liberty. Revised extract. *Int J Sociol Law.* **27**: 379–99.
- Fleming JM (1997) Prevalence of childhood sexual abuse in a community sample of Australian women. *Med J Aust.*; http://www.mja.com.au
- Ghate D and Spencer L (1995) *The Prevalence of Child Sexual Abuse in Britain.* HMSO, London.
- Gutteridge KEA (2001) Failing women: the impact of sexual abuse on childbirth. *Br J Midwifery.* **9**: 312–15.
- Hallett C (1995) Child abuse: an academic overview. In: P Kingston and B Pen-hale (eds) *Family Violence and the Caring Professions.* Macmillan, Basingstoke.
- Hendricks-Matthews MK (1993) Survivors of abuse: health care issues. *Prim Care.* **20**: 391–406.

- Herman JL, Russell DEH and Trochi K (1986) Long-term effects of incestuous abuse in childhood. *Am J Psychiatry.* **143**: 1293–6.
- Holz KA (1994) A practical approach to clients who are survivors of childhood sexual abuse. *J Nurse Midwifery.* **39**: 13–18.
- Home Office, Department of Health, Department of Education and Science and Welsh Office (1991) *Working Together Under the Children Act 1989.* HMSO, London.
- Horan DL, Hill LD and Schulkin J (2000) Childhood sexual abuse and pre-term labor in adulthood: an endocrinological hypothesis. *Women's Health Issues.* **10**: 27–33.
- Jackson H and Nuttall R (1997) *Childhood Abuse: effects on clinicians' personal and professional lives.* Sage Publications, London.
- Jehu D (1988) *Beyond Sexual Abuse: therapy with women who were childhood victims.* John Wiley & Sons, Chichester.
- Kendall-Tackett K (1998) Breastfeeding and the sexual abuse survivor. *J Hum Lactation.* **14**: 127–30.
- Kitzinger S (1992) Birth and violence against women. Generating hypotheses from women's accounts of unhappiness after childbirth. In: H Roberts (ed.) *Women's Health Matters.* Routledge, London.
- Koss MP and Heslet L (1992) Somatic consequences of violence against women. *Arch Fam Med.* **1**: 53–9.
- Mullen P, Martin J, Anderson J, Romans S and Herbison G (1993) Childhood sexual abuse and mental health in adult life. *Br J Psychiatry.* **163**: 721–32.
- Nagy S, DiClemente R and Adcock A (1995) Adverse factors associated with forced sex among Southern adolescent girls. *Pediatrics.* **96**: 944–6.
- National Center on Child Abuse and Neglect (1978) *Child Sexual Abuse. Incest, assault and sexual eploitation: a special report.* National Center on Child Abuse and Neglect, Washington, DC.
- Parratt J (1994) The experience of childbirth for survivors of incest. *Midwifery.* **10**: 26–39.
- Petersen AC (1993) (chair) *Understanding Child Abuse and Neglect.* National Academy Press, Washington, DC.
- Polusny MA and Follette VM (1995) Long-term correlates of child sexual abuse: theory and review of the empirical literature. *Appl Prev Psychol,* 4: 143–66.
- Rhodes N and Hutchinson S (1994) Labor experiences of childhood sexual abuse survivors. *Birth.* **21**: 213–21.
- Rouf K (1999) Child sexual abuse and pregnancy: a personal account. *Pract Midwife.* **2**: 29–31.
- Saradjian J (1996) *Women Who Sexually Abuse Children: from research to clinical practice.* John Wiley & Sons, Chichester.
- Scott A (1996) *Real Events Revisited: fantasy, memory and psychoanalysis.* Virago, London.
- Sedlack AJ and Broadhurst DD (1996) *Third National Incidence Study of Child Abuse and Neglect.* Department of Health and Human Services, Washington, DC.
- Simkin P (1994) Memories that really matter. *Childbirth Educ Magazine.* **Winter Issue**: 23–7.
- Simkin P (1996) Childbirth education and care for the childhood sexual abuse survivor. *Int J Childbirth Educ.* **11**: 31–3.

- Smith M (1998) Childbirth in women with a history of sexual abuse. 1. *Pract Midwife.* **1**: 20–3.
- Smith P (1993) *Childhood Sexual Abuse, Sexuality, Pregnancy and Birthing. A life history study.* Inside-Out Books, Palmerston North, New Zealand.
- Stevens-Simon C and McAnarney ER (1994) Childhood victimization: relationship to adolescent pregnancy outcome. *Child Abuse Neglect.* **18**: 569–75.
- Stevens-Simon C and Reichert S (1994) Sexual abuse, adolescent pregnancy and child abuse. A developmental approach to an intergenerational cycle. *Arch Pediatr Adolesc Med.* **148**: 23–7.
- Stevens-Simon C, Kaplan DW and McAnarney ER (1993) Factors associated with preterm delivery among pregnant adolescents. *J Adolesc Health.* **14**: 340–2.
- Tilley J (2000) Sexual assault and flashbacks on the labour ward. *Pract Midwife.* **3**: 18–20.
- Wallace H (1999) *Family Violence: legal, medical and social perspectives* (2e). Allyn and Bacon, London.
- Walling MK, Reiter RC, O'Hara MW, Milbourn AK, Lilly G and Vincent SD (1994) Abuse history and chronic pain in women. 1. Prevalences of sexual abuse and physical abuse. *Obstet Gynecology.* **84**: 193–9.
- Yellowlees PM and Kaushik AV (1994) A case–control study of the sequelae of childhood sexual assault in adult psychiatric patients. *Med J Aust.* **160**: 408–11.
- Young L (1992) Sexual abuse and the problem of embodiment. *Child Abuse Neglect.* **16**: 89–100.

CHAPTER 16

The new reproductive technologies: threat or opportunity?

Marilyn Crawshaw

This chapter looks at the use of medically assisted conception treatments within a medical, legal and social framework. The author seeks to separate the facts from both the ways in which those facts have been interpreted and the ways in which practices in the field of medically assisted conception treatments have developed. Certain areas of practice have been considered in more detail, namely access to treatments, and the treatments themselves and their aftermath. Within this framework, statutory requirements with regard to 'the welfare of the child', counselling, the licensing of treatments, the inspection process, and preparation for parenthood are discussed. The author concludes that there is a potential for prejudicial professional practice and policies to develop, that critical awareness of the social context of developments in the new reproductive technologies is essential to counteract this, and that the separate influences of the medical, legal and social frameworks can be diluted or reinforced when they interweave with each other.

Introduction

People who enter the world of assisted conception treatments as patients may find themselves faced with medically, ethically and socially complex decisions about treatments, and they do so within a context of intense media interest. The treatment decision that they face today may be the subject of a documentary or magazine article tomorrow. A decision to withdraw from treatment and 'move on' with their lives may be thrown into turmoil when the newspaper headline the following week claims an exciting new breakthrough.

As people move from the private world of 'trying for a baby' to the public world of seeking medical assistance with conception, they little know how extended their transition to parenthood may become, if indeed it ever culminates in parenthood. For those who achieve parenthood, their fertility impairment is rarely altered but only circumvented.

It is not just people who are experiencing difficulty in conceiving who struggle to make sense of the world of reproductive technology. The confusion and ambivalence that many individuals experience will reflect their thoughts and feelings about the relationship between medicine, science and human reproduction. While they welcome some interventions as offering hope for people who find the route to parenthood blocked, uneasy visions of 'Frankenstein monsters' may lurk in the shadows. We use terms like 'designer' babies to express our revulsion at the notion of pre-selecting for 'social' characteristics in our offspring. Yet no equivalent value-laden term is accorded to the process of pre-implantation genetic diagnosis (PGD) or antenatal screening, reflecting our dual standards when the selection aims to eliminate individuals with certain hereditary impairments.

As a result of assisted conception techniques, new family forms are created for which our cultural, emotional and social understanding lags behind the scientific understanding. Women have acted as surrogates for their daughters and given birth to their own grandchildren. Twins have been born years apart from frozen embryos. Men have fathered children after their death through posthumous conception. Reproductive tissue from young children undergoing treatment for cancer is stored for possible maturation and use in many years' time. New techniques offer the possibility of individuals being conceived using the gametes of two females alone. Finally, scientists in the USA have announced that they will shortly clone a human being (Borger, 2001). Babies can now be conceived who have up to four parents and 12 or more grandparents at birth — if the genetic mother donates her egg, the genetic father donates his sperm, and the embryo which is created is donated to a couple in which the woman carries the fetus and gives birth to the baby for whom she and her partner will be the social parents (four parents). If each of the social parents has two genetic parents, each of whom is with a new partner, there is the potential for the baby to have four genetic grandparents (from their gamete donors) and eight social grandparents. Previously simple classroom tasks in which children are asked to draw their family tree may now present some unexpected challenges for the unsuspecting teacher! And such challenges will become more commonplace given that the number of people conceived using donated gametes each year (approximately 2000 in the UK) is now approaching the number being adopted from the care system (approximately 2200 in England alone) (Ivaldi, 2000).

Health professionals who are providing a service to women (and their partner, if they have one) in the antenatal and postnatal period following assisted conception treatment have to manage their own feelings and views about the treatments in order to be emotionally impartial and factually clear enough to provide an appropriate service. Some may have personal experiences either from their own lives or from their circle of family or friends. Others may hold strong views due to religious, moral or political standpoints. All of these may prove unexpectedly difficult to sustain when faced with the immediate pain (or joy) that an individual or couple bring to the professional encounter.

It is important to be aware of one's personal values and the way in which they interact with the professional task. Equally, it is important to be clear about one's factual knowledge base, in order to keep the boundaries between fact and opinion clear. Finally, this needs to be encompassed by the development and maintenance of a rigorous and reflective critical awareness of the influence of the social context in which the new reproductive technologies have been developed. A framework which may assist with this is outlined below.

A framework for understanding medically assisted conception

The term 'the new reproductive technologies' is used to encompass new forms of intervention with regard to human reproduction, including medically assisted conception. This chapter will focus on two aspects of assisted conception treatments. However, the framework for this critical appraisal is potentially applicable to the whole field.

Medically assisted conception can be analysed within three main frameworks – medical, legal and social. By considering how their interrelationship affects the construction of and discourse on our understanding and experience, we can become clearer about their effects on the individuals who are providing, using and being affected by treatment services.

Medical framework

This seeks to understand difficulties in conceiving primarily in terms of bodily malfunction, with a view to repairing or circumventing the malfunctioning parts. It fuels the drive to acquire new information about the functioning of the human reproductive system, with the body and body parts being the main site for technical exploration. It uses determinants of success which have clear parameters, usually the achievement of a pregnancy and, more specifically, the birth of a single live baby who is free of any impairment and a birth mother who remains physically healthy. This approach allows unsuccessful treatments to continue if they hold the promise of greater rewards. Thus the (relatively) low success rates of *in-vitro* fertilisation (IVF) (when measured by live birth rates as in the annual HFEA *Patients' Guides*) (Human Fertilisation and Embryology Authority, 2000) can be defended on the basis that improved knowledge about reproductive function might lead to lowered miscarriage rates, improved preventative work, and increased understanding of genetics. At its most reductionist, humans are seen as the sum of their body parts, and as increasingly determined by their genetic make-up. This potentially allows an individual's function within the medical process to be given primacy over them as a whole person. For example, they may be seen primarily in their role as providing gametes for donation (biological function), obscuring the fuller picture in which they are also engaged in a complex social and emotional donation transaction.

Legal framework

This seeks to regulate the way in which society manages matters (primarily but not exclusively) in the public domain. It does so by administering and interpreting a codified set of rules that are determined in the first place by Parliament. Regulatory mechanisms may be proactive or reactive.

- *Proactive mechanisms*: these include inspection systems designed to ensure that standards are maintained or promoted. They are invested in bodies such as the

Human Fertilisation and Embryology Authority (HFEA), the regulators of professional conduct (e.g. the General Medical Council) and the Care Standards Commission and National Health Service (NHS) clinical governance frameworks.

- *Reactive mechanisms*: these include the courts of law, and ethics committees which are used when rules are breached or adjudication is sought.

Interpretation of the law also takes place within policy-making forums (e.g. health authorities), within individual professional practices and elsewhere.

The legal framework is premised on the belief that the common good can be determined in a civilised society by using rational analysis that is based on a set of rules.

Social framework

This seeks to understand human actions at individual, group and societal levels, by considering the extent to which they are affected by the wider social context in which they occur. This is achieved through a variety of routes, including the following:

- data collection based on social characteristics (e.g. identifying patients by age, gender, marital status, ethnicity, impairment or sexual orientation)
- research, discussion and development of theoretical constructs on psychosocial issues.

The social framework aims to identify the presence of patterns emerging from individual (patient, professional and lay) actions and experiences which might potentially be understood in psychosocial terms. An illustration of this is the way in which recent developments in genetics have been accompanied by changes in the ways in which relationships are described. For example, where one might previously have said '*x is y's biological father*', one may now say '*x is y's genetic father*'. A social framework approach considers the significance of such a change in discourse, particularly in relation to kinship (Franklin, 1997), and encourages consideration of the interrelationship between scientific developments and the way in which we think about relationships between prenatal genetic predisposition and postnatal socialisation.

Using the framework to aid professional interventions

By separating factual information from interpretation within this framework and considering the reinforcing or diluting influence of each component on the other, professionals can better understand their own reactions in this complex area, and can hopefully increase their potential for offering a more patient-centred approach to their service.

This can be illustrated by two key aspects of medically assisted conception services.

1 Who gains access to treatments?
2 What do the treatments involve and what happens when they end in pregnancy?

Who gains access to treatments?
What does the law say?

The relevant legal framework is mainly to be found in the Human Fertilisation and Embryology Act 1990 (HFE Act) and the subsequent Code of Practice drawn up by the Human Fertilisation and Embryology Authority (HFEA). The HFEA was established in 1991 (with publicly appointed members, a Chairperson and a small paid staff under a Chief Executive) in order to:

- set standards and license and regulate clinics where licensed treatments are offered, where gametes are stored and/or where certain specified research is being undertaken
- publish a Code of Practice
- monitor new developments internationally and consult with both professional and patient groups and the general public to determine whether to license new treatments
- publish information for patients
- maintain the confidential Register of Information, whose purpose is to enable people over the age of 18 years (or 16 years if they are contemplating marriage) to find out, after appropriate counselling, whether they were born as a result of licensed fertility treatment, and whether they are related to someone whom they intend to marry or with whom they wish to establish a sexual relationship. (Note that although this Act was passed as recently as 1990, and this clause was inserted because of concerns about consanguinity, there is currently no provision for anyone contemplating entering a sexual relationship who is under the age of 18 years to gain access to the Register.)

The Act itself does not restrict treatments to any category of individual, and this is reinforced in the Code of Practice (Section 3.10). However, the interpretation of these legal facts has the potential to allow selection on non-medical grounds, although no official figures are available.

There are three key gate-keeping points for entry into treatment.

1 At the point of referral for those NHS patients whose health authority has drawn up eligibility criteria – that is, *political practice*. Note that a major cause of controversy with regard to the funding of assisted conception treatments is the regional variation in NHS provision. This impacts most heavily on people from low-income groups, who may thus be completely excluded from treatment. Anyone accessing private health facilities may incur very considerable costs. This aspect will not be dealt with in detail here, but further information and discussion of the issues can be obtained from the National Infertility Awareness Campaign (*see* Useful addresses section).

2 At the point of referral, where individual referring doctors may operate their own (unpublished) criteria – that is, *professional practice.*
3 At the point of entry into treatment, when some clinics have selection criteria (published or otherwise) – that is, *political or professional or commercial practice.*

It is noteworthy that the HFEA has never withdrawn a clinic's licence on the grounds that its selection criteria prohibit access to specific social groups, such as single women and lesbian couples (even though some clinics do operate such a policy). Despite the wording of the HFE Act, there does not appear to be any obligation for clinics to treat those referred, and this is perhaps compounded by the fact that much treatment takes place in private health facilities. However, fear that automatic refusal to treat certain patient groups may be challenged under the Human Rights Act 1998 has led some clinics to modify their practice by removing overt reference to such exclusions from their patient information.

In drawing up eligibility criteria, policy makers make interpretations of the Act's stipulations, which include the following:

1 'a woman shall not be provided with treatment services unless account has been taken of the welfare of any child who may be born as a result of the treatment (including the need of that child for a father), and of any child who may be affected by the birth' (Section13(5))
2 people must be given 'a suitable opportunity to receive proper counselling about the implications of taking the proposed steps' (Section 13(6); Schedule 3 paragraph 3(1)(a)).

This is the only area of law where such conditions apply in relation to medical treatments or entry into parenthood, perhaps reflecting the unease with which this area of work was viewed in Parliament.

What does the 'welfare of the child' mean?

The Code of Practice sets out the areas that must be covered in the assessment of *all* prospective parents with regard to the 'welfare of the children' (Sections 3.8 to 3.34), and lists additional requirements where the use of donated gametes is proposed (3.14). As it does not publish the evidence base that was used to draw these up, practitioners and others are left to interpret the reasons for their inclusion and the weight that should be afforded them in risk assessments.

The Code states that, among other things, prospective parents should:

• show commitment to having a child
• be able to provide a stable and supportive environment
• be in a state of health and of an age that is conducive to looking after or providing for a child
• not pose any risk to the child through neglect or abuse.

In cases where the use of donated gametes is proposed, prospective parents must, among other things:

- be able to cope with any questions that the growing child may have about his or her origins
- be able to cope with the attitudes of family members to that child.

The Code of Practice requires clinics to have a written procedure in place for such assessments and for dealing with any issues that arise. Many clinics routinely ask the patients themselves and, with their permission, their GPs for any relevant information. The majority of assessments end at this point and thus involve nothing more than the requesting of information. Some clinics routinely conduct fuller assessments on certain groups of patients (e.g. lesbian couples, single women). Others only move on to fuller assessments if a member of the clinic team (or individuals consulted) expresses concerns.

The first step in fuller assessments may be to seek additional information (e.g. from psychiatrists, Social Services, and so on). Some clinic counsellors agree to conduct at least part of these fuller assessments, whereas others regard this as contrary to their counselling role. The Code stipulates that the distinction between assessment and counselling should be made clear to the patient(s) (although how achievable this is remains in doubt).

Each clinic must have an ethics committee or access to a forum at which ethically complex cases can be discussed. Such committees and forums may become involved either routinely with certain groups of patients or only with specific requests. Here again, practice varies. There is no statutory requirement for professional child welfare expertise to be included in ethics committees' membership.

Whatever the nature of the risk assessment, the final decision always rests with the clinician who is responsible for administering the treatment.

One can immediately see that there is ample opportunity for facts and opinion to become blurred, especially in the fuller assessments, and for the grounds on which risk is assessed to become open to challenge. Within child protection work, full risk assessments in relation to an unborn child are among the most complex to undertake, and are always conducted by a team of social workers and other professionals who are trained and skilled in such work. If the recommendation is that prospective parents should be denied the opportunity to have care of their baby, the decision is made at a multi-disciplinary, multi-agency Child Protection Case Conference, and may be open to the independent scrutiny of the courts. In the assisted conception setting, risk assessments are undertaken before a pregnancy is even achieved, there is no statutory requirement for multi-disciplinary and multi-agency involvement in the decision, and no route for independent scrutiny through the courts.

Now it could be argued that the two situations are very different, and at one level they are. However, the current system in assisted conception clinics has two areas in which potential flaws can arise.

1   The facts on the basis of which decisions are made might not hold up under scrutiny according to an accepted child welfare evidence base.
2   Decisions will usually be made by professionals who are not trained in child welfare risk assessments.

The potential for prejudicial situations to arise is worrying, and there is at least anecdotal evidence that some groups may be particularly vulnerable, including those whose lifestyle (e.g. sex workers, drug users), physical attributes (e.g. wheelchair users, people with HIV), learning difficulties or sexual orientation may be deemed unsuitable to equip them to be parents (Campion, 1995; Saffron, 2001).

Given the additional conditions to be met in cases where the use of donated gametes is proposed, one might assume that good parental practice is thought to include making offspring (and family members) aware of the nature of their genetic origins. It would therefore be difficult to imagine how prospective parents could be assessed as being of low or no risk if they have a stated intention of secrecy. Yet this is the case. One is left to speculate about the extent to which here, too, the professionals' personal views affect the conduct of assessments.

What are the requirements with regard to counselling?

Although the offer of counselling is a legal requirement, the way in which it is offered and provided is open to interpretation. The Code of Practice states that, where this is practicable, at least one of the counselling staff should hold a recognised qualification. In practice, this has proved difficult to verify, given the number of unregulated general counselling awards that are now available (readers who are interested in the longstanding discussions and developments with regard to infertility counselling qualifications and training should refer to the British Infertility Counselling Association (BICA) *Journal of Fertility Counselling*). The Code also allows for the requirement about qualification to be dispensed with, provided that such a qualified person is available as an adviser to other (unqualified) counselling staff and available to clients 'as required' (Section 1.10).

The Code specifies the following different types of counselling that should be available (Part 8):

- *implications counselling* – to enable the person concerned to understand the implications of the proposed course of action for themselves, their family and any children who are born as a result
- *support counselling* – to offer emotional support at times of particular stress (e.g. failure to achieve a pregnancy)
- *therapeutic counselling* – to help people to cope with the consequences of infertility and treatment and to help them resolve any problems that these may cause. It includes helping people to adjust their expectations and to accept their situation.

Only implications counselling *must* be offered; provision of the other types of counselling carries a lower mandate. Perhaps because it is offered at the same time as the patient is being considered for treatment, and may be seen by some professionals and patients as an indication of poor coping ability or emotional instability (even though the Code stresses that it should not be seen in this light), the uptake of implications and other types of counselling remains low unless attendance is a condition of treatment (Boivin *et al.*, 1999). Moreover, many clinics only provide a small number of free sessions, and the financial pressure on couples who are accessing private treatment may preclude them from engaging in further contact. Counselling should also be made available at different stages in the process, including when treatment ends and at points in the future, but the Code makes it clear that clinics are required to assist people in *obtaining* counselling, but not necessarily to *provide* it (for a fuller review of counselling provision, *see* Jennings, 1995; Read, 1995; Lee, 1996; for a review of the research into the emotional effects of infertility, *see* Burns and Covington, 1999; Eugster and Vingerhoets, 1999; for a review of gender effects, *see* Monach, 1993; for a review of the effects on couples, *see* Pengelly *et al.*, 1995; Cooper-Hilbert, 1998).

So how is the quality of services assured?

'Welfare of the child' assessments, the provision of counselling and all other requirements of the Code must be carried out to the satisfaction of HFEA Inspectors. Annual inspections are conducted by a team drawn from appointed clinical, scientific and social and ethical inspectors, or by an HFEA Inspector Co-ordinator working alone. Inspection reports are then prepared for the HFEA Licensing and Fees Committee, where the final decision is made about renewal of licences and any imposition of conditions or recommendations.

The inspection process has not been without criticism, both from those who are opposed to it and from those who consider that it should be more rigorous (Crawshaw, 1999). Indeed, even the system for appointing inspectors has been criticised. For all areas except counselling that are required by law to be inspected (i.e. the medical and scientific aspects), teams of inspectors with the relevant qualifications were appointed. However, for inspecting the counselling services there was no such requirement, and social and ethical inspectors were appointed who could be drawn from any area.

The work of inspectors and the HFEA is further hindered by the lack of comprehensive published standards. Although the Code can be argued to have set out some standards, it is unclear which of them are mandatory, which are for guidance only and which carry sanctions. The difficulty for treatment providers and regulators alike is that there is no public forum for debate and little or no involvement of the courts in creating case law to guide future actions. Not surprisingly, there are wide interpretations of acceptable practice in controversial areas such as 'welfare of the child' and counselling. For example, clinics where the provision of (free) counselling by an independent training counsellor is virtually non-existent may be inspected and deemed to be as acceptable as those where there is unlimited free counselling. Even in areas where there may be more so-called 'hard' evidence to draw upon (e.g. with regard to the number of embryos to transfer in order to reduce the risk of multiple births), reaching a consensus remains difficult.

Developments within NHS services in the aftermath of the Bristol Inquiry and the Alder Hey scandal, including the introduction of NHS and Care Standards Commission requirements around clinical governance procedures in both NHS and private facilities, add weight to the demands for change. Consistent with this, the recent Quinquennial Review of the HFEA by the Department of Health will lead to inspections being more rigorous and transparent, to the inspection requirements in relation to the welfare of the child being afforded particular scrutiny, and to the work of the authority in general being more open (Department of Health, 2001).

What do the treatments involve and what happens when they end in pregnancy?

What is classed as a licensed treatment?

Treatments fall into two categories with regard to their regulation under the HFE Act.

1   Licensed treatments include the following:
   • *in-vitro* fertilisation (IVF), including that with donor sperm, eggs or embryo
   • intra-cytoplasmic sperm injection (ICSI)
   • donor insemination (DI)
   • pre-implantation genetic diagnosis (PGD).
2   Non-licensed treatments include the following:
   • gamete intra-fallopian transfer (GIFT)
   • ovulation induction
   • intrauterine insemination with husband's/partner's sperm (IUI).

Although it is not a medical treatment, surrogacy is also subject to regulation either through the surrogacy legislation alone where licensed treatment is not involved (in particular, the Surrogacy Arrangements Act 1995, Parental Orders (Human Fertilisation and Embryology) Regulations 1994 and Parental Orders (Human Fertilisation and Embryology) (Scotland) Regulations 1994) or, where it is involved, through both these and the HFE Act.

What do the treatments entail?

There are many texts on the market that explain medical interventions from the perspective of those administering them (Winston, 1996; Balen and Jacobs, 1997). There is also a growing number of publications which offer accounts from the perspective of individuals who have undergone the interventions (Mason, 1993; Barnby, 1995; Benson and Robinson-Walsh, 1998; Brian, 1998).

   One of the key features of fertility treatments is that, regardless of whether or not the woman has any fertility impairment herself, she will (invariably) be centrally involved in undergoing treatment. She will therefore be exposed to the associated risks from drug regimes, anaesthetics, surgical procedures, and any emotional risk of achieving pregnancy through a medically assisted procedure. This is a not inconsiderable fact that has to be managed by the woman and her partner (if she has one), given that only approximately 30% of impairments are located in the female partner alone. This is one of the few areas in which treatments are undergone by a non-impaired individual in order to 'overcome' the impairment of another person.

Why are some treatments licensed and not others?

Some interesting decisions were made by Parliament about which treatments were to be licensed. This led to a two-tier system whereby health facilities which only offer non-licensed treatments (e.g. GIFT, IUI and ovulatory treatments) are not required to be licensed or inspected by the HFEA. Where such treatments are offered alongside licensed treatments, *all* of the treatments are inspected!

The yardsticks for determining which treatments to include were not apparently related to the complexity or innovatory nature of the treatments. Bennett and Harris (1999) have suggested that they may have had more to do with how closely the treatments mimic the natural process. Thus they argued that GIFT, IUI and ovulation induction remain unlicensed because fertilisation does not take place outside the body. However, this does not account for the inclusion of DI, perhaps the oldest (and previously unregulated) form of treatment, and surrogacy via other regulatory legislation. For these treatments one can only conclude that it was the presence of a genetic parent who does not become the social parent that led Parliament to favour external regulation.

Where similarly constituted families are formed *as a result of professional involvement* (e.g. adoption, fostering), there has also traditionally been a legal framework to regulate professional involvement and to monitor the children's well-being. However, there are important differences from the HFE Act which may reflect the medical rather than the non-medical professional involvement and setting. In mainstream children's legislation (Children Act 1989, which interestingly went through Parliament at almost the same time as the Human Fertilisation and Embryology Act 1990 under the same Government; proposed changes to adoption law that are currently before Parliament) and surrogacy arrangements:

- the welfare of the child has paramountcy over that of all other interested parties
- children have the right, at the age of majority, to have access to their public agency records, including identifying information about their genetic parents.

In the HFE Act, these principles do not apply even when, as is the case with the use of donated embryos, neither of the social parents has a genetic link to the child. There is no legal requirement for parents to inform their children of their origins, and indeed the HFE Act made it legal for the non-genetic father to be named on the birth certificate.[16.1] Unlike the situation with surrogacy or adoption, there is nothing on the birth certificate to alert the person to their genetic origins and therefore no independent way for them to find out. For example, in surrogacy a Section 30 Parental Order is applied for between 6 weeks and 6 months after the birth and a new birth certificate is issued. However, ironically, if surrogacy takes place in a licensed centre and involves the use of a donated egg, the offspring may gain access to their original birth certificate, but this will *not* tell them that their birth mother was not their genetic mother.

There are no sanctions against clinics which do not insist on prospective parents discussing their strategies for dealing with the needs arising with regard to openness with their child and with family members (see above), as it is only the *offer* of

---

[16.1] If a man who is being treated with a woman signs written consent to treatment, the HFE Act considers him to be the 'legal father', even if the woman is married to someone else. However, if the couple are not married, he will not have legal 'parental responsibility' unless he applies for a parental responsibility agreement or order after the birth. It is only the woman who gives birth who is considered to be the legal mother, even if she has no genetic relationship to the child, as would be the case with a donated embryo.

implications counselling which is mandatory. Thus donor offspring can only find out if they were donor conceived if someone chooses to tell them this in either a planned or an unplanned way.

This raises the question of why such differences were enacted. If one were to ask the general public whether it is emotionally healthy or morally acceptable for parents to keep such key information secret from their children, the answer would probably be 'no'. Yet the culture of secrecy surrounding the use of donated gametes remains pervasive in the legislation, in the practices of many centres and professionals, and among some prospective parents.

- The HFE Act makes donor offspring the only group of people in the country who are excluded by law from access to identifying information about their origins.
- Delays continue to occur in drawing up the Regulations to govern the use of the Register of Information, even though in 2008 the first person will be eligible to approach it, and consultation on the Regulations has been promised since the late 1990s. Enquirers may thus find that only very limited non-identifying information about their origins has been stored, as the current requirement for records is minimal. In addition, due to the lack of Regulations or guidance there may be no record on the Register of any additional information from the donor(s) that may have been acquired by the clinics during the years following donation.
- Patients undergoing (licensed) treatment are probably the only group of people who have to sign consent to disclosure before any information about their treatment can be given to any health professional outside the centre (thus ensuring privacy with regard to the use of donated gametes).
- Current HFEA guidance is, controversially, that neither the woman donating eggs nor the woman receiving them in an egg-sharing arrangement should be told the outcome. Apparently this is on the grounds that the woman who is providing the eggs may be distressed if the other woman achieves a pregnancy when she does not, thus giving paramountcy of welfare to the former (Human Fertilisation and Embryology Authority, 2001). (Egg-sharing arrangements are primarily intended to reduce the waiting-list for egg donation by offering reduced-cost treatments to women who are willing to share their eggs with another.)
- According to a recent statement from the British Fertility Society, 'Anonymous donation is encouraged in accordance with sperm donation practice ... at present, a majority view favours secrecy' (Aird *et al.*, 2000: 162).
- The policy of anonymity and payment of donors has been defended on the grounds that removal of either might lead to a reduction in the number of donors who come forward (Aird *et al.*, 2000).

It has been suggested that not giving paramountcy to the welfare of children allows the welfare of the adults who are present at the time of decision making to take precedence (Freeman, 1996; Douglas *et al.*, 1998; Speirs, 1998). It also allows any roots for secrecy in social stigma to remain unchallenged, as in the early days of adoption (Harper, 1993). Evidence from the limited number of adult donor offspring who come forward and from parents who are committed to openness is putting increasing pressure on this situation. It appears that at least some donor offspring and their parents want to know the full details of their genetic origins and consider that there is indeed an emotional and medical significance to the nature of their conception (Donor Conception Support Group of Australia, 1997; Blyth *et al.*, 1998; Whipp, 1998; Cordray, 1999; Turner and Coyle, 2000) hitherto denied by some professionals and policy makers (Deech, 1998; Shenfield, 1999; Aird *et al.*, 2000).

One is drawn to consider the impact of the context within which this is taking place (i.e. the medical context). People may remain in treatment for extended periods of time, and there is a danger that their transition to parenthood will become reframed as a medical event that requires a medical solution, rather than a social and emotional one. Scant attention may then be paid to their psychosocial needs as prospective parents. It is to this topic that we shall now turn.

What help do people receive in preparing for parenthood?

Elsewhere, health professional involvement in the transition to parenthood is restricted to monitoring of the pregnancy (although this is becoming increasingly intrusive) and to helping the prospective parents to *prepare* for the parenting tasks ahead. In the non-medical arena, this element of preparation is maintained, for example, in adoption preparation.

However, there is no requirement for assisted conception clinics to provide help with preparation for this particular form of parenthood, even in cases where donated gametes are used. Indeed, the emphasis on 'welfare of the child' assessments may actually marginalise preparation needs. Patients who achieve a pregnancy are usually transferred early on to the care of antenatal services who may or may not be aware of the particular circumstances of the conception. Although the Code of Practice states that clinics should be prepared for future contact from donors, parents, offspring or others affected by the treatment, the difficulties with regard to inspection outlined earlier make it difficult to enforce this or to prescribe minimum standards. The clinic's only further involvement may therefore be to notify the HFEA Register of Information when the woman informs them of the birth. (Note that when the woman gives birth, she is required to notify the Centre where she had the treatment so that they in turn can notify the HFEA Register of Information. There are no penalties attached to failure to notify, and there is no official system for monitoring how often this actually happens.)

Parents, offspring and others are therefore left to manage the resulting personal and family dynamics unaided, with no publicly funded specialist service taking ongoing responsibility for them. This is of concern when one considers the potential vulnerabilities of these family members, including the following:

- research evidence which suggests that some adults will continue to have (and possibly repress) unresolved feelings about the use of donated gametes (Daniels and Taylor, 1993; Daniels *et al.*, 1995; Snowden and Snowden, 1998)
- research evidence that parents who use donated gametes are more likely to downplay the importance of genetic material than parents with genetically related offspring (Van den Akker, 2000)

- the lack of biographical and identifying information available to parents who choose to be open in order to help their child to integrate the facts of his or her identity
- the potential medical disadvantages of not having full access to information about, or even awareness of, genetic heritage (Simpson, 1998)
- the dangers associated with accidental disclosure, as are apparent from adoption research (Ryburn, 1994; Triseliotis et al., 1997)
- the socially isolating effect of the culture of secrecy, which means that family members will have reduced access to support systems
- the psychological effect of managing any stigma that is felt in relation to coming to parenthood through medically assisted conception

If indeed it is the medicalisation of the process, possibly combined with social stigma surrounding the process (especially where this involves the use of donated gametes), that has silenced or at least delayed the debate about parenthood, then the diluting of its influence is imperative.

Conclusion

This chapter has considered the use of medically assisted conception treatments and sought to identify the medical, legal and social frameworks within which they are practised. It has suggested that midwives who are working with women in the antenatal and postnatal period need to be vigilant about the potential for their personal values and experiences to affect professional tasks. It has argued that the development of a clear factual base means separating fact from opinion. This needs to be encompassed by a rigorous and reflective critical awareness of the influence of the social context in which new developments arise. Awareness of the diluting or reinforcing effect of the interweaving of medical, legal and social frameworks can better enable the professional to maintain a patient-centred approach to their work, where the uniqueness of the patient's situation is viewed against this backdrop.

Specific aspects of the new reproductive technologies have been considered in order to illustrate both their complexities and their potential for social manipulation. In particular, the position of people who are conceived by the use of donated gametes has been highlighted. The media tend to express opposition to the new reproductive technologies too simplistically as arising *either* from a religious standpoint *or* from people who have not yet fully understood these technologies. This brief examination makes it clear that it is infinitely more complex to try to answer the question of whether the new reproductive technologies represent a threat or an opportunity.

- Personal values and experiences can prejudice the performance of professional tasks.
- Critical awareness of the social context of developments in the new reproductive technologies is essential.
- The separate influences of medical, legal and social frameworks can be diluted or reinforced when they interweave with each other.

Useful addresses

Patient organisations

CHILD (The National Infertility Support Network)
Charter House
43 St Leonards Road
Bexhill on Sea
East Sussex TN40 1JA
Tel: 01424 732 361

DC Network
PO Box 265
Sheffield S3 7YX
Information line: 020 8245 4369

Issue (National Fertility Association Ltd)
114 Lichfield Street
Walsall WS1 1SZ
Tel: 01922 722888

Other organisations

British Infertility Counselling Association
69 Division Street
Sheffield S1 4GE
Helpline: 01342 843880

Human Fertilisation and Embryology Authority
Paxton House
30 Artillery Lane
London E1 7LS
Tel: 020 7377 5077

National Gamete Donation Trust
PO Box 62
Bury BLO 9GE
Tel: 01706 829428

National Infertility Awareness Campaign (NIAC)
PO Box 2106
London W1A 3DZ
Tel: 0207 439 3067

References

- Aird I, Barratt C, Murdoch A and the British Fertility Society Committee (2000) BFS recommendations for good practice on the screening of egg and embryo donors. *Hum Fertility*. **222**: 162–5.
- Balen A and Jacobs HS (1997) *Infertility in Practice*. Churchill Livingstone, Edinburgh.

- Barnby K (1995) *Labours of Eve: women's experiences of infertility*. Boxtree Ltd, London.
- Bennett R and Harris J (1999) Restoring natural function: access to infertility treatments using donated gametes. *Hum Fertility.* **2**: 18–21.
- Benson J and Robinson-Walsh D (1998) *Infertility and IVF: facts and feelings from patients' perspectives*. Scarlet Press, London.
- Blyth E, Crawshaw M and Speirs J (eds) (1998) *Truth and the Child 10 Years On: information exchange in donor-assisted conception*. BASW Publications, Birmingham.
- Boivin J, Scanlan LC and Walker SM (1999) Why are infertile patients not using psychosocial counselling? *Hum Reprod.* **14**: 1384–91.
- Borger J (2001) Maverick scientists promise a human clone. *Guardian.* **8 August**: 1.
- Brian K (1998) *In Pursuit of Parenthood: real-life experiences of IVF*. Bloomsbury Publishers Ltd, London.
- Burns LH and Covington SN (1999) *Infertility Counselling. A comprehensive handbook for clinicians*. Parthenon Publishing Group, Carnforth.
- Campion MJ (1995) *Who's Fit to be a Parent?* Routledge, London.
- Cooper-Hilbert B (1998) *Infertility and Involuntary Childlessness: helping couples cope*. WW Norton & Co, New York.
- Cordray W (1999) A survey of people conceived through donor insemination. *Donor Conception Support Group of Australia Newsletter.* **September issue**: 13–15.
- Crawshaw MA (1999) What do BICA-licensed centre counsellors think should be covered as part of a good-quality HFEA inspection of counselling services? *J Fertil Counsel.* **6**: 21–4.
- Daniels KR and Taylor K (1993) Secrecy and openness in donor insemination. *Politics Life Sci.* **12**: 155–70.
- Daniels KR, Lewis GM and Gillett W (1995) Telling donor insemination offspring about their conception: the nature of couples' decision making. *Soc Sci Med.* **40**: 1213–20.
- Deech R (1998) Family law and genetics. *Modern Law Rev.* **61**: 697–715.
- Department of Health (2001) HFEA Quinquennial Review 2001: executive summary. *J Fertil Counsel.* **8**: 23.
- Donor Conception Support Group of Australia (1997) *Let the Offspring Speak: discussions on donor conception*. Donor Conception Support Group of Australia, Georges Hall, New South Wales, Australia.
- Douglas G, Lavery R and Plumtree A (1998) Truth and the child: the legal perspective. In: E Blyth, M Crawshaw and J Speirs (eds) *Truth and the Child 10 Years On: information exchange in donor-assisted conception*. BASW Publications, Birmingham.
- Eugster A and Vingerhoets AJJM (1999) Psychological aspects of *in vitro* fertilisation: a review. *Soc Sci Med.* **48**: 575–89.
- Franklin S (1997) *Embodied Progress: a cultural account of assisted conception*. Routledge, London.
- Freeman M (1996) The new birth right: identity and the child of the reproduction revolution. *Int J Child's Rights.* **4**: 273–97.
- Harper J (1993) What does she look like? What children want to know about their birth parents. *Adoption Fostering.* **17**: 27–9.
- Human Fertilisation and Embryology Authority (2000) *Patients' Guides*. Human Fertilisation and Embryology Authority, London.

- Human Fertilisation and Embryology Authority (2001) *Code of Practice* (5e). Human Fertilisation and Embryology Authority, London.
- Ivaldi G (2000) *Surveying Adoption. A comprehensive analysis of local authority adoptions, 1998–1999 (England).* British Agencies for Adoption and Fostering, London.
- Jennings SE (ed.) (1995) *Infertility Counselling.* Blackwell Science, Oxford.
- Lee S (1996) *Counselling in Male Infertility.* Blackwell Science, Oxford.
- Mason MC (1993) *Male Infertility. Men talking.* Routledge, London.
- Monach JH (1993) *Childless: no choice.* Routledge, London.
- Pengelly P, Inglis M and Cudmore L (1995) Infertility: couples' experiences and the use of counselling in treatment clinics. *Psychodynam Counsel.* **1**: 507–25.
- Read J (1995) *Counselling for Fertility Problems.* Sage Publications, London.
- Ryburn M (1994) *Open Adoption: research, theory and practice.* Avebury, Aldershot.
- Saffron L (2001) Decision making among lesbians wishing to get pregnant. *J Fertil Counsel.* **8**: 31–5.
- Shenfield F (1999) Truth or dare – anonymity: the case for. *Prog Reprod.* **3**: 24.
- Simpson S (1998) Truth and the child: a genetic perspective. In: E Blyth, M Crawshaw and J Speirs (eds) *Truth and the Child 10 Years On: information exchange in donor-assisted conception.* BASW Publications, Birmingham.
- Snowden R and Snowden E (1998) Families created through donor insemination. In: KR Daniels and E Haimes (eds) *Donor Insemination. International social science perspectives.* Cambridge University Press, Cambridge.
- Speirs J (1998) Children's rights or adult's rights? In: E Blyth, M Crawshaw and J Speirs (eds) *Truth and the Child 10 Years On: information exchange in donor-assisted conception.* BASW Publications, Birmingham.
- Triseliotis J, Shireman J and Hundleby M (1997) *Adoption: theory, policy and practice.* Cassell, London.
- Turner AJ and Coyle A (2000) What does it mean to be a donor offspring? The identity experience of adults conceived by donor insemination and the implications for counselling and therapy. *Hum Reprod.* **15**: 2041–51.
- Van den Akker O (2000) The importance of a genetic link in mothers commissioning a surrogate baby in the UK. *Hum Reprod.* **15**: 1855–9.
- Whipp C (1998) The legacy of deceit: a donor offspring's perspective on secrecy in assisted conception. In: E Blyth, M Crawshaw and J Speirs (eds) *Truth and the Child 10 Years On: information exchange in donor-assisted conception.* BASW Publications, Birmingham.
- Winston RML (1996) *Infertility: a sympathetic approach.* Optima, London.

CHAPTER 17

Fetal surveillance

Christine Grabowska

This chapter will challenge accepted opinion on fetal screening and ask the reader to explore the wider, covert issues related to the production of human beings. Eugenics and politics will be discussed in an attempt to highlight some of the reasons for the availability and eventual outcomes of screening. This chapter will consider the acceptance of tests on the fetus, mainly using the ideas of Foucault and Parsons for sociological interpretation. An explanation of the social influences both on the individual and on the organisation will lead to a discussion of the possibilities for the future. These theories are applied to practice. The chapter challenges the practitioner to explore why screening is adhered to routinely. It asks who is in control of the process (the woman or the doctor) and what the actual purpose of screening is (to create a uniformity of human beings or reduce suffering). It briefly asks the moral questions of whether the fetus is entitled to life and whether society is at liberty to choose a suitable commodity in the form of a child. It demonstrates that women, although they are at the centre of the screening process, have little say about screening and even less about the outcomes.

Introduction

The fetus is open to the perfect system of surveillance, namely one that observes the silent body of the non-consenting fetus – a body that cannot object or eagerly participate. Its mother, who is obeying social norms or accepted practice, regards the surveillance as 'normal'. The question of normality is explored to the conclusion that it is a social convention. It has no meaning other than that it is happening to the majority of people. Normality knows no boundaries, and society can push its meaning in any direction. It is only morality that puts a stop to the proceedings.

What is surveillance?

To keep something under surveillance, simply defined, means nothing more than to keep a close eye, or the definition according to *Collins English Dictionary and Thesaurus* (5th edition) is 'to keep watch'. The word may conjure up images of closed-circuit television (CCTV) within shops and other public places. The idea of 'Big Bother is watching you' has less meaning today than when Aldous Huxley wrote *Brave New World*, which was published in 1932, or George Orwell wrote *Nineteen Eighty-Four*, which was published in 1949. It is the age of technology, machinery and gadgets. People have been subsumed to the mechanistic era and have integrated 'Big Brother' as part of their existence. It has become normal and is therefore no longer seen or acknowledged as untoward. The maternity contract between hospital providers and users may be said to have the same implicit message.

Fetal surveillance may be considered to be overrated because it would be negligent and untrue to suggest that we have the technology to prevent fetal 'abnormalities'. Yet somehow the public are led to believe that this is possible and they have the expectation that this will be the result. If the system fails them, litigation or revenge is often the next step. This is the system of fetal surveillance at present. Is this desirable? Should society be free of so-called 'abnormalities'? Control over genetics now resides with scientists, doctors, insurance companies, medical suppliers and the Government.

What are the consequences of fetal surveillance?

Fetal surveillance has enhanced the personal blame culture of the materialist world. In other words, the individual is directly responsible within a world where monetary profit is a priority. Because 'abnormalities' can be destroyed, it is up to the individual to take on the responsibility to do this. The popular culture is one in which the facilities and resources for caring for the 'disabled' are decreasing, and there is a social stigma and stereotype surrounding disability. The fetus can thus become a commodity like anything else that can be purchased, and it depends on surveillance to be accepted or rejected. Parenting for a child becomes conditional until the quality is approved through technology. People, including mothers and practitioners, are now secondary in the process.

The emergence of surveillance

Foucault (1973) considers that medicine has moved away from listening and seeing to the three-dimensional examination involving physical, technical and laboratory aspects. Classically, the doctor would listen to the patient and base the diagnosis on their 'story'. The treatment would be based on the traditional fifteenth-century diagnosis of 'humours', which included 'blood', 'black/green bile' or 'mucous'. Finally, with the introduction of the post-mortem into the medical school curricula, the doctor could discover the body away from the patient. Post-mortems moved 'life, disease and death' to a technical arena (Eribon, 1989: 153). The doctor learned about non-living tissue – tissue that could not tell its 'story' and tissue that was abstracted from life. This is often the place where doctors start their careers today.

The three-dimensional examination takes on objectivity, as the doctor does not have to be influenced by the patient. It becomes truly objective when the specimen can be removed from the patient and tested in the laboratory, so that a diagnosis can be made without the patient ever being present. Align this with the fetus under the ultrasound scan, the fetus being the specimen under observation. Tissue or fluid can be removed, and the specimen has no choice and no say in the matter. The diagnosis that is made on this specimen often leaves two choices – one of life and the other of death.

Foucault (1972) would liken fetal surveillance to the *panopticon* – the perfect system of surveillance. He takes his ideas from the model of a prison that Jeremy Bentham described in 1786 (Boyne, 2000). This is an eight-sided building with two windows to each cell. The prison warder is able to view each prisoner from a central area. The light from the window would mean that the warder could view each prisoner, but the prisoners could not see the warder. The warder could stand in one place and view those all around. Foucault called this 'the gaze', whereby everyone could be viewed from one vantage point. He suggested that hospitals and schools, as well as prisons, have been built so as to incorporate 'the gaze', and he called this *institutional surveillance*. The nurse in a hospital could view everyone from the middle of a nightingale ward, and the teacher in a school could view all of the pupils in their rows from the podium. However, the patients or pupils did not have the same vantage point as the nurse or teacher in that they could not gaze upon all of the other patients or pupils.

The ultimate purpose of 'the gaze' is to reduce deviancy by means of self-conformity. Consider a prisoner who is planning an escape but does not know when he is being gazed upon. Foucault calls this mechanism that produces conformity through observation the *disciplinary power*. 'What is being punished is non-conformity which the exercise of disciplinary power seeks to correct' (Smart, 1985: 86).

Rajchman (1985: 56) notes that society itself is 'one big panopticon', and certainly with the use of CCTV, laser scanning in shops and payment by means of credit cards, everyone is being surveyed and gazed upon.

> A gaze which each individual under its weight will end by interiorising to the point that he is his own overseer, each individual thus exercising this surveillance over and against himself.
> (Foucault, 1972: 155)

Thus, the gaze is turned in on the person him- or herself, and this results in self-discipline or conformity. Surveillance has made it possible to change medicine from being involved with sickness alone to having the potential to discover abnormality and thus to blame the victim – in this instance, the mother (Petersen and Bunton, 1997).

In health promotion, the message is that health deviance can be avoided and the potential for choice is given to the mother. Katz-Rothman (1986: 14) suggests that choice is an illusion because the mother ends up 'taking the least awful choice'. She is 'trapped, caught … in a nightmare' (Katz-Rothman, 1986: 189). The 'forced choice' is that of whether she will devote her life to caring for a handicapped child, in the midst of social disapproval, or whether she will destroy the life.

Who is making choices?

The gaze is extended into all areas of life – for example, the male gaze on the female body. Males have culturally developed an 'appetite' for certain bodily characteristics by gazing upon models. Females, on the other hand, on seeing the same media propaganda aspire to copy the body image so that they, too, will be gazed upon. The increase in cosmetic surgery supports the notion that people are aiming to be similar (King, 1999). The gaze is so strong that society is trying to improve its so-called 'health', with the aim of trying to look similar to an established norm. This 'looking similar' appears to boost the ego. The way in which this is achieved is often through 'healthy' living, which would include working out, dieting, liposuction, and so on (Frank, 1991).

The gaze will produce uniformity (and thus conformity) of looks and expectations. 'Because most people don't want to become delinquent, they accept normative values that are supposed to make them "good" citizens' (Danaher *et al.*, 2000: 60). However, this leads to self-punishment, when the gaze is turned in upon the self, and at the extreme it causes eating disorders, excruciating workouts and subjecting the body to cosmetic surgery. Equally, women will tolerate pain (e.g. via an amniocentesis or vaginal ultrasound scan) in order to gaze upon the fetus. Screening is seen as demanded by women themselves. Therefore the choices that women make are socially created as well as socially constrained. However, when the gaze is applied to the fetus it will be possible to reject not only the sex of the child but also their height, weight, eye, hair and skin colour. Again, this will achieve uniformity. If this appears abhorrent, consider the following. The orthodox church in Cyprus, prior to marrying a couple, asks them to provide evidence of their thalassaemia carrier status. The church will only marry couples who are both carriers, on the premise that they will use prenatal diagnosis and abortion. The church does not condone abortion for other reasons (Richards, 1993; Statham *et al.*, 2000). The point is that thought originates in culture (Foucault, 1974) and it can then become normalised.

The pregnant woman conforms by considering that the fetus is to be gazed upon. She knows that the fetus is being surveyed, but she does not know everything that is seen. The technician who has this information therefore wields power. Merquior (1985) tells us that power is associated with repression. Power allows people to exploit others for their own gain (Brewis, 2001). Cousins and Hussain (1984) suggest that power is not always confined to an individual, but may originate from the needs of capitalism, so that people express this in the power exerted. It is the Marxist notion that women will reproduce according to the capitalist needs, and therefore the woman will be alienated from the end-product, just like the car-assembly worker who only has a small part to play in the car's production. She is the commodity that serves political and economic needs.

> The biological traits of a population become relevant factors for economic management, and it becomes necessary to organize around them an apparatus which will ensure not only their subjection but the constant increase of their utility.
>
> (Foucault, 1972: 172)

Materialism is promoted by capitalism. Machinery manufacturers continuously create ever more 'precise' equipment (e.g. ultrasound), which is welcomed by the maternity services.

It can be seen that the technology which is established to further the capitalist economy holds a powerful footing. The problem with power is that it can be belittled or removed, and therefore to prevent this from happening it becomes important to subordinate women and create a continuous struggle to develop 'secret' knowledge (which is expressed through the manipulation of machinery, technology and gadgets) (Smart, 1985). According to Nola (1998), Foucault recognises that knowledge creates and results in domination. Subordination is evident not just in hospitals, but in every area of society where power is to be maintained, including even the microstructure of the family. In general, what is observed during an ultrasound scan examination is a subordinate woman lying (often silently) and looking at the screen, hoping to feel pleasure in response to what she sees.

Foucault (1972) acknowledges that the ultrasound scan will produce knowledge which in turn 'produces discourse'. The discourse or discussion is usually among professions, and it is this discourse which increases the body of knowledge. The doctor's gaze puts symptoms into signs, through language and meaning, and the description of the dis-ease is then formulated (Cousins and Hussain, 1984). Foucault (1974) simply says that language is the basis of knowledge. Language 'is a necessary medium for any scientific knowledge that wishes to be expressed in discourse' (Foucault, 1974: 296). It is the medically formulated language of the uncertain, or previously unknown, that is translated as knowledge (Cousins and Hussain, 1984).

Without language the dis-ease could not be labelled and therefore could not be treated or obliterated. Therefore the label that is given allows the doctor to reason and create what is acceptable or not. Merquior suggests that 'reason itself is a technology of power, science and an instrument of domination' (Merquior, 1985: 146). Thus if women questioned the dis-ease, they would be driven into subordination by the act of reasoning. The reasoning will validate surveillance which will have included machinery, technology or gadgets (which are venerated with the truth).

The creation of knowledge, which is often an agreed opinion, gives power and status not to the specimen that was gazed upon, but to those who created the label to describe what was gazed upon. 'Knowledge is inextricably entwined with relations of power and advances in knowledge associated with advances and developments in the exercise of power' (Smart, 1985: 64). Nola (1998) goes one step further to suggest that the subjects of truth, knowledge and what is considered right are all creating power. It is power that creates what is then accepted as truth.

The Human Genome Project creates the perfect objective gaze, because in order to know the truth of a pathological fact the doctor must abstract the patient (Foucault, 1973). Danaher et al. state that 'one of discipline's concerns is with producing docile healthy bodies' (Danaher et al., 2000: 50). Ultimately the production of designer children will be possible if this trend is continued, thereby creating children who conform to ethnocentric ideas of normality and desirability.

Foucault (1973) describes how at the end of the eighteenth century the life/death continuum started to change from being normal to abnormal. The only abnormal deaths prior to this time resulted from murder or war. Birth and death now occur mainly in hospital. The hospital depicts Max Weber's 'ideal type' of institution (Andreski, 1983) – that is, a rational, hierarchical, bureaucratic structure in which everyone performs a unique function or skill with a minimum cost to the organisation. To ensure efficiency, everyone is overseen and will thus be subordinated to some part of the hierarchy: 'the hierarchy established to provide a progression

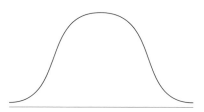

Figure 17.1 Histogram for a representative population.

towards the more complex and the less exact' (Foucault, 1974: 246). It can be seen from this that allowing birth/death to occur naturally can overturn the 'ideal type', and therefore both ends of the continuum are manipulated with the help of machinery, technology and gadgets. This change is regarded as normal.

Normality is therefore socially constructed. The statistical norm and its place in the histogram (or bell-shaped curve) are shown in Figure 17.1.

The norm is a line drawn down the middle to represent the greatest number of the population. Therefore if this is a representation of pregnant women who are undergoing ultrasound scans in the UK, the majority will actually have a scan and the 'bell' of the curve will be very narrow, as shown in Figure 17.2.

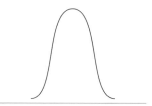

Figure 17.2 Histogram for a similar population.

It can thereby be concluded that it is *normal* for women to have ultrasound scans during pregnancy. However, this is very different to it being *natural*.

Consider the difference between a natural birth and a normal birth. What is now regarded as normal cannot be termed natural. Most normal births will have occurred as a result of the use of machinery, technology and gadgets. Equally, death that has occurred with the use of technology involving drugs cannot be thought of as natural. This is easier to see in the fetus than in the adult. For instance, some might argue that injecting potassium chloride into the fetal heart with the intention of committing fetocide is not different to offering morphine as 'pain relief' to the terminally ill adult.

The changing social view of normality may originate in the scientific or technocratic community. Doctors today speak in terms of a 'normal' or 'abnormal' baby. A technological diagnosis is made on the basis of chromosome analysis, for example, and if the result is 'abnormal' the doctor offers the option of death of the fetus to the parents. This is termed a 'therapeutic abortion', but for whom is it therapeutic? A similar option would not be given to the parents if a doctor deemed the baby to be 'normal'. Foucault considers that 'the hospital is more the seat of death for the cities where it is sited than a therapeutic agent for the population as a whole' (Foucault, 1972: 177). Informed choice includes looking at all of the options, yet the options appear to be limited when that of termination of the pregnancy dominates the conversation. This might be argued to be the present-day form of eugenics.

Eugenics

Historically, eugenics might have been said to originate in order to prevent the higher social classes being burdened with 'social problems'. In 1919, Marie Stopes, one of the original eugenicists, wrote that she developed contraception in order to produce 'more children from the fit, less from the unfit' (cited in Kelves, 1985: 90). However, it was Francis Galton, a statistician, who founded the Eugenics Society and first used the term 'eugenics' in 1883 (Wikler, 1999). He developed an interest in obtaining 'good human stock'. He observed that farmers and horticulturists could obtain a permanent species of animal or plant, and he saw a normal development of applying this process to human beings. Thus developed the Eugenics Society, which included such members as Charles Darwin's nephew, Leonard Darwin, who in 1926 suggested ways of getting rid of the inferior by 'the lethal chamber, murder, segregation by imprisonment, confinement and supervision, sterilization and family limitation by contraception or abstinence'.

Publishing one's thoughts was considered 'normal' in the 1920s, and the notion of political correctness certainly did not prevail at the time. Therefore it is easier to see how Adolf Hitler and his ideas about producing the Aryan race did not cause a public outcry. Considering a historical eugenicist example will enlighten us about where present-day practices may lead. Eugenics and 'racial hygiene' were introduced into the medical school curricula in Germany by 1933. It could be argued that Nazi racial policy thus originated from the scientific community (Annas and Grodin, 1992). Galton had introduced pedigrees into England prior to this time, but Nazi Germany introduced them under the race laws. On 14 July 1937, the sterilisation law was passed for the prevention of genetically diseased offspring, and hundreds of thousands of people were sterilised under these laws. Euthanasia was made legal for the mentally ill, handicapped and infirm, which meant that homes and hospitals could be closed down. The war years brought mass extermination of human beings to prevent their reproduction. This potted history misses much but allows us to visualise the 'slippery slope'.

After World War Two, the majority regarded eugenics as abhorrent, and in the USA the word 'eugenics' was interpreted as racism. The eugenicist publications were changing the name to 'genetics' in their titles, and interestingly the first genetic advisory clinic in Britain was set up in 1946. It used pedigrees in the history-taking process, as do present-day genetic counsellors.

Fetal surveillance took on a different meaning in 1967, when abortion first became legally available. Although amniocentesis was a technique with which the medical profession was familiar prior to 1967, it did not become available to pregnant women until 1967, when a fetus that was deemed to be 'abnormal' could be terminated – a procedure termed (as already mentioned) therapeutic abortion. Is this therapeutic for the fetus or for society?

The Human Genome Project could be said to represent the continuation of eugenics. It identifies all of the material in the 23 pairs of chromosomes that gives information about a person, and which is possibly, as yet, unknown and unseen. It was Watson amd Crick who discovered the double-helix structure of DNA in 1953, and this initiated the Human Genome Project. It is now known that there are three billion base pairs in the human genome (Conrad and Gabe, 1999). The question remains as to what will be done with all of this information. It will be expensive to buy the information on one individual. However, it is thought that some employers would be willing to pay the price in order to avoid a 'bad' risk. Equally, insurance companies may choose to do the same (Nuffield Council on Bioethics, 2001). This could work either to their advantage or to their disadvantage. The companies may not insure 'bad' risks, but then people with 'good' health may decide that they do not need the insurance. The premiums would therefore increase dramatically, so people who required insurance would not be able to afford it (Kaufert, 2000).

The Human Genome Project is funded by the United States Department of Energy and the National Institutes of Health, together with other government agencies worldwide, and by private biotechnology companies. Blood samples for testing/experimentation are obtained from the poorer populations of the world. Although these individuals may receive a small sum of money for their participation, there do not appear to be any plans for a return or direct benefit to the people who contributed to the discovery of the genome.

Ethical considerations

Jackson (2000) tells us that the fetus has no rights as a person in the law and therefore cannot have full moral status (Gillam, 1999). Today, as a result of the 1990 Human Fertilization and Embryology Act, termination of pregnancy can be performed at any gestation if there is a serious fetal handicap.

Kuhse and Singer (1999) have asked whether abortion for fetal abnormality is any different to paediatric euthanasia. At present the latter is not a 'normal' or legal procedure, whereas fetal euthanasia is an acceptable and legal practice. Ethically, Kuhse and Singer (1999) cannot quantify a difference. Gillam (1999) suggests that selective abortion is equivalent to non-voluntary euthanasia. However, the challenge is to question the moral outrage that this can engender (until the time when it becomes 'normal'). Since January 1995, the Government in China has forbidden couples with a serious genetic disease to have children, and this is enforced through abortion. The GMTV poll on 15 February 1995 asked the public whether doctors should kill 'abnormal' babies, and the majority of respondents were in agreement with this. The social conventionist view is that it is humans who determine normality, not nature.

Destruction of life because of 'abnormalities' can be traced back to classical times. Aristotle suggested that in his politics the ideal legislation was to destroy deformed infants. Plato not only agreed with Aristotle, in *The Republic*, but added that the destruction of babies who were the result of 'unfit' parents, or who were produced by parents past the ideal childbearing age, would also be beneficial (Tooley, 1983).

Analysis of the reasons for fetal surveillance poses the following question. Is its purpose to remove genetic defects or to produce individuals with more desirable qualities? Given that fetuses have been killed, for example, because they have cleft lips or are female, it may well be the latter. From an ethical viewpoint it could be argued that the removal of pain and suffering from the potentially disabled child through prevention of their life is beneficence. Associated with this is the belief that no harm is caused. Equally, a child who is born disabled could sue his or her parents for a tort of wrongful life. However, none of this can be enforced on moral grounds (Clarkeburn, 2000). Is it the parents who are making the decision about what is genetically worthy? Or is it the doctor, on behalf of society, who first acts as the detective in the technical screening process and then acts within the eugenicist principles of enforcing abortion through social control? Mendonca (2000) suggests that leadership, as in the case of the doctor, can only be ethical if it is based on altruism and not egotism.

However, the Abortion Act (1967) reiterates the doctor's choice (as two doctors have to sign it – not the woman). If women's autonomy is to be respected, then medicine cannot be paternalistic. Autonomy is a person's ability to make their own decisions and act upon them. In order to be able to fulfil the individual requirement of autonomy, obtaining informed consent before submission to any medical procedure is essential. Therefore, women who freely 'choose' the option of abortion are also willing to accept responsibility for this decision, which would include the possibility of sterility.

The technology behind surveillance cannot be neutral. There is an argument which would suggest that:

* from a feminist point of view the technology is sexist
* from a disabled rights point of view the technology is able-ist
* from a race relations point of view the technology is racist.

1   Some feminists view technology as abusing women and their bodies. Women tend to accept the procedural norms of the maternity system, often neither questioning nor receiving sufficient information (Denny, 1994; Press and Browner, 1997). Information has to be given in order to avoid litigation, but enough can be withheld to ensure compliance. Women are coerced (by the doctor, their family, the genetic counsellor or the midwife) to have an abortion because there is a fetal abnormality, while believing that they have made the choice themselves. The technology can be seen as a form of harassment which is formulated by the male-gendered medical profession against women (Brewis, 2001).
2   Disabled rights organisations acknowledge that, due to the increase in the number of abortions, there are dwindling resources to support disability in society, and with a gradual removal of disabled rights, there is less likelihood of trying to find a cure (Jackson, 2000). This is probably the result of cause and effect. In most cases, prenatal diagnosis and abortion are cheaper than financially supporting an 'abnormal' person. Disability is seen as undesirable, whereas able people are viewed as desirable, and therefore by implication people who already exist with a disability are also undesirable. However, prenatal diagnosis and selective abortion are juxtaposed with an increasing number of people who are surviving with 'abnormalities' such as diabetes or cardiac disease. They would otherwise not have been conceived, or would have been miscarried, been a stillbirth or died early in life. These people now survive because of the efforts of technology. It is also inconsistent when able-bodied people are being sent to wars to be killed or maimed, and thus disabled.
3   Racism arises from the issue of trying to narrow the gene pool or promote a certain genetic stock, in principle suggesting that every other resulting human being is unworthy of human status (Nuffield Council on Bioethics, 2001). Caplan *et al.* (1999) argue that eugenics is producing a desirable phenotype or genotype which is different to what the parents would choose (thus overriding

individual choice). This is racist. What does this say about a society that will not tolerate differences? And is there not a duty to allow all humans to live (Persson, 1999)?

Who has the power?

Talcott Parsons (1951), a structural functionalist, was clear that power resided with the doctor. He recognised that the pregnant woman had an obligation to obey the doctor. Parsons considered that the doctor had social influence and that this alone would ensure that patients would carry out their duties and obligations. The mother is seen to have a duty to subordinate her own interest of having a child to that of the greater interest of the society in the creation of 'normality' (Robertson and Turner, 1991).

Parsons considered that the woman would not be able or competent to make a technical decision. In fact, he alluded to her subjectivity and thus her irresponsibility. It is important to view this in context. Consider the role of women in the 1950s in the USA. The social expectation was that women would be mothers and housewives. Value was placed on the capitalist ethic of economic productivity, as it is today, and therefore women who were unpaid for their work derived low status and often felt disempowered. However, Parsons saw the doctors gaining the empowerment and economic reward, and it is from this social context that he was able to write the following:

> Birth and the rearing of a child constitutes a 'cost' to the society, through pregnancy, childcare, socialisation, formal training and many other channels. Premature death, before the individual has had the opportunity to play out his full quota of social roles, means that only a partial 'return' for this cost has been received.
>
> (Parsons, 1951: 430)

Parsons, it could be argued, was a linear reductionist in that he was able to 'box everything' simply or put it in its place. All human beings were shown to have social roles which defined their existence. Parsons was literally able to discuss one set of human activities and show how it would go on to affect another set of human activities. However, he only dealt with the external environmental role (or how the individual interacted in society), and he did not explore internal issues (Menzies, 1976). Parsons, before Foucault, considered the sick role as one of a disciplinary process: 'The sick role allowed exemption from normal responsibilities but [the individual had] an obligation to seek medical help' (Frank, 1991: 207). Again, like Foucault, Parsons recognised that there is a choice between obeying procedural norms and an alternative of punishment. Choice is not available when one is carrying out an obligation.

Parsons regards handicap as dysfunctional, as it cannot fit into the scheme of society. Handicap is being labelled as 'useless' to society and therefore has to be obliterated. The human activity associated with handicap is not seen as productive to society from a capitalist perspective, and therefore it would not set off the linear set of human activity associated with capitalism. One way of obliterating handicap is through socialising women into accepting fetal surveillance. On entering the hospital and the maternity system, there is for the majority of women an unspoken contract to obey procedural norms, and, according to Parsons, women should have no say.

The hospital is an institution of social control. Medicine can label our dis-eases and make them real. The technology originated not as a result of public demand, but as a response to demand from doctors, scientists and large multinational pharmaceutical and technical equipment companies (Parsons and Atkinson, 1993), thus promoting the capitalist ethos. Parsons might say that the institutionalisation and therefore normalisation of fetal surveillance means that women will find the procedure comforting and thus worthwhile. Women want confirmation of normality (Menzies, 1976; Press and Browner, 1997). However, if the sick role is to become the health role, then the domination of the doctors will take on less importance, while there will be an engendering of self-interest and responsibility by the woman (Frank, 1991).

Prevention

The majority of 'abnormalities' in fact result from the environment and not from the gene pool. Genetic disorders account for 3–5% of handicap, and 2% of individuals are born with a congenital abnormality (Green and Statham, 1993). Perhaps, in an effort to prevent 'abnormality', attention needs to be directed towards the prevention of war, poverty, environmental hazards/pollutants, accidents and disease (Wertz, 1997). Within the capitalist economy that exists, large multinational companies may consider profit before health, and thus handicap will result from food pollution, chemical contamination, nuclear power, the effects of acid rain on fish, and so on. Policies to change employment, state benefit, housing and taxation are some areas that need to be addressed in order to prevent 'abnormality' and gain the long-term benefit of the production of healthy children.

The prevention of poverty and deprivation would be costly and have less effect on the development of careers and personal interests. Fetal surveillance is given preference because it is cheaper than social welfare. For instance, nutrition affects our cell production, and social pressure can affect our immune response. Social policy to improve our nutritional status, housing and economic support can be ignored if the origins of 'abnormality' are cast back on the individual, as is happening in this victim-blaming society. The victim-blaming perspective could be used to provide an elitist model, which would make use of a person's genetic profile to determine his or her 'worthiness' for different jobs, insurance risks, reproductive mates and material wealth. Clearly this is a huge political issue which, if tackled, would need to change the ethos in society from the 'I'm all right, Jack' culture to developing a sense of community which has been lost in many major cities of the world.

Conclusion

Surveillance has become normalised through the ritual of maternity care. Merquior notes that where rituals contain within them observation and supervision, the 'right to punish [is] deeply entwined' (Merquior, 1985: 94). How many women 'give in' to the ritual for fear of being reprimanded? Will the 'slippery slope' develop the continuum of what is genetically worthy based on the scientific community's opinion? Or is it possible that, on the other hand, the nature of society will change from a competitive, materialist culture to an acceptance of diversity and improvement of the environment which will enhance the lives of all human beings?

- Fetal normality is defined within the scientific community.
- Eugenics originated within the scientific community.
- Technology originates from the needs of capitalism.
- Technology can be viewed as sexist, able-ist and racist.
- Fetal surveillance is a process designed to select desirable individuals.

References

- Andreski A (1983) *Max Weber*. George Allen and Unwin Ltd, London.
- Annas GJ and Grodin L (1992) *The Nazi Doctors and the Nuremberg Code*. Massachusetts Open University Press, New York.
- Boyne R (2000) Post panopticism. *Econ Society*. **29**: 285–307.
- Brewis J (2001) Foucault, politics and organizations: (re)-constructing sexual harassment. *Gender Work Organization*. **8**: 37–60.
- Caplan AL, McGee G and Magnus D (1999) What is immoral about eugenics? *BMJ*. **319**: 1284–5.
- Clarkeburn H (2000) Parental duties and untreatable genetic conditions. *J Med Ethics*. **26**: 400–3.
- Conrad P and Gabe J (1999) Sociological perspectives on the new genetics: an overview. *Sociol Health Illness*. **21**: 505–16.
- Cousins M and Hussain A (1984) *Michel Foucault*. Macmillan Education Ltd, Basingstoke.
- Danaher G, Schirato T and Webb J (2000) *Understanding Foucault*. Allen & Unwin, Cambridge, MA.
- Darwin L (1926) *The Need for Eugenic Reform*. John Murray, London.
- Denny E (1994) Liberation or oppression? Radical feminism and *in vitro* fertilization. *Sociol Health Illness*. **16**: 63–80.
- Eribon D (1989) *Michel Foucault*. Harvard University Press, Cambridge, MA.
- Foucault M (1972) *Power and Knowledge*. Harvester Press Ltd, Brighton.
- Foucault M (1973) *The Birth of the Clinic: an archaeology of medical perception*. Tavistock, London.
- Foucault M (1974) *The Order of Things: an archaeology of the human sciences*. Tavistock, London.
- Frank AW (1991) From sick role to health role: deconstructing Parsons. In: R Robertson and BS Turner (eds) *Talcott Parsons: theorist of modernity*. Sage Publications, London.
- Gillam L (1999) Prenatal diagnosis and discrimination against the disabled. *J Med Ethics*. **25**: 163–71.
- Green J and Statham H (1993) Testing for fetal abnormality in routine antenatal care. *Midwifery*. **9**: 124–35.

- Jackson E (2000) Abortion, autonomy and prenatal diagnosis. *Soc Legal Stud.* **9**: 467–94.
- Katz-Rothman B (1986*) The Tentative Pregnancy*. Pandora, London.
- Kaufert PA (2000) Health policy and the new genetics. *Soc Sci Med.* **51**: 821–9.
- Kelves DJ (1985) *In the Name of Eugenics*. Penguin, Harmondsworth.
- King DS (1999) Pre-implantation genetic diagnosis and the 'new' eugenics. *J Med Ethics.* **25**: 176–82.
- Kuhse H and Singer P (eds) (1985*) Bioethics: an anthology*. Blackwell Science, Oxford.
- Mendonca M (2000) Personal mastery in ethical leadership. *Med Law.* **19**: 855–62.
- Menzies K (1976) *Talcott Parsons and the Social Image of Man*. Routledge and Kegan Paul, London.
- Merquior JG (1985) *Foucault*. Fontana, London.
- Nola R (1998) *Foucault*. Frank Cass, London.
- Nuffield Council on Bioethics (2001*) Genetics and Human Behaviour: the ethical context*. Nuffield Council on Bioethics, London.
- Parsons E and Atkinson P (1993) Genetic risk and reproduction. *Soc Rev.* **41**: 679–706.
- Parsons T (1951) *The Social System*. Routledge and Kegan Paul, London.
- Persson I (1999) Equality and selection for existence. *J Med Ethics.* **25**: 130–6.
- Petersen A and Bunton R (1997) *Foucault, Health and Medicine*. Routledge, London.
- Press N and Browner CH (1997) Why women say yes to prenatal diagnosis. *Soc Sci Med.* **45**: 979–89.
- Rajchman J (1985) *Michel Foucault: the freedom of philosophy*. Columbia University Press, New York.
- Richards MPM (1993) The new genetics: some issues for social scientists. *Sociol Health Illness.* **15**: 567–86.
- Robertson R and Turner BS (1991) *Talcott Parsons: theorist of modernity*. Sage Publications, London.
- Smart B (1985) *Michel Foucault*. Ellis Horwood Publishers, Chichester.
- Statham H, Solomon W and Chitty L (2000) Prenatal diagnosis of fetal abnormality: psychological effects on women in low-risk pregnancies. *Clin Obstet Gynaecol.* **14**: 731–47.
- Tooley M (1983) *Abortion and Infanticide*. Oxford University Press, Oxford.
- Wertz D (1997) Society and the not-so-new genetics: what are we afraid of? Some future predictions from a social scientist. *J Contemp Health Law Policy.* **13**: 299–345.
- Wikler D (1999) Can we learn from eugenics? *J Med Ethics.* **25**: 183–94.

CHAPTER 18

Breastfeeding: a natural phenomenon or a cultural construct?

Cathryn Britton

There can be no dispute that breastfeeding can enhance the health of babies and their mothers. Yet despite the evidence of its health-enhancing properties, women in the UK often either choose not to breastfeed or curtail the activity after a relatively short time. Traditionally, health professionals have considered health promotion to be an important aspect of encouraging more women to breastfeed. There is an assumption that imparting knowledge may change attitudes and beliefs. However, it is naive to assume that if women are simply given more information about breastfeeding, the rates of breastfeeding might increase. The majority of women in the UK are not ignorant of the health benefits of breastfeeding. However, a variety of influences affect their infant feeding decisions. The main focus of this chapter will be on the social and cultural influences that exist within the UK which might help or hinder breastfeeding.

Introduction

It is generally accepted that most women, after giving birth, are physiologically able to lactate. The biology of lactation has been well described elsewhere (e.g. Wool-ridge, 1995; Stables, 1999). Women, like all female mammals, have breasts in order to suckle their young. There is an implied natural law and naturalness with regard to breastfeeding. Lactation occurs without question – women expect their breasts to produce breast milk. However, in many societies in the world breastfeeding is not only performed by the infant's mother, but might be shared by other members of the kin group (Hrdy 2000). This type of 'wet-nursing' has an important function in strengthening kin ties. It might be considered that breast milk will transmit important qualities to the infant (Skeel and Good, 1988; Creyghton, 1992). In Mali, a mother who does not breastfeed her infant is considered to have relinquished kin ties to her baby (Dettwyler, 1988). In those societies where breastfeeding of the infant is not confined to the infant's mother, milk kinship might be formed with the other women who feed the infant (Khatib-Chahidi, 1992; Harrison *et al.*, 1993).

The breastfeeding woman might not be biologically related to the infant but, through the breastfeeding act, a powerful bond is created where the term 'second mother' might be bestowed on the woman (Vincent, 1999).

Around the world women breastfeed without question. There is a natural assumption that the breast will be offered to the newborn infant and that breast milk will nourish the infant until weaning. In many societies there is little discourse on the health benefits of breastfeeding, because the latter is fundamental to child survival. There is one exception to this, namely the ingestion of colostrum. Vincent (1999) provides many examples of negative health beliefs associated with colostrum. Commonly quoted views are that colostrum is 'dirty', 'bad for the baby' and 'old and stale'. It is difficult to explain why these beliefs about colostrum exist. Kitzinger (1995) suggests that these customs reinforce the relationships between women by engaging other women in the active care of both mother and baby.

However, in the UK the dominant discourse of breastfeeding relies on promoting the activity by emphasising the health benefits to be gained by breastfeeding.

Health benefits

There are many health benefits to be gained by a mother breastfeeding her baby. Many research studies have demonstrated a positive correlation between breastfeeding and subsequent health in childhood. These include studies which have shown a reduction in gastrointestinal infections (Howie et al., 1990), respiratory infections (Wilson et al., 1998), ear infections (Duncan et al., 1993; Aniansson et al., 1994), allergic diseases (Lucas et al., 1990; Saarinen and Kajosaari, 1995) and insulin-dependent diabetes mellitus (Virtanen et al., 1991; Karjalainen et al., 1992; Gerstein, 1994). There is also evidence that infant–parent co-sleeping and breastfeeding may reduce the risk of sudden infant death syndrome (McKenna and Bernshaw, 1995; McKenna, 1996; Gordon et al., 1999). Other studies have demonstrated that breastfed children achieve higher scores in standardised tests of mental development than do children who have been fed artificial formula milk (Lucas et al., 1992; Rogan and Gladen, 1993; Temboury et al., 1994).

Although breastfeeding is usually promoted as an infant health issue, there is little doubt that there are health benefits for women, too (Dermer, 1998; Labbok, 2001). For women who have a history of breastfeeding, scientific studies have demonstrated a lower incidence of premenopausal breast cancer (Chilvers, 1993; Newcomb et al., 1994), ovarian cancer (Gwinn et al., 1990; Rosenblatt et al., 1993), and hip fractures in older women (Cumming and Klineberg, 1993).

Despite the evidence that breastfeeding is a health-enhancing activity, the breastfeeding rates in the UK are disappointing. In the recent *Infant Feeding* report, the prevalence of breastfeeding at birth was 66%, followed by a steep decline in breastfeeding during the first week of birth and a steady decline to 27% by the time the baby was 4 months old (Foster et al., 1997).

So the question that needs to be asked is this. If breastfeeding is so good for the infant and the mother, why do more women not do it?

If it is accepted that most women are able to lactate and understand the health benefits of breatfeeding, it is essential to look at those forces which affect the everyday life of breastfeeding women in the UK and consider what makes them decide to breastfeed initially and what makes them give up or continue breast-feeding. However, before considering the contemporary life of women in the UK, it is useful to discuss the historical context of infant feeding which has affected modern practices.

Historical influences

It is useful to consider breastfeeding within an historical context in order to understand the prevailing attitudes towards infant feeding. Giving an infant nourishment other than their mother's milk is not a new phenomenon. Throughout world history there are accounts of infants being given breast milk from other women (wet-nursing) or milk from animals (Fildes, 1986, 1988). Between 1500 and 1900 the use of wet-nurses in England was commonplace, especially among the wealthy. Although it later became uncommon in England, some industrialised nations (e.g. Austria, Italy and the USA) were using wet-nursing as an alternative to maternal breastfeeding until at least the 1940s (Fildes, 1988). Historical records suggest that infants were commonly given foodstuffs such as bread and broth as a complement to or substitute for breast milk (Fildes 1986; Apple 1987). Artificially formulated milk from animals became widely available in Europe, Australia and the Americas during the late 1800s, when the scientific community became interested in the subject of infant nutrition (Apple, 1987; Latteier, 1998). During the Second World War, national dried milk was introduced to encourage women into the workplace, and following the war the infant formula industry became very com-petitive, with intense marketing strategies equating bottle-feeding with affluence and consumerism. The marketing of artificial formula milk has received considerable attention as a major cause of the global decline in breastfeeding (Van Esterik, 1989; Palmer, 1993;). Human lactation as an unreliable body function became a cultural truth that has persisted to the present day (Wolf, 2000).

The 'bottle-feeding culture' became a part of the medicalisation of infant feeding, where scientists and doctors became 'the experts'. Various practices were intro-duced to control and regulate infant feeding, whereby predictability and measuring the baby's intake became important, which arose from the bottle-feeding culture (Dykes, 1997). As women were encouraged to approach the management of breastfeeding from a scientific paradigm, this caused a lack of confidence in their ability to nourish their babies. This lack of confidence in breastfeeding persists in the UK today (Renfrew *et al.*, 2000). Despite the known health benefits of breastfeeding, prejudicial attitudes against breastfeeding in the UK still remain. Many of the people with whom a woman comes into contact during her repro-ductive life have been exposed to the 'norm' of bottle-feeding, and it is clear that the social milieu is a major influence on women's ability to breastfeed.

The social experience of breastfeeding

The breastfeeding experience is not an isolated event but one that exists in a social context. Not only does a woman have to choose whether she will initially breastfeed her infant, but she may also need to consider the length of time for which she will breastfeed, how she will incorporate breastfeeding into her everyday life, where she will breastfeed, in whose company she feels comfortable breastfeeding, whether she will breastfeed during the weaning process and whose advice and opinions will guide her (e.g. family, friends and/or health professionals). These decisions are likely to be shaped by political, economic, social and cultural influences. In most societies there will be political influences which drive child health issues. In the UK the public health message is that 'breast is best' and Government guidelines suggest that the optimal duration of breastfeeding is 4 to 6 months. Economic factors concern the necessity to work during the breastfeeding period, which might raise issues about access to a breastfeeding child in the workplace and the acceptability of breastfeeding or expressing the breasts during work-time. Social and cultural factors will determine the norms of behaviour with regard to breastfeeding – that is, what is tolerated, what is not, and how behaviour might be regulated.

In many societies in the world breastfeeding is commonly continued into toddlerhood (Dettwyler, 1995a). This does not mean that these women are *exclusively* breastfeeding 2- or 3-year-old children, but they continue to provide breast contact in some form along with other foodstuffs. This practice is not confined to 'other' societies – it also occurs in the UK (Britton, 2000). It is difficult to determine the extent of long-term breastfeeding in the UK because national infant feeding statistics are not collected after the infant reaches 9 months of age. Breastfeeding a toddler is not generally a publicly visible activity, as most women choose to confine the activity to the home (Britton, 2000). In babyhood, breastfeeding is promoted as being the best form of nutrition for an infant, but as the child grows older, breastfeeding might become problematic in social situations. The mother might find herself having to defend her breastfeeding activity if others comment on the appropriateness of breastfeeding an older child. A range of opinions might be vocalised about *when is too old to breastfeed a child.* For some people there is a notion of what can be expected of a child at certain ages, and a child who is breastfeeding once they are wearing shoes, can articulate what they want or have 'a mouthful of teeth' might be deemed too old to breastfeed (Britton, 2000).

The public health message produced by the UK Government and reinforced by health professionals is that breastfeeding is right and proper until 4 months of age, after which the child should be encouraged to take supplementary foodstuffs, and they should 'weaned' by 6 months of age (Health Education Authority, 1992; Department of Health, 1994). The most recent *Infant Feeding* report (Foster *et al.*, 1997) confirms that the majority of infants aged 4 to 6 months are not receiving any breast milk. Yet this is at odds with the World Health Organization (WHO) recommendation, which suggests that infants should be breastfed *and* given appropriate and nutritionally adequate complementary foodstuffs until the age of 2 years or beyond (World Health Organization, 1989). Although the WHO has publicly supported the continuation of breastfeeding for at least the first 2 years of an infant's life, this has been ignored in the public health discourse on breastfeeding.

The concept of 'success' in breastfeeding

Although the policy discourse encourages the notion that successful breastfeeding equates to following the guidelines, it is important to gauge what constitutes success from the woman's perspective. The term *successful breastfeeding* is a value-laden term, as one person's view about successful breastfeeding may not be shared by another. For example, if a woman has breastfed an infant for over a year, her concept of success might be to suckle subsequent children for at least one year. However, another woman might feel successful if she has breastfed her infant for a few weeks prior to returning to work. Health professionals also have their own ideas about optimal breastfeeding and might assume that a woman who starts to breastfeed is committed to do so for as long as possible. Therefore care needs to be taken to ensure that assumptions are not made.

Why (not) breastfeed?

The reasons why some women either do not breastfeed or else breastfeed for only a limited period of time are multiple and complex. Breastfeeding is socially constructed and exists within a woman's social world. It is not an isolated event that can be readily assigned to scientific reasoning alone. Other issues which affect women's lives and have received little attention in the medical approach to breast-feeding are societal and cultural influences that will influence a woman's choice with regard to initiating and sustaining breastfeeding. A woman may experience con-flicting roles as mother, wife and wage earner. Women who feel unsupported by their partners with regard to their breastfeeding decision are less likely to be successful in breastfeeding (Palmer, 1993; Isabella and Isabella, 1994). In the UK many women return to work after the birth of their baby. For some the return to the workplace makes breastfeeding problematic, as the promotion of breastfeeding in the workplace is not seen as a priority for employers. The absence of breastfeeding facilities during the working day, limited or no access to the infant and difficulties in expressing and storing breast milk all contribute to the early cessation of breast-feeding for most working women. Many women believe that if they do not continue to express their breasts during the day their milk supply will cease. In the policy discourse the promotion of breastfeeding is focused on the early weeks of the activity, not on long-term breastfeeding. The promotion of breastfeeding is targeted at the infant's first 6 months. From the time when supplementary foods are expected to be introduced there is little attention given to promoting the continu-ation of breastfeeding activities.

Research has been conducted to investigate why women choose not to breastfeed at all or else give up early (Wylie and Verber, 1994; Clements *et al.*, 1997; Foster *et al.*, 1997; Hoddinott, 1998). A key focus of the research studies has been to investigate the link between sociodemographic variables and the decline in breastfeeding. The outcomes of these studies demonstrate that women who are in the higher social classes, who have remained in full-time education until 18 years of age, and who live in south-east England, are all more likely to breastfeed. Although statistical analyses can be useful for detecting associations between sociodemographic factors and infant feeding choices, they are unable to explain the choices that are made by individual women. Differences in breastfeeding uptake cannot be explained by sociodemographic variables alone. Social and cultural factors may be important, but they have received little attention.

Social and cultural influences

Women are exposed to a variety of social and cultural factors which influence their chosen feeding method (Morse, 1990; Isabella and Isabella, 1994; Hall, 1997). The attitudes and opinions of family members, friends and health professionals are likely to affect the uptake and continuation of breastfeeding (Giugliani *et al.*, 1994; Humenick *et al.*, 1998; Hoddinott and Pill, 1999). Health professionals have traditionally encouraged women to breastfeed their babies, by giving information about its benefits. However, there may be other social and cultural values which affect the breastfeeding event, such as the dominant societal and media representations of breastfeeding, and feeling able to breastfeed in public.

These issues are influenced and underpinned by the way in which others regulate the body of an individual. Within each society an individual learns the cultural norms with regard to their body in everyday life (e.g. bodily adornment, private and public parts of the body, interpretation of bodily functions). The way in which the body is managed in everyday life and the impact that it has on others must also be considered. For example, both emotional and physical control of the body will gain meaning from and be interpreted within cultural norms (Featherstone and Hepworth, 1991; Lupton, 1998).

Religious beliefs may also impact on the reproductive life of some women. There are several instances where control of women's bodies has been driven by religious ideology. For example, the Catholic Church does not support contraception and abortion. The everyday life of women may be controlled by religious teachings such as the seclusion of women from public view (e.g. *purdah* in many Islamic societies). Breastfeeding may be affected by religious ideology with regard to maintaining modesty during the act of breastfeeding, and by doctrines in religious texts (e.g. the Koran, which recommends that women should breastfeed their infants for 2 years) (Schott and Henley, 1996).

In recent years the reproductive body has been a focus of attention in the disciplines of anthropology and sociology. The medicalisation of childbirth has been widely debated (Davis-Floyd, 1992; Kitzinger, 1992), where childbirth has been defined as a 'problem' which needs to be controlled by experts and monitored by technology. Turner (1992) suggests that medicine, law and religion are preoccupied by the regulation of the body. In the UK there is no law regulating breastfeeding practices, although this has happened elsewhere. In the USA there are many legal cases involving breastfeeding, such as the effect of breastfeeding on custody and visitation rights, the right to breastfeed at work, and breastfeeding in public places. Consequently, breastfeeding legislation in the USA has been developed in order to promote and encourage breastfeeding (Baldwin, 2000; Baldwin and Friedman, 2000).

In UK society, individuals learn from an early age that the body needs to be managed and disciplined (Shilling, 1993). Drawing on the work of Elias (1982), the body has been subjected to the 'civilising process'. During the course of socialisation most natural functions have been classified as offensive and distasteful. Body fluids fit into this category very well – the sight or smell of body fluids such as urine, faeces or menstrual blood may be seen as 'matter out of place' (Douglas, 1984). People expect to be in charge of their bodies, so if the body goes out of control it can be viewed as problematic – not only for others, but by the self as well. Women have been socialised to control their body fluids and render them invisible (Britton, 1996). For example, during breastfeeding the leaking milk is contained by the use of breast pads. The control of decency may also be an issue when the breasts become 'public' during breastfeeding. However, concern about the public display of the breast during breastfeeding seems to be in direct contradiction to the media representation of the breasts in the popular press.

Societal notions of the breast and breastfeeding

Societal notions of the breast and breastfeeding in the UK are embedded in a cultural context which shapes people's opinions about the breast and attitudes towards breastfeeding activities. The visual and print media in any culture depict the 'desirable' female body, such as the appropriate shape and size of the breast (Thapan, 1997). Those women who are dissatisfied with their breasts have sought assistance from surgeons with regard to reconstructive surgery to enable them to achieve the desired shape and size of breast. The breast may also be perceived as an erotic body part, where it is represented both in pornography and in the media as an essential feature for attracting heterosexual men.

Cross-cultural accounts provide evidence of societies, such as the UK and North America, where there is a strong association of the breast with sex (Anderson, 1983; Van Esterick, 1989; Dettwyler, 1995b). The sexual nature of the breast in the UK means that breastfeeding is ultimately linked with female sexuality, and this might be an important factor influencing a woman's success in breastfeeding. At the other end of the spectrum there are societies, such as Mali, where the breast is not considered to be sexually arousing during sexual intercourse (Latteier, 1998). There are those societies in which the breast is regarded as both sexual and maternal, which enables a breastfeeding culture to exist within a society that sexualises the breast (Latteier, 1998).

The media has the ability to influence public opinion. Breastfeeding women are acutely aware of the media's interest in aspects of breastfeeding (Britton, 2000). The sexualisation of the breast through the media image has become commonplace in UK society, with various newspapers, magazines and television programmes portraying the female breast as sexual. In the UK there is a strong cultural preference for sexualised breasts. When women breastfeed they may be seen as transgressing the boundary between motherhood and sexuality (Young, 1998). The media can also influence attitudes to breastfeeding (Henderson, 1999). The media interest in breastfeeding often focuses on problems associated with breastfeeding in the social world. There have been several examples of ways in which the media has encouraged public debate about the issue of breastfeeding in public. The results of opinion polls have been published in magazines such as *Bella* which are targeted at female readers, and they reported that most people do not think that breastfeeding is an activity that should be witnessed. The British Tourist Authority (1996) gave official advice to tourists visiting the UK that breastfeeding in public was not acceptable in this country.

Breastfeeding in everyday life: the public dimension

In everyday life a breastfeeding woman will breastfeed on someone's territory, whether it be a public place or in her own domestic space. In many societies breastfeeding in public is not an issue — the breastfeeding act is incorporated into everyday life without question. In the UK, breastfeeding in public has become a topic of debate. In recent years there has been a plethora of newspaper and media

---

Box 18.1 Examples of newspaper articles debating breastfeeding in public spaces

Breast is best but not in public
Independent on Sunday 1996

Women breastfeeding in a mall in Belfast were seen on CCTV and asked to move as they were embarrassing others.

Getting abreast of the new laws
The Daily Telegraph 1997

Report on legislation that was passed to make it legal for a woman to breastfeed in public.

SHAME – I just wanted to breastfeed my baby, but this man threw dirty water at us
The Express 1997

A shopkeeper threw water over a breastfeeding woman and her baby because he claimed the wall she was sitting on was his. He felt breastfeeding in public spaces was unacceptable, similar to urinating in front of others.

What they say about breastfeeding in public
The Times Magazine 1998

Demonstrates contrasting opinions of support and contempt for the issue

Feeding frenzy
The Guardian 1999

The editor of *Debrett's Guide to Etiquette* claims that 'it is bad manners to expel any liquid from any orifice in public, and breastfeeding is no different'.

---

articles questioning its appropriateness (*see* Box 18.1). The very fact that it has become an issue for public debate indicates that it is a problematic activity for society in general. Many women in the UK find it difficult to breastfeed in public places (Foster *et al.*, 1997; Britton 2000), and their concerns are reinforced when the media highlight their plight.

If women feel concerned about incorporating breastfeeding into their social life, they will give up breastfeeding in public or quickly develop an awareness of appropriate facilities, such as mother-and-baby rooms, which are regarded as areas of 'safe refuge'. Mother-and-baby facilities can offer women a place which is frequented by other women with children, which provides privacy away from the public gaze, and where their mothering capabilities are not on public display. However, the environment within such mother-and-baby rooms is not always ideal. Often the space is cramped, and chairs for breastfeeding may be placed next to nappy bins. If mother-and-baby facilities are not available, then women might find other 'safe' areas in which to breastfeed, such as restaurants and cafes, or they might negotiate an area with shop assistants. However, they may go to some length to create a safe space within these settings by placing themselves away from others in order to avoid the public gaze. When seeking a safe, private area in which to breastfeed their baby, a public toilet might be the only readily available place, which women loathe, as they equate breastfeeding with nourishment rather than with excretion (Britton, 2000). Although 'safe refuges' are welcomed by most women, their presence can reinforce the social concerns about breastfeeding in public by reducing it to a clandestine activity.

In the early weeks of motherhood, women may express anxiety about going away from the home, because they will have to manage and regulate their baby in a social setting among strangers. First-time mothers in particular are conscious of their new role and have differing degrees of confidence in handling and managing a young baby. For some women, the public display of mothering is an anxious time if they believe that others might monitor their skills. The act of breastfeeding might be regarded as a public demonstration of how the woman copes with her baby and attends to its needs appropriately.

Breastfeeding in everyday life: the domestic dimension

The home is usually regarded as a safe, private place in which breastfeeding can take place. However, the presence of others within this space may impose a reordering of the place to breastfeed. Those women who would normally breastfeed in a 'day' area, such as a living-room, may retreat to a more private area, such as a bedroom, rather than breastfeed in the view of others in their domestic space.

In the domestic setting, public and private demarcations of space may change according to whether the woman is breastfeeding in front of friends and family. She may manage breastfeeding on her own, with her partner present, or in front of friends and family in different ways, depending on how comfortable she feels breastfeeding in front of these individuals. The domestic space may usually be regarded as private space in which a breastfeeding woman can choose where to feed her child. However, this may become disrupted when the domestic arena becomes public (e.g. when guests are invited into the home). A demarcation of public and private space might occur, with the woman removing herself to a private space should breastfeeding be necessary. What is interesting here is that for some breastfeeding women their domestic space has different meanings depending on who is present. This issue becomes complicated by factors that influence the woman's choice of feeding venue, namely her relationship to the guest, the sex of the guest, and her partner's view on breastfeeding in front of 'others'. The woman's personal preferences also have to be considered, as well as those of the individuals who were invited into the home, and consequently a re-evaluation of the use of private and public domestic space may occur.

Conclusion

The results of scientific research can improve our understanding of the biological benefits of breastfeeding and influence the development of strategies to increase the number of women who initiate breastfeeding. However, the social context of breastfeeding must be considered in order to gain an improved understanding of the conflicts and dominant forces that shape breastfeeding for many women.

The reasons why some women do not breastfeed at all, or only breastfeed for a limited time, are multiple and complex. The predominant societal and cultural influences will affect a woman's decision as to whether to initiate and sustain breastfeeding. By examining these forces, health professionals can identify how they may better support women who choose to breastfeed and appreciate the constraints to breastfeeding that women might encounter.

In the UK, the medical/scientific approach to breastfeeding in policy discourse is dominant, and little attention is given to the social and cultural values which underlie a woman's reasons for breastfeeding. Nevertheless, there is evidence that without an understanding of cultural attitudes the medical message is often unable to permeate to the wider audience. Despite women's knowledge that breastfeeding can be health enhancing, some women choose not to breastfeed. In order to promote breastfeeding, health professionals have used the dominant discourse of medicine to encourage an increase in the number of women who breastfeed. The strategies that they use are the provision of information about the health benefits and the use of scientific research to underpin advice about appropriate management of breastfeeding concerns. However, this is not enough – it is essential to acknowledge the cultural and social influences which might help or hinder the act of breastfeeding.

- Lactation is universal, but the act of breastfeeding is socially constructed.
- Breastfeeding does not take place as an isolated event, but is influenced by the social world of the woman.
- Political, economic, social and cultural influences may shape breastfeeding decisions.

Useful addresses

The Breastfeeding Network
PO Box 11126
Paisley PA2 8YB
Supporter line: 0870 900 8787

La Leche League (GB)
PO Box 29
West Bridgeford
Nottingham NG2 7NP
Tel: 0207 242 1278

National Childbirth Trust
Alexandra House
Oldham Terrace
Acton
London W3 6NH
Tel: 0870 444 8707

Baby Milk Action
23 St Andrew's Street
Cambridge CB2 3AX
Tel: 01223 464420

References

- Anderson P (1983) The reproductive role of the human breast. *Curr Anthropol.* **24**:1 25–45.
- Aniansson G, Alm B, Andersson B *et al.* (1994) A prospective cohort study on breastfeeding and otitis media in Swedish infants. *Pediatr Infect Dis J.* **13**: 183–8.
- Apple R (1987) *Mothers and Medicine: a social history of infant feeding, 1890–1950.* University of Wisconsin Press, Madison, WI.
- Baldwin E (2000) *Extended Breastfeeding and the Law.* La Leche League website; www.lalecheleague.org/Lawextended.html
- Baldwin E and Friedman K (2000) A current summary of breastfeeding legislation in the US. La Leche League website; www.lalecheleague.org/LawBills.html
- British Tourist Authority (1996) *Days Out.* British Tourist Authority, London.
- Britton C (1996) Learning about 'the curse': an anthropological perspective on experiences of menstruation. *Women's Stud Int Forum.* **19**: 645–53.
- Britton C (2000) *Women's experiences of early and long-term breastfeeding in the UK.* Unpublished PhD thesis, University of Durham, Durham.
- Chilvers C (1993) Breastfeeding and risk of breast cancer in young women. *BMJ.* **307**: 17–20.
- Clements M, Mitchell E, Wright S *et al.* (1997) Influences on breastfeeding in south-east England. *Acta Paediatr.* **86**: 15–6.
- Creyghton M (1992) Breast-feeding and *baraka* in Northern Tunisia. In: V Maher (ed.) *The Anthropology of Breastfeeding.* Berg Publishers, Oxford.
- Cumming RG and Klineberg RJ (1993) Breastfeeding and other reproductive factors and the risk of hip fractures in elderly women. *Int J Epidemiol.* **22**: 684–91.
- Davis-Floyd R (1992) *Birth as an American Rite of Passage.* University of California Press, Berkeley, CA.
- Department of Health (1994) *Weaning and the Weaning Diet. Report of the Working Group on the Weaning Diet of the Committee on Medical Aspects of Food Policy.* HMSO, London.
- Dermer A (1998) Breastfeeding and women's health. *J Women's Health.* **7**: 427–33.
- Dettwyler K (1988) More than nutrition: breastfeeding in urban Mali. *Med Anthropol Q.* **2**: 172–83.
- Dettwyler K (1995a) A time to wean: the hominid blueprint for the natural age of weaning in modern human populations. In: P Stuart-Macadam and K Dettwyler (eds) *Breastfeeding: biocultural perspectives.* Aldine de Gruyter, New York.

- Dettwyler K (1995b) Beauty and the breast: the cultural context of breast-feeding in the United States. In: P Stuart-Macadam and K Dettwyler (eds) *Breastfeeding: biocultural perspectives.* Aldine de Gruyter, New York.
- Douglas M (1984) *Purity and Danger: an analysis of the concepts of pollution and taboo.* Ark Paperbacks, London.
- Duncan B, Ey J, Holberg C *et al.* (1993) Exclusive breastfeeding for at least 4 months protects against otitis media. *Pediatrics.* **5**: 867–72.
- Dykes F (1997) Return to breastfeeding: a global health priority. *Br J Midwifery.* **5**: 344–9.
- Elias N (1982) *The Civilising Process.* Basil Blackwell. Oxford.
- Featherstone M and Hepworth M (1991) The mask of ageing and the post-modern lifecourse. In: M Featherstone, M Hepworth and B Turner (eds) *The Body: social processes and cultural theory.* Sage Publications, London.
- Fildes V (1986) *Breasts, Bottles and Babies: a history of infant feeding.* Edinburgh University Press. Edinburgh.
- Fildes V (1988) *Wet Nursing: a history from antiquity to the present.* Basil Black-well. Oxford.
- Foster K, Lader D and Cheesborough S (1997) *Infant Feeding 1995.* The Stationery Office, London.
- Gerstein HC (1994) Cow's milk exposure and type 1 diabetes mellitus. *Diabetes Care.* **17**: 13–19.
- Giugliani E, Caiaffa W, Vogelhut J, Witter F and Perman J (1994) Effect of breastfeeding support from different sources on the mother's decisions to breastfeed. *J Hum Lactation.* **10**: 517–61.
- Gordon A, Saadi A, Mackenzie D *et al.* (1999) The protective effect of breastfeeding in relation to sudden infant death syndrome (SIDS): detection of IGA antibodies in human milk that bind to bacterial toxins implicated in SIDS. *FEMS Immunol Med Microbiol.* **25**: 175–82.
- Gwinn M, Lee N, Rhodes P, Layde P and Rubin G (1990) Pregnancy, breast-feeding and oral contraceptives and the risk of epithelial ovarian cancer. *J Clin Epidemiol.* **43**: 559–68.
- Hall J (1997) Breastfeeding and sexuality: societal conflicts and expectations. *Br J Midwifery.* **5**: 350–54.
- Harrison G, Zaghoul S, Galal O and Gabr A (1993) Breastfeeding and weaning in a poor urban neighbourhood in Cairo, Egypt: maternal beliefs and percep-tions. *Soc Sci Med.* **36**: 1–10.
- Health Education Authority (1992) *Birth to Five.* Health Education Authority, London.
- Henderson A (1999) Mixed messages about the meanings of breastfeeding representations in the Australian press and popular magazines. *Midwifery.* **15**: 24–31.
- Hoddinott P (1998) *Why don't some women want to breastfeed and how might we change their attitudes?* MPhil Thesis. University of Wales College of Medicine, Cardiff.
- Hoddinott P and Pill R (1999) Qualitative study of decisions about infant feeding among women in the east end of London. *BMJ.* **318**: 30–4.
- Howie P, Forsyth S, Ogston S, Clark A and Florey C (1990) Protective effect of breastfeeding against infection. *BMJ.* **300**: 11–16.
- Hrdy SB (2000) *Mother Nature.* Vintage, London.

- Humenick S, Hill P and Spiegelberg P (1998) Breastfeeding and health professionals' encouragement. *J Hum Lactation.* **14**: 305–10.
- Isabella P and Isabella R (1994) Correlates of successful breastfeeding: a study of social and personal factors. *J Hum Lactation.* **10**: 257–64.
- Karjalainen J, Martin J, Knip M *et al.* (1992) A bovine albumin peptide as a possible trigger of insulin-dependent diabetes mellitus. *NEJM.* **327**: 302–7.
- Khatib-Chahidi J (1992) Milk kinship in Shi'ite Islamic Iran. In: V Maher (ed.) *The Anthropology of Breastfeeding.* Berg Publishers, Oxford.
- Kitzinger S (1992) Birth and violence against women: generating hypotheses from women's accounts of unhappiness after childbirth. In: H. Roberts (ed.) *Women's Health Matters.* Routledge, London.
- Kitzinger S (1995) Commentary. In: P Stuart-Macadam and K Dettwyler (eds) *Breastfeeding: biocultural perspectives.* Aldine de Gruyter, New York.
- Labbok M (2001) Effects of breastfeeding on the mother. *Pediatr Clin North Am.* **48**: 143.
- Latteier C (1998) *Breasts: the women's perspective on an American obsession.* Harrington Park Press, New York.
- Lucas A, Brooke G, Morley R, Cole T and Bamford M (1990) Early diet of preterm infants and development of allergic or atopic disease: randomised prospective study. *BMJ.* **300**: 837–40.
- Lucas D, Morley R, Cole T *et al.* (1992) Breast milk and subsequent intelligence quotient in children born preterm. *Lancet.* **339**: 261–64.
- Lupton D (1998) Going with the flow: some central discourses in conceptualising and articulating the embodiment of emotional states. In: S Nettleton and J Watson (eds) *The Body in Everyday Life.* Routledge, London.
- McKenna J (1996) Sudden infant death syndrome in cross-cultural perspective: Is infant–parent co-sleeping protective? *Annu Rev Anthropol.* **25**: 201–16.
- McKenna J and Bernshaw N (1995) Breastfeeding and infant–parent co-sleeping as adaptive strategies: are they protective against SIDS? In: P Stuart-Macadam and K Dettwyler (eds) *Breastfeeding: biocultural perspectives.* Aldine de Gruyter, New York.
- Morse J (1990) 'Euch, those are for your husband!': examination of cultural values and assumptions associated with breastfeeding. *Health Care Women Int.* **11**: 223–32.
- Newcomb P, Storer B, Longnecker M *et al.* (1994) Lactation and a reduced risk of premenopausal breast cancer. *NEJM.* **330**: 81–7.
- Palmer G (1993) *The Politics of Breastfeeding.* Pandora Press, London.
- Renfrew M, Woolridge M and Ross Mcgill H (2000) *Enabling Women to Breastfeed.* The Stationery Office, London.
- Rogan W and Gladen B (1993) Breastfeeding and cognitive development. *Early Hum Dev.* **31**: 181–93.
- Rosenblatt KA, Thomas DM, Berry G *et al.* (1993) Lactation and the risk of epithelial ovarian cancer. The WHO collaborative study of neoplasia and steroid contraceptives. *Int J Epidemiol.* **22**: 499–503.
- Saarinen UM and Kajosaari M (1995) Breastfeeding as prophylaxis against atopic disease: prospective follow-up study until 17 years old. *Lancet.* **346**: 1065–9.
- Schott J and Henley A (1996) *Culture, Religion and Childbearing in a Multiracial Society.* Butterworth-Heinemann, Oxford.
- Shilling C (1993) *The Body and Social Theory.* Sage Publications, London.

- Skeel L and Good M (1988) Mexican cultural beliefs and breastfeeding: a model for assessment and intervention. *J Hum Lactation.* **4**: 4.
- Stables D (1999) *Physiology in Childbearing with Anatomy and Related Biosciences.* Baillière Tindall, London.
- Temboury M, Otero A, Polanco I and Arribas E (1994) Influence of breast-feeding on the infant's intellectual development. *J Pediatr Gastroenterol Nutrition.* **18**: 32–6.
- Thapan M (1997) Femininity and its discontents: the woman's body in intimate relationships. In: M Thapan (ed.) *Embodiment: essays on gender and identity.* Oxford University Press, Delhi.
- Turner B (1992) *Regulating Bodies: essays in medical sociology.* Routledge, London.
- Van Esterik P (1989) *Motherpower and Infant Feeding.* Zed Books, London.
- Vincent P (1999) *Feeding our Babies: exploring traditions of breastfeeding and infant nutrition.* Hochland and Hochland Ltd, Hale.
- Virtanen SM, Rasanen L, Aro A *et al.* (1991) Infant feeding in children <7 years of age with newly diagnosed IDDM. *Diabetes Care.* **14**: 415–17.
- Wilson AC, Forsyth S, Greene S, Irvine L, Hau C and Howie P (1998) Relation of infant diet to childhood health: seven-year follow-up cohort of children in Dundee infant feeding study. *BMJ.* **316**: 21–5.
- Wolf J (2000) The social and medical construction of lactation pathology. *Women Health.* **30**: 93–110.
- Woolridge M (1995) Breastfeeding: physiology into practice. In: D Davis (ed.) *Nutrition in Child Health.* Royal College of Physicians, London.
- World Health Organization (1989) *Innocenti Declaration.* World Health Organization, Geneva.
- Wylie J and Verber I (1994) Why women choose not to breastfeed. *Matern Child Health.* **19**: 76–80.
- Young I (1998) Breasted experience: the look and the feeling. In: R Weitz (ed.) *The Politics of Women's Bodies: sexuality, appearance and behaviour.* Oxford University Press, New York.

Glossary

Determinism   The theory that human sexuality is determined by a necessary chain of causation.

Discourse   A term used to describe a domain of language that is unified by common assumptions and ideologies and is likely to preserve a particular distribution of power and exclude other ways of thinking.

Enlightenment   A philosophical and social movement, often referred to as the 'Age of Reason', that developed in Europe in the eighteenth century. Enlightenment philosophers developed a range of progressive ideas, including freedom of thought and expression, a criticism of religion, the value of rational thinking and science, a commitment to social progress, and the significance of the individual. These critical and secular concepts played a crucial role in the emergence of modern societies.

Essentialism   The theory that gender and biological sex are synonymous.

Modernity   A term used to describe the specific attributes of modern societies. Much of the work in human sciences is based on the assumption that a clear divide exists between pre-modern and modern societies. There is considerable debate over the nature of these two types of societies, as well the precise time when Western societies became modern. Modernity is defined on economic, political, social and cultural grounds. There is controversy over the temporalisation of modernity, some equating it with the emergence and spread of capitalism from the fourteenth century onwards, some linking it to religious changes from the fifteenth century, some associating it with the onset of industrialisation in the late eighteenth and nineteenth centuries, and other linking it with cultural transformations occurring from the end of the nineteenth century onwards.

Social constructionism   The theory that society and social roles are constructed/shaped by interest groups/people in society.

Universalism   The theory that women's oppression is common to all women.

Index